Medical Emergency Teams

Michael A. DeVita, M.D.
Associate Professor of Critical Care Medicine and Internal Medicine,
University of Pittsburgh School of Medicine, Associate Medical Director,
UPMC Presbyterian Hospital, Pittsburgh, Pennsylvania

Kenneth Hillman, M.D.
Co-Director of Critical Care, Simpson Centre for Health Services Research,
Liverpool Hospital, Liverpool, New South Wales, Australia

Rinaldo Bellomo, M.D.
Director of Intensive Care Research, Department of Intensive Care, Austin
Hospital, Heidelberg, Victoria, Australia

Editors

Medical Emergency Teams

Implementation and Outcome Measurement

With a Foreword by Ake Grenvik, M.D., Ph.D.

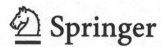 Springer

Michael A. DeVita, M.D.
Associate Professor of Critical Care
    Medicine and Internal Medicine
University of Pittsburgh School of Medicine
Associate Medical Director
UPMC Presbyterian Hospital
Pittsburgh, PA 15213-3404
USA

Kenneth Hillman, M.D.
Co-Director of Critical Care
The Simpson Centre for
Health Services Research
Liverpool Hospital
Liverpool
New South Wales 1871
Australia

Rinaldo Bellomo, M.D.
Director of Intensive Care Research
Austin Hospital
Heidelberg, Victoria 3084
Australia

Library of Congress Control Number: 2005932106

ISBN-10: 0-387-27920-2
ISBN-13: 978-0387-27920-6

Printed on acid-free paper.

Printed in the United States of America.   (BS/MVY)

9 8 7 6 5 4 3 2 1

springeronline.com

Foreword
Why Critical Care Evolved METs?

In early 2004, when Dr. Michael DeVita informed me that he was considering a textbook on the new concept of Medical Emergency Teams (METs), I was surprised. At Presbyterian-University Hospital in Pittsburgh we introduced this idea some 15 years ago, but did not think it was revolutionary enough to publish. This, even though, our fellows in critical care medicine training were all involved and informed about the importance of "Condition C (Crisis)," as it was called to distinguish it from "Condition A (Arrest)." We thought it absurd to intervene only after cardiac arrest had occurred, because most cases showed prior deterioration and cardiac arrest could be prevented with rapid team work to correct precluding problems.

The above thoughts were logical in Pittsburgh, where the legendary Dr. Peter Safar had been working since the late 1950s on improving current resuscitation techniques, first ventilation victims of apneic from drowning, treatment of smoke inhalation, and so on. This was followed by external cardiac compression upon demonstration of its efficiency in cases of unexpected sudden cardiac arrest. Dr. Safar devoted his entire professional life to improvement of cardiopulmonary resuscitation. He and many others emphasized the importance of getting the CPR team to out-of-hospital victims of cardiac arrest as quickly as possible. Similarly, much attention was given to identify other crisis situations in which trained ambulance personnel and other responders could reach the victims quickly to treat and preferably prevent threatening cardiac arrest by appropriate interventions.

Similar systems would have been logical and easy to arrange within hospitals for admitted patients. But such arrangements would collide with conventional training of physicians. In teaching hospitals, the tradition has been first to engage the intern to recognize all problems and treat the patients accordingly. If not successful, he or she would call on the assigned resident, leaving the attending physician out of the loop, frequently until too late to save a patient in crisis. Only recently has it become obvious that such a system fails. Training must be secondary to optimal and immediate care in evolving crisis.

Because of the above roadblocks, implementation of our Condition C team was not easy. The problem was frequently discussed in our Hospital's ICU Committee but the idea was considered too contrary to traditional clinical education and the concept was not accepted. After two years of ICU Committee debate in the 1980s, seemingly heading nowhere, as Chairman of this Committee, I received an emergency call one day from the chairman of the Surgical Department. He had a patient who was hypotensive and in respiratory distress on the "Gold Coast" ward after drainage of a malignant pleural effusion. We called our first team together, intubated the patient for mechanical ventilation, inserted a chest tube to drain a large hemopneumothorax that was obvious on chest x-ray, infused lactated Ringer's solution intravenously because of hypotension, and admitted her to the ICU. She could be extubated and returned to her ward the following day. This patient never developed cardiac arrest because of rapid resuscitation, workup, and indicated therapy without delay. It was nothing heroic, but it was such a convincing demonstration of the value of Condition C that the next ICU Committee Meeting unanimously approved the system for immediate implementation.

Using METs should be a mandatory requirement for all hospitals. This system significantly reduces the frequency of cardiac arrest among hospitalized patients. Consequently, many lives are saved. The traditional medical culture must change to earliest possible involvement of a well-trained and experienced team preventing evolving crisis from developing into lethal consequences.

Michael DeVita and his excellent group of editors successfully present the introduction of METs in medicine to prevent unnecessary hospital deaths, first discussing why the current system fails and then describing system-wide approaches, the challenge of implementation, and finally the evaluation of hospital patient safety initiatives. In all, some thirty chapters by carefully selected authors provide a thriller-like and fascinating story of MET development in modern hospital patient management at a time when patient safety and appropriate timely care is recognized to be our most important obligation. Interestingly, the byproduct is improved educational experiences for both physician trainees, nurses, and other health care providers. This is clearly opposite to the anticipated effect of using METs.

In conclusion, this book may very well become a bestseller. Readers are likely to include not only physicians and nurses, but also hospital administrators, insurance agents and government representatives. The message is clear and the editors and authors are to be congratulated to so successfully completing their most important task.

Ake Grenvik, M.D., Ph.D.
Distinguished Service Professor
of Critical Care Medicine
University of Pittsburgh School of Medicine

Preface

As the editors of *Medical Emergency Teams* and as clinicians, we have been working on improving hospital responses to crises for more than ten years. We have learned the hard way how not to build the wrong response, how not to step on toes, how not to intimidate people from calling for help, and how not to lose focus when energizing hospital personnel to prevent deaths by responding early and in a systematic fashion. We have had to convince people to work for and fund the program initially using only enthusiasm and logic. One of us applied for a grant to implement METs only to hear from the agency that not only were such teams impractical, no one would want to do the extra work they required!

We worked in isolation for a period of time, first winning over our own organization, and then, through stronger and stronger evidence of benefit, beginning to convince others of the need for and potential impact of medical emergency teams. Each of us has developed a new culture in our hospital, one that attempts to prevent cardiac arrests rather than responding to them. It a culture that is focused on the patient and on safety. It is a culture that constantly asks what is required for medical crises to be recognized early and reliably, for help to be requested promptly, and for well-designed systematic response to the call for help to arrive quickly and act effectively. Our hospitals had come to learn that mortality can be decreased dramatically, work days become more stable, and job satisfaction improve due to a reduction of perceptions of abandonment and a rise in empowerment. Each on us has begun to try to move this new culture of hospital medicine elsewhere.

The culture that needed to be changed was one that accepted sudden and unexpected death as a status quo event in a hospital. The culture that needed to be created was to one where unexpected death was systematically reduced by the creation of a planned system to respond to crisis: the Medical Emergency Team (MET). The MET goes by many names including a Rapid Response Team (RRT), critical care outreach team, and the Condition C (for Crisis) team. They amount to the same thing: a well-designed institutional plan for trained health care professionals to come to the aid of patients in distress.

In early 2004, we met and shared our experiences and determined to join forces to create a medical revolution of sorts. There were three things that were needed to change the culture of medicine. First, we need greater recognition that a MET response existed and that METs might be helpful. Until recently, few people had even heard of MET responses. Second, there must be a greater understanding of what METs can do: even if people knew about them, many were skeptical about their merit or outcome benefit. Third, people need a reference manual that includes information (and advice) on how to implement such a team. We have come to learn that even when people are aware and convinced of the benefits of METs, they had no map for implementing a MET response in their hospital.

Therefore, we chose to have a three-fold strategy to change international culture. First: we would hold an international conference to raise awareness. Second, we would bring together the world's experts in MET responses to discuss the quality of the data and determine the best methodology to move the science forward. And third, we would create a manual for those who might want to implement a MET program. This book is that manual.

Chapters 1 to 7 discuss patient safety in hospitals and provides a context for how a MET system fits into the patient safety rubric. Chapters 8 to 19 devoted to the logistics of developing a system. How to create a team, alternatives methodologies for responding to patients in crisis, how to train team members, and how such teams impact important medical and nursing functions like education, staff recruitment and retention, and finally how to identify and overcome political hurdles. Finally, Chapters 20 to 25 describe how to measure the impact of these teams in hospitals: from improved mortality data to reduction in errors and finally to staff satisfaction.

We have assembled the authors who have been most successful in developing a MET (or similar systems) program and who have been prolific in writing about their experiences. We have also attempted to bring authors from a variety of disciplines and geographically far flung areas of the globe in an attempt to create a manual for anyone interested in METs. This book is a "How-To," "Why-Do It," and "Prove-It" manual. We feel it is a tool that can be used by administrators to help convince skeptical staff, for staff to convince unwilling administrators, and for all to use to work through the nuts and bolts of introducing and sustaining a MET response program.

We believe the concept of hospital-wide early recognition of management of seriously ill patients will facilitate a much needed revolution in hospital patient safety by breaking down current professional and geographical barriers and concentrating on systematic patient centered identification and resuscitation of the seriously ill at an early stage in their deterioration. The MET system links real time incident monitoring and response, as well as providing a basis for measuring and comparing hospital quality. While the glamour of METs is in the rapid response to crisis, perhaps the power is in the way analysis of events preceding them can feed into a process improvement metric.

We recognize that there is some redundancy among chapters. This is to some extent intentional. Our intention is to create a manual wherein each chapter can stand on its own. This design allows the reader to skip between chapters or even read just one or two and still understand the context and importance of the content as it relates to METs. Having said this, we have also tried to create a textbook that the reader can study from beginning to end, with earlier chapters laying the foundation for later ones.

We have truly learned a lot in writing this textbook. We hope the readers will not only likewise become more knowledgeable about METs, but also carry around the manual as they develop their own program and hopefully create a change in culture in their own institution. If clinician investigators from the early 1990s are correct, some 80% of hospital unexpected deaths are preventable. We believe this is unacceptable and have seen the MET system reduce this dramatically first hand. We can yet do better. Patient safety is an agenda with no end. Thus there is much to learn and much more to do. This book we hope is a start.

Michael A. DeVita, M.D.
Kenneth Hillman, M.D.
Rinaldo Bellomo, M.D.

Contents

SECTION THREE   MEASURING OUTCOMES

Contributors

Rinaldo Bellomo, M.D.
Department of Intensive Care, Austin Hospital, Heidelberg, Victoria 3084, Australia

Daniel Brown, M.D.
Modality Manager—Critical Care, South East Asia, Draeger Medical, Singapore

Michael Buist, M.B.Ch.B.
Department of Critical Care, Dandenong Hospital, Victoria 3175, Melbourne, Australia

Donald Campbell, M.D.
Monash Institute for Health Services Research, Monash University, Melbourne, Victoria 3168, Australia

Lakshmipathi Chelluri, M.D.
Department of Critical Care Medicine, University of Pittsburgh Medical Center, Pittsburgh, PA 15261, USA

Jack Chen, Ph.D.
The Simpson Centre for Health Services Research, Liverpool Hospital, Liverpool, New South Wales 1871, Australia

Michelle Cretikos, M.D.
The Simpson Centre for Health Services Research, Liverpool Hospital, Liverpool, New South Wales 1871, Australia

Brian Currie, M.D.
Department of Epidemiology, Montefiore Medical Center, Bronx, New York 10467, USA

Edgar Delgado, R.R.T.
Respiratory Care Department, University of Pittsburgh Medical Center, Pittsburgh, PA 15213, USA

Michael A. DeVita, M.D.
Departments of Critical Care Medicine and Internal Medicine, University of Pittsburgh School of Medicine, Associate Medical Director, UPMC Presbyterian Hospital, Pittsburgh, PA 15213, USA

Kathy D. Duncan, R.N.
Critical Care Services, Baptist Memorial Hospital, Memphis, TN 38120, USA

Melinda Fiedor, M.D.
Department of Critical Care Medicine, University of Pittsburgh Medical Center, Pittsburgh, PA 15213, USA

Arthas Flabouris, F.J.F.I.C.M.
Intensive Care Unit, Royal Adelaide Hospital, Adelaide, South Australia 5000, Australia

Donna Goldsmith, M.N.
Department of Intensive Care, Austin Hospital, Heidelberg, Victoria 3084, Australia

John Gosbee, M.D.
National Center for Patient Safety, United States Department of Veterans Affairs, Ann Arbor, MI 48108, USA

Wendeline J. Grbach, R.N.
Department of Nursing Education, University of Pittsburgh Medical Center, Shadyside School of Nursing, Pittsburgh, PA 15206, USA

Ake Grenvik, M.D., Ph.D.
Department of Critical Care Medicine, University of Pittsburgh Medical Center, Pittsburgh, PA 15261, USA

Scott R. Gunn, M.D.
Department of Critical Care Medicine, University of Pittsburgh Medical Center, Pittsburgh, PA 15261, USA

Kenneth Hillman, M.D.
The Simpson Centre for Health Services Research, Liverpool Hospital, Liverpool, New South Wales 1871, Australia

David T. Huang, M.D.
Department of Emergency Medicine, University of Pittsburgh Medical Center, Pittsburgh, PA 15261, USA

Elizabeth A. Hunt, M.D.
Department of Anesthesiology & Critical Care Medicine, The Johns
Hopkins University School of Medicine, Baltimore, Maryland 21205, USA

Daryl Jones, M.D.
Department of Intensive Care, Austin Hospital, Heidelberg, Victoria 3084,
Australia

Juliane Kause, M.B.B.S.
Department of Critical Care Medicine, Portsmouth Hospitals National
Health Service Trust, Portsmouth, Hampshire, PO6 3LY, United Kingdom

Joanne Kowiatek, M.P.M., R.Ph.
Department of Pharmacy and Therapeutics, University of Pittsburgh
Medical Center, Pittsburgh, PA 15213, USA

Vladimir Kvetan, M.D.
Department of Critical Care Medicine, Montefiore Medical Center, Bronx,
New York 10467, USA

Stephen W. Lam, M.B.B.S.
Intensive Care Unit, Royal Adelaide Hospital, Adelaide, South Australia
5000, Australia

Geoffrey K. Lighthall, M.D., Ph.D.
Department of Anesthesia, Palo Alto Veteran Affairs Medical Center, Palo
Alto, CA 95304, USA

David J. McAdams, M.D.
Division of Internal Medicine, University of Pittsburgh Medical Center,
Pittsburgh, PA 15213, USA

Marlene Miller, M.D.
Department of Pediatrics, The Johns Hopkins University School of
Medicine, Baltimore, Maryland 21205, USA

Nicolette C. Mininni, R.N.
Department of Critical Care, University of Pittsburgh Medical Center,
Shadyside School of Nursing, Pittsburgh, PA 15232, USA

Andrew W. Murray, M.B., Ch.B.
Department of Anesthesiology, University of Pittsburgh Medical Center,
Pittsburgh, PA 15213, USA

Helen Ingrid Opdam, M.D.
Department of Intensive Care, Austin Hospital, Heidelberg, Victoria 3084,
Australia

Peter J. Pronovost, M.D., Ph.D.
Department of Anesthesiology and Critical Care Medicine, The Johns Hopkins University School of Medicine, Baltimore, Maryland 21205, USA

Emanuel P. Rivers, M.D.
Department of Emergency Medicine, Wayne State University, Detroit, MI 48202, USA

John J. Schaefer III, M.D.
Department of Anesthesiology, University of Pittsburgh Medical Center, Pittsburgh, PA 15213, USA

Carole C. Scholle, R.N., M.S.N.
Director, Critical Care Services, University of Pittsburgh Medical Center, Pittsburgh, PA, USA

Gary B. Smith, F.R.C.A., F.R.C.P.
Department of Critical Care Medicine, Portsmouth Hospitals National Health Service Trust, Portsmouth, Hampshire, PO6 3LY, United Kingdom

Craig White
Department of Intensive Care, Austin Hospital, Heidelberg, Victoria 3084, Australia

Brad Winters, M.D., Ph.D.
Department of Anesthesiology and Critical Care Medicine, The Johns Hopkins University School of Medicine, Baltimore, Maryland 21205, USA

Lis Young, M.A., C.C.M.
The Simpson Centre for Health Services Research, Liverpool Hospital, Liverpool, New South Wales 1871, Australia

1
Measuring and Improving Safety

PETER J. PRONOVOST, MARLENE MILLER, BRAD WINTERS, and ELIZABETH A. HUNT

Introduction

November 2004 marked the 5-year anniversary of the Institute of Medicine's landmark report *To Err Is Human*, which revealed a significant problem with patient safety in the United States and presented a call to action (1). In response to this report, many health care leaders actively addressed patient safety. Segments of the health care community have educated themselves on methods to improve safety, and some—although not nearly enough—have executed interventions toward this goal (2,3). However, few health care organizations have evaluated the impact of their efforts. Thus, 5 years later, it is difficult to answer the question, "Are patients safer?"

Sorrel King, the mother of Josie King, who died at the age of 18 months from mistakes at the Johns Hopkins Children's Center, asked if Josie would be less likely to die today, 5 years after *To Err Is Human*. She did not want just our perceptions of whether Josie would be less likely to die; rather, she wanted evidence. How do we *know* that our patients are safer and our efforts to improve patient safety are working?

Measuring and improving safety is difficult. Not all safety measures lend themselves to rates. We have come to understand that a critical factor for success in improving patient safety is to actively change the culture of the institution. Considering these challenges, how will we answer the tough question asked by Sorrel King, "How do we know patients are safer?" (2,3)

This chapter provides an overview of the issues in measuring patient safety, and presents a framework for measuring and improving safety. It is important to recognize that safety is a component of the broader concept of "quality," which includes care that is effective, efficient, patient-centered, timely, and equitable (4). The boundaries between these concepts are unclear, and measures can often fall in more than 1 category. For example, is the failure to use an evidence-based therapy a safety measure—a mistake of omission—or an effectiveness measure? Is a complication, such as a catheter-related bloodstream infection that also increases length of stay,

1

a safety or effectiveness measure? The distinction is less important than having a valid measure. Thus, in this chapter, we will use the term "safety" to refer to both safety and effectiveness.

Approach for the Organizational Evaluation of Patient Safety

Donabedian's approach to measuring quality of care—evaluating how we organize care (the structures), what we do (the processes), and the results we obtain (the outcomes)—also provides a framework for institutions to measure safety (5). Many institutional efforts to improve safety focus on structural measures, such as policies and procedures (6). Institutions may also measure processes and outcomes, although these are generally more difficult to develop and collect than structural measures. For example, organizations may measure how often certain aspects of safe and effective care were performed (a process), or how often certain complications occurred (an outcome) (7,8).

While process and outcome measures are generally preferable to structural measures, they are not sufficient. Generally, process and outcome measures are rates that include a numerator and denominator, but not all measures of safety can, or should, be presented as rates. For example, a single episode of potential harm or actual harm (such as the death of Josie) may be statistically insignificant but sufficient to trigger an organizational change. If organizations do not recognize and learn from such single episodes, they fail to maximize opportunities to improve safety. In addition, measurement of rates is resource-intensive and not feasible for every type of medical error.

Along with the ability to learn, many other aspects of an organization's culture have a significant impact on safety (9,10). In aviation, changes in culture have been responsible for most of the advancements in safety over the last 2 decades (9,11). Within health care, communication failures are a common cause of sentinel events, both at Johns Hopkins and at other institutions across the United States (12) (www.jcaho.org). Indeed, communication patterns within an organization are an important aspect of culture. Thus, the measure of both organizational learning and culture may provide insight into an organization's measure of safety.

W. Edwards Deming once said, "There is no true value of anything that is measured; change the method of measurement and you change the result." The same concept applies to measuring safety. In the absence of standard definitions and methods to measure patient safety, including methods for risk adjustment (e.g. health care–acquired infections) (13), it is unlikely that national measures of patient safety will be achieved.

There are multiple ways to measure each area of patient safety. Consider medication safety: we can have a structural measure, such as the presence of computerized physician order entry; a process measure, such as pre-scribing errors; or an outcome measure, such as adverse drug events. More-over, each category (structure, process, or outcome) can be measured in multiple ways. For example, the methods of surveillance for evaluating adverse drug events—many of which use self-reported events, with the numerator being how the adverse event is defined and the denominator being either patient, number of patient days, or dose—vary widely (Table 1.1)(14–18). Which method provides the "correct" rate of medication safety? They all may. In the absence of standardized definitions, compar-isons within and among institutions is problematic (19,20). Even with stan-dard definitions, there is concern that comparing outcomes among hospitals is not scientifically sound, with differences influenced by insufficient risk adjustment and random error rather than variations in patient safety (8, 19–21).

Based on this background, our approach to evaluating patient safety at the organizational level has 4 components and prompts the institution to answer the following 4 questions: (1) how often do we harm patients; (2) how often do patients receive the interventions they should; (3) how often do we learn from our mistakes; and (4) how well have we created a culture of patient safety. This framework is presented in Table 1.2.

Measuring Defects

To measure safety, we often estimate reliability in defects per unit, or Sigma, with 1 Sigma defined as defects per units of 10, 2 Sigma as defects per unit of hundreds, 3 Sigma defects per thousand, 4 Sigma defects per ten thou-sand, 5 Sigma defects per hundred thousand, and 6 Sigma defects per million. Measuring safety is difficult, and the methods are evolving (8). Often we are not clear regarding the unit of analysis for the denominator—in anesthesia, for example, is the appropriate denominator the minutes of anesthesia, or the number of times we induce anesthesia? The defect rate can be influenced significantly by the chosen denominator.

Moreover, often measures are easy to collect yet lack meaning for the frontline staff expected to use the measure to improve safety. For example, at many health care organizations, the staff is not aware of the quality and safety measures collected by the central administration (often done to satisfy regulatory requirements). System-level measures need to be mean-ingful to the workers in their local areas.

In our zeal to create measures of safety, we have often compromised validity and viewed the goal as increasing the number of identified defects rather than learning from those defects. Many organizations use rates of self-reported adverse drug events as a measure of safety without recogniz-ing that, as for all outcome measures, variations in the method of data collection/definition/data quality, case-mix, and quality, as well as chance, influence outcomes (19). Moreover, variations in data quality and case-mix

TABLE 1.1. Sample of methods to measure medication

Study	Number studied	Numerator	Denominator	Assessed by	Rate of events
Leape, et al. NEJM 1991	30 195 records	Disabling adverse events	Per record reviewed/admission	Physician Reviewer	3.7 per 100 admissions
Lesar, Briceland JAMA 1990	289411 medication orders/1 yr.	Prescribing errors	Number of Orders written	Physicians	3.13 errors for each 1000 orders
Lesar, Briceland Stein JAMA 1997	1 year of prescribing errors detected and averted by pharmacist	Prescribing errors	Per medication orders written	Pharmacists, retrospectively evaluated by a physician and 2 pharmacists	3.99 errors per 1000 orders
Cullen, et al. Crit Care Medicine 1997	4031 adult admissions over 6 months.	Adverse drug events	Number of patient days	Self report by nurse and pharmacists, daily review of all charts by nurse investigators.	19 events per 1000 ICU patient days

TABLE 1.2. Framework for an institutional scorecard for patient safety and effectiveness

Domain	Definition	Example from department of anesthesiology
How often do we harm patients?	Measures of health care–acquired infections	Bloodstream infections Surgical site infections
How often do patients receive the interventions they should?	Using either nationally validated process measures, or a validated process to develop a measure, what percentage of patients receive evidence-based interventions	Use of perioperative beta blockers Elevation of head of bed in mechanically ventilated patients Rates of postoperative hypothermia
How often do we learn from our mistakes?	What percentage of months does each area learn from mistakes	Monitor percentage of months in which the department creates a shared story, as in Figure 1.1
How well have we created a culture of patient safety?	Annual assessment of safety culture at the unit level	Percentage change in culture scores for each care area

are likely to be far greater than the variation in safety, which limits our ability to make inferences about quality of care from these measures.

Measures of safety and quality must be important, scientifically sound, feasible, and usable. Important and usable are value judgments that are typically made by the group, institution, or organization that decides to measure a particular area. Scientifically sound refers to validity and reliability. An indicator is deemed valid if the following criteria are met (www.rand.org) (22):

- Adequate scientific evidence or professional consensus exists supporting the indicator.
- There are identifiable health benefits to patients who receive care specified by the indicator.
- Based on experience, health professionals with significantly higher rates of adherence to an indicator would be considered higher-quality providers.
- Most factors that determine adherence to an indicator are under the control of the health professional (or are subject to influence by the health professional, such as smoking cessation).

An indicator is considered to be feasible if (22):

- The information necessary to determine adherence is likely to be found in a typical medical record.

- Estimates of adherence to the indicator based on medical record data are likely to be reliable and unbiased.
- A reliable measure produces similar results when measurement is repeated.

In many efforts to measure quality of care and safety, the measures are collected without the support of additional staff. As such, the feasibility of a measure figures prominently in its success. Finally, a measure must be usable—that is, it must be useful to the people who are expected to improve quality.

To measure quality, we need valid numerators (defects) and denominators (risk pool). To be scientifically sound, both the numerator and denominator must be valid and reliable. Yet there are challenges in measuring both. Most health care areas have not defined what a defect is, limiting the ability to measure a numerator. For example, substantial evidence suggests that controlling blood sugar in patients in an intensive care unit (ICU) reduces mortality, yet we do it infrequently. What might be a defect in glucose control? Is it 1 high blood sugar, 2 high sugars, or the average sugar over some period above a defined threshold?

In addition, it is unclear what the unit of analysis should be for the denominator. The choice of denominator can change performance by several Sigmas. For example, aviation and anesthesia changed its denominators from minutes flown to takeoffs and landings, and anesthesia from minutes of care to a case. Thus, if an average flight was over 100 miles, or an average anesthesia case 100 minutes, the defect rate would change 2 Sigmas without any change in safety. Consider also ways to measure rates of failed extubation: should the denominator be the patient, the ventilator day, or an attempted extubation? There are often tradeoffs between validity and feasibility of data collection.

It is also important to distinguish whether we are measuring the reliability of a process (what we do) or an outcome (the results we get). While commercial aviation is believed to perform at 6 Sigmas for crashes (outcome), it performs at 1 or 2 Sigmas for on-time departures. Intuitively, outcome measures are more appealing than process measures, yet measuring outcomes pose added risk for bias that often leads to little or no useful information (19,23). Reliability of an outcome measure can be influenced by variations in the methods of surveillance, in methods of data collection and definitions, in case-mix, in true variation in safety, and random error (23). Among institutions, variation in quality is often significantly smaller than variation of other variables. In health care, we need to work toward standardized measures of reliability. The gold standard, and perhaps the only valid outcome measure, is the National Nosocomial Infections Surveillance (NNIS) program that provides standardized methods to monitor health care–acquired infections (13).

Evidence-based processes of care (defects of omission) lend themselves to monitoring rates. However, we currently only have a handful of validated process measures, and these are mainly limited to internal medicine. A more diverse group of quality measures is needed. These measures must be appropriately monitored as defect rates.

In addition, health care organizations need to recognize that the value of some defects lies solely in learning from the numerator; the costs of obtaining an appropriate denominator, even if methodologically feasible, would be prohibitive. For example, methods to monitor health care–acquired infections, commonly reported as measures of safety, evolved over 20 years, include rigorous and detailed specifications, and are supported by an entire department devoted to collecting and monitoring the rates of these infections. Even so, data collection is commonly limited to a few areas—will we create departments to monitor medication safety, complications, or other outcomes? Measures of safety need to be valid, yet we can learn from defects that lack denominators.

How might measures be selected? Deming provides some guidance. Measures should be selected to optimize learning: that is, ensure the measure has face validity—does the person expected to use the data to measure specifications believe it measures something important? To develop measures that are clinically meaningful, we need the combined input of frontline staff and researchers with methodological rigor. For example, the exposure risk for a failed extubation is an attempted extubation. Yet rates of failed extubation are often presented using patients or ventilator days as the denominator (24). To estimate feasibility, first test-run the data collection tools. Moreover, the measurement of safety should be approached with the same rigor as that applied in clinical research. Whether we are measuring bloodstream infections as part of a federally funded trial or for hospital safety efforts, we need a valid measure of infections. Much research is needed to advance the science of measuring defects.

Given this, what are some measures of safety for Medical Emergency Teams (METs)? Although ICU admission and number of codes called are common measures, they lack validity. We do not know whether an increase or decrease in the rate of ICU admission is high-quality care. The measure does not differentiate between patients who required ICU care and those who did not, or who may have had a preventable reason for admission. On the other hand, use of chest compressions or intubations may be an appropriate numerator for defects. Deaths may also be an informative numerator.

In addition to the numerator, we need to consider an appropriate denominator or risk group. Although patients are used commonly as the denominator, patient days may be a more valid denominator. A patient's risk for arrest is influenced by, among other things, the length of time they are in the hospital. The longer a patient is in the hospital, the greater the risk.

Hospital mortality and length of stay may be measures of safety for METs but, as with all outcome measures, case-mix will significantly influence these outcomes making comparisons among hospitals difficult to interpret (23). As long as a hospital does not add or drop a product line, case-mix within a hospital is relatively constant, making changes in mortality rate within a hospital potentially important and measurable. Much more effort is needed to produce scientifically sound and feasible measures of safety for METs.

How Might We Improve Safety?

Recently, one of the authors went to the circus with his wife and 2 children. It was both exhilarating and exhausting: 3 rings of nonstop activity, noise, and motion. He noticed how flawless all of the interventions were; the circus functioned without a hazardous event. Trapeze artists flew through the air with perfect timing, and men on motorcycles rode around in a metal globe, perilously missing each other by inches. As he watched the show, he esti-mated that the number of critical processes was probably equivalent to about a week's worth of activities in 30 operating rooms, yet no defects occurred. He wondered how the circus performed with such high reliabil-ity, and noticed that everything was scripted down to the tiniest detail. All the processes were standardized. The cleanup crews in ring 1 did the same things in ring 2. All the events were timed and sequenced by what they were doing and when it was done. One act ended and the next began, flawlessly.

How might this circus performance inform patient safety? It appears that most organizations are aware of the need to improve patient safety, and many have committed to doing so. Yet only a small number have a clear plan of attack to accomplish this goal and even fewer have actually improved safety. This should not be surprising. The drive to improve patient safety is new in health care, and we must view health care delivery as a science as well as an art if we are to improve safety. Here we present an overview of measuring and reducing defects in health care and suggest some potential system-level measures of safety.

A Framework to Improve Reliability

In health care, most of our processes are between 1 and 2 Sigma. For a wide variety of processes, patients can rely on receiving the interventions they should half the time, or 1 Sigma (25). For some outcomes, defects are 2 to 3 Sigmas—for example, catheter-related bloodstream infection rates and rates of ventilator-associated pneumonia are typically between 1 to 20 per 1000 catheter or ventilator days (13,26). Nevertheless, there are some notable exceptions in anesthesia in healthy patients and in blood banking that are estimated to be 4 or 5 Sigma (defects per 10000 or 100000) (27,28).

Caregivers in these areas, and multiple other non-health care organizations, deliver high-reliability care because they are standardized. To improve reliability, we need to create a culture of safety first, where the entire care team makes the patient their "North Star" according to which they create and implement common goals. A culture of safety allows all members of the care team to speak up when they have concerns and listen when others voice concerns. Next comes standardization, specifying what is done and when it should be done (29–31). This contrasts with current practice in which the art of medicine trumps the science—individual caregiver practice is unstructured and at times appears chaotic (i.e., caregivers do what they want, when they want). In the ICU, the therapies that a patient receives depend more on who is making the rounds, rather than what the evidence suggests. Without standardization, reliability will remain at 10^{-1} imparting a significant toll on patients.

An important aspect of standardization is to simplify or reduce complexity. Every step is a process that has an independent probability of failure. As such, processes that have 5 steps are more likely to fail than those that have 4, 3, or 2 steps. An analogy is the telephone game, in which a story is told through a series of people: the risk factors for getting a garbled story (a defect) at the end are defined by how complex the story is and how many people it passes through. If we reduce the number of steps in a process, we have a higher probability of improving reliability. Undoubtedly this is an oversimplification, since there are feedback loops that may catch mistakes. Nevertheless, it is helpful to consider simplification when we examine our work processes.

Let us give you an example of reducing complexity. We had a mistake with transvenous pacing. The physician attempting the procedure had to obtain a sheath (Cordis) and a pacing wire. The wire goes through the sheath, note there are different sizes and types for both sheaths and wires. Unfortunately, the equipment needed for transveous pacing is not packaged together, and physicians need to obtain the equipment through different steps. Predictably, the physician grabbed the wrong combination of pacing wire and sheath, and the patient suffered an air embolism. To reduce complexity and the potential for another mistake, we now have Central Supply package all pieces of equipment for specific procedures together.

Third, we need to identify and learn from defects. This involves creating independent checks to identify defects. A significant challenge we face in health care is a shared definition or concept of a defect. To illustrate, Johns Hopkins developed a glucose protocol in the ICU. Like most protocols, we were only capturing about 80% of patients. To improve reliability, we needed an independent check to identify defects. The problem was that we had not defined a defect. Although we could have defined it in multiple ways, we decided that in the morning during the shift change, the nurses would review a patient's glucose and if 2 blood sugars were out of range, they would talk to the physician and implement the protocol. We defined the defect first and then created an independent check to identify it. Nurses in the ICU now present a patient's last 3 glucose measures each morning on rounds. If a defect is identified—that is, the sugar levels are out of range—the patient is placed back on another protocol.

To learn from defects, we need to investigate what went wrong and make recommendations for improvement. In the related example, the ICU nurse manager did this beautifully. After implementing the glucose control protocol, she started to hold glucose rounds with the nurses, during which they discussed any patient who was on but then fell off the glucose protocol. These discussions would often surface a variety of system factors that posed barriers to improving glucose care; some were beliefs and attitudes among nurses, some dealt with the availability of supplies to measure glucose hourly, and others involved communication with physicians. We have developed a tool kit to learn from a defect. This tool kit (Table 1.3) helps uncover what happened, why it happened, and what must be done to fix the defect.

These steps—(1) create a culture of safety, (2) standardize what and when actions are done, and (3) identify and learn from defects—provide a framework to improve reliability. Transfusion medicine offers an example of how the application of these principles created a high reliability process: using discharge data, the estimated incidence of a transfusion reaction in health care is 4 per 100000. How did they achieve such success? They standardized, created independent checks for key processes, and learned from defects (Figure 1.1).

Physicians often resist standardization. I asked several blood bank directors how they achieved their degree of standardization. They uniformly replied that the threat of a Food and Drug Administration sanction created the culture. Several felt they would not have the authority to standardize physician practice without the backing of federal regulation. Although regulations may be an important vehicle for standardization, there are far too many processes for regulators to standardize. Indeed, we need the courage of leaders within our health care systems to support standardization.

TABLE 1.3. How to investigate a defect

Problem statement: Health care organizations could increase the extent to which they learn from defects.

What is a defect? A defect is any clinical or operational event or situation that you would not want to happen again. These could include incidents that you believe caused a patient harm or put patients at risk for significant harm.

Purpose of tool: The purpose of this tool is to provide a structured approach to help caregivers and administrators identify the types of systems that contributed to the defect and follow up to ensure safety improvements are achieved.

Who should use this tool?
• Clinical departmental designee at morbidity and mortality rounds
• Patient care areas as part of the Comprehensive Unit-based Safety Program (CUSP)

TABLE 1.3. *Continued*

All staff involved in the delivery of care related to this defect *should be present when this defect is evaluated.* At a minimum, this should include the physician, nurse, and administrator, and others as appropriate (e.g. medication defect includes pharmacy, equipment defect includes clinical engineering).

How to Use This Tool: Complete this tool on *at least 1 defect per month.* In addition, departments should investigate all of the following defects: liability claims, sentinel events, events for which risk management is notified, case presented to morbidity and mortality rounds and health care–acquired infections.

Investigation Process

I.   Provide a clear, thorough, and objective explanation of *what happened.*
II. Review the list of factors that contributed to the incident and check off those that negatively contributed and positively contributed to the impact of the incident. *Negative contributing factors* are those that harmed or increased risk of harm for the patient; *positive contributing factors* limited the impact of harm.
III. Describe how you will reduce the likelihood of this defect happening again by completing the table. List *what* you will do, *who* will lead the intervention, *when* you will follow up on the intervention's progress, and *how* you will know risk reduction has been achieved.

Investigation process

I. What happened? (Reconstruct the timeline and explain what happened. For this investigation, put yourself in the place of those involved in the event as it was unfolding, to understand what they were thinking and the reasoning behind their actions/decisions when the event occurred.)
An African American male >65 years old was admitted to a cardiac surgical ICU in the early morning hours. The patient was status-post cardiac surgery and on dialysis at the time of the incident. Within 2 hours of admission to the ICU it was clear that the patient needed a transvenous pacing wire. The wire was threaded using an IJ Cordis sheath, which is a stocked item in the ICU and standard for pulmonary artery catheters, but not the right size for a transvenous pacing wire. The sheath that matched the pacing wire was not stocked in this ICU, because transvenous pacing wires are used infrequently. The wire was threaded and placed in the ventricle but staff soon realized that the sheath did not properly seal over the wire, thus introducing risk of an air embolus. Since the wire was pacing the patient at 100%, there was no possibility for removal at that time. To reduce the patient's risk of embolus, the bedside nurse and resident sealed the sheath using gauze and tape.
II. Why did it happen? Below is a framework to help you review and evaluate your case. Please read each contributing factor and evaluate whether it was involved, and if so, whether it contributed negatively (increased harm) or positively (reduced impact of harm) to the incident.

Contributing factors *(example)*	Negatively contributed	Positively contributed
Patient factors		
Patient was acutely ill or agitated *(Elderly patient in renal failure, secondary to congestive heart failure.)*		
There was a language barrier *(Patient did not speak English.)*		
There were personal or social issues *(Patient declined therapy.)*		
Task factors		
Was there a protocol available to guide therapy? *(Protocol for mixing medication concentrations is posted above the medication bin.)*	XX	

Table 1.3. *Continued*

Contributing factors *(example)*	Negatively contributed	Positively contributed
Were test results available to help make care decision? *(Stat blood glucose results were sent in 20 minutes.)*		
Were tests results accurate? *(Four diagnostic tests done; only magnetic resonance imaging [MRI] results needed quickly—results faxed.)*		
Caregiver factors		
Was the caregiver fatigued? *(Tired at the end of a double shift, nurse forgot to take a blood pressure reading.)*		
Did the caregiver's outlook/perception of own professional role impact on this event? *(Doctor followed up to make sure cardiac consultation was done expeditiously.)*		
Was the physical or mental health of the caregiver a factor? *(Caregiver was having personal issues and missed hearing a verbal order.)*		
Team factors		
Was verbal or written communication during handoff clear, accurate, clinically relevant, and goal-directed? *(Oncoming care team was debriefed by outgoing staff regarding patient's condition.)*		
Was verbal or written communication during care clear, accurate, clinically relevant, and goal-directed? *(Staff was comfortable expressing concern regarding high medication dose.)*		
Was verbal or written communication during crisis clear, accurate, clinically relevant and goal-directed? *(Team leader quickly explained and directed the team regarding the plan of action.)*		
Was there a cohesive team structure with an identified and communicative leader? *(Attending physician gave clear instructions to the team.)*		
Training and education factors		
Was the caregiver knowledgeable, skilled, and competent? *(Nurse knew dose ordered was not standard for that medication.)*	XX	
Did the caregiver follow the established protocol? *(Provider pulled protocol to ensure steps were followed.)*		
Did the caregiver seek supervision or help? *(New nurse asked preceptor to help mix medication concentration.)*		
Information technology/computerized physician order entry factors		
Did the computer/software program generate an error? *(Heparin was chosen, but Digoxin printed on the order sheet.)*		
Did the computer/software malfunction? *(Computer shut down in the middle of provider's order entry.)*		
Did the user check what was entered to make sure it was correct? *(Caregiver initially chose .25 mg, but caught error and changed it to .025 mg.)*		

TABLE 1.3. *Continued*

Contributing factors *(example)*	Negatively contributed	Positively contributed
Local environment factors		
Was adequate equipment available and was it working properly? *(There were 2 extra ventilators stocked and recently serviced by clinical engineering.)*	XX	
Was operational (administrative and managerial) support adequate? *(Unit clerk out sick, but extra clerk sent to cover from another unit.)*		
Was the physical environment conducive to enhancing patient care? *(All beds were visible from the nurse's station.)*		
Was enough staff on the unit to care for patient volume? *(Nurse ratio was 1:1.)*		
Was there a good mix of skilled and new staff? *(A nurse orientee was shadowing a senior nurse and an extra nurse was on to cover the senior nurse's responsibilities.)*		
Did workload impact the provision of good care? *(Nurse caring for 3 patients because nurse went home sick.)*		
Institutional environment factors		
Were adequate financial resources available? *(Unit requested experienced patient transport team for critically ill patients, and one was made available the next day.)*		
Were laboratory technicians adequately in-serviced/educated? *(Lab technician was fully aware of complications related to thallium injection.)*		
Was there adequate staffing in the laboratory to run results? *(There were 3 dedicated laboratory technicians to run stat results.)*		
Were pharmacists adequately in-service/educated? *(Pharmacists knew and followed the protocol for stat medication orders.)*		
Did pharmacy have a good infrastructure (policy, procedures)? *(It was standard policy to have a second pharmacist do an independent check before dispensing medications.)*		
Was there adequate pharmacy staffing? *(There was a pharmacist dedicated to the ICU.)*		
Does hospital administration work with the units regarding what and how to support their needs? *(Guidelines established to hold new ICU admissions in the emergency department when beds are not available in the ICU.)*		

III. How will you reduce the likelihood of this defect happening again?

Specific things to be done to reduce the risk of the defect	Who will lead this effort?	Follow-up date	How will you determine the risk is reduced? (action items)
Bedside nurse called Central Supply and requested pacing wires and matching sheaths be packaged together.	Bedside nurse	1 week	Supplies are packaged together

Safety Tips:
· Label devices that work together to complete a procedure

Case in Point: An African American male ≥ 65 years of age was admitted to a cardiac surgical ICU in the early morning hours. The patient was status-post cardiac surgery and on dialysis at the time of the incident. Within 2 hours of admission to the ICU it was clear that the patient needed a transvenous pacing wire. The wire was threaded using an IJ Cordis sheath, which is a stocked item in the ICU and standard for PA caths, but not the right size for a transvenous pacing wire. The sheath that matched the pacing wire was not stocked in this ICU since transvenous pacing wires are used infrequently. The wire was threaded and placed in the ventricle and staff soon realized that the sheath did not properly seal over the wire, thus introducing risk of an air embolus. Since the wire was pacing the patient at 100%, there was no possibility for removal at that time. To reduce the patient's risk of embolus, the bedside nurse and resident sealed the sheath using gauze and tape.

System Failures: Opportunities for Improvement:

Knowledge, skills & competence. Care providers lacked the knowledge needed to match a transvenous pacing wire with appropriate sized sheath.

Regular **training and education**, even if infrequently used, of all devices and equipment.

Unit Environment: availability of device. The appropriate size sheath for a transvenous pacing wire was not a stocked device. Pacing wires and matching sheathes packages separately… increases complexity.

Infrequently used equipment/devices **should still be stocked** in the ICU. Devices that must work together to complete a procedure should be packaged together.

Medical Equipment/Device. There was apparently no label or mechanism for warning the staff that the IJ Cordis sheath was too big for the transvenous pacing wire.

Label wires and sheaths noting the appropriate partner for this device.

ACTIONS TAKEN TO PREVENT HARM
The bedside nurse and resident were alert enough to realize the sheath was too big and used their knowledge and skills to seal the sheath with gauze and tape to reduce the risk of an air embolus.

The bedside nurse contacted central supply and requested that pacing wires and matching sheaths be packaged together.

FIGURE 1.1. Case summary.

To date, most efforts to improve reliability of evidence-based therapies in health care have focused on practice guidelines: a series of conditional probability, or "if yes then 'x'" statements (32). The Centers for Disease Control and Prevention's (CDC's) guidelines for preventing catheter-related bloodstream infections, a nearly 100-page document (www.cdc.gov), is one example. It is not surprising that the use of guidelines alone has met with little success (32,33). Under time pressure, it is difficult for caregivers to think in terms of conditional probabilities (34). An additional problem is that most guidelines have been developed for physicians, ignoring other members of the care team who could provide an independent check.

A checklist is one tool to help standardize work processes and increase reliability. Checklists have led to significant improvements in aviation, nuclear power, and rail safety. For checklists to be useful, they need to transform a complex diagnostic/therapeutic decision into a series of simple yes/no tasks. It is first necessary to identify which parts of a task are "mission critical," especially those supported by strong evidence, and develop measures for those tasks. For example, staff from hospital epidemiology and infection control and our ICUs culled a list of 5 key processes from the CDC guidelines for preventing catheter-related infections: ensure you need the central line, wash your hands, use full barrier precautions, clean the skin with chlorhexadine, and avoid the femoral site if possible (26). This kind of checklist can then be used to monitor performance, with each item serving as a process measure of quality of care (7,35,36). Measurement becomes a tool to improve performance, rather than a tool for historical data collection.

Why METs Might Improve Safety

METs are well grounded in the science of safety outlined above. In many, and perhaps even most, sentinel events, someone either did not speak up, or spoke up but was not heeded because of a hierarchical or punitive culture (people had previously been reprimanded when they spoke up). With METs, frontline staff are empowered—indeed encouraged—to call the MET when they are concerned. This requires a strong culture of safety. Frontline staff is also trained to call for a standardized set of parameters, in the absence of which the trigger for calling someone is generally a code. The MET identifies problems early, when there is still time to recover from them. As such, METs are based on sound safety theory and would be expected to improve safety.

Conclusion

The science of measuring safety is gradually maturing. Some measures of safety lend themselves to rates, while others do not. We have described an approach for organizations to answer the question, "Are patients safer?" We also have summarized the issues regarding measuring and improving reliability, and provided a framework for improving safety. With these measures, we defer to the wisdom of caregivers and administrators to identify and mitigate safety concerns, but also attempt to provide a framework to assist the caregiver with safety efforts. The need to improve quality and safety is significant, and hospitals are learning how to accomplish this goal. METs are grounded in safety theory and offer the promise to reduce patient harm. We hope practical strategies such as those proposed here help move safety and quality efforts forward.

Acknowledgments. We acknowledge Sorrel King for her tireless work to help improve patient safety and for being the guiding light in our work and in representing patients and their families.

References

1. Kohn LT, Corrigan JM, Donaldson MS, eds. *To Err Is Human: Building a Safer Health System.* Washington, DC, National Academies Press; 2000.
2. Altman DE, Clancy C, Blendon RJ. Improving patient safety—5 years after the IOM report. *N Engl J Med.* 2004;351:2041–2043.
3. Wachter RM. The end of the beginning: patient safety five years after "To Err Is Human." *Health Affairs.* 2004;1–12.
4. Committee on Quality of Health Care in America, Institute of Medicine. *Crossing the Quality Chasm: a New Health System for the 21st Century.* Washington, DC: National Academies Press; 2001.
5. Donabedian A. Evaluating the quality of medical care. *Millbank Mem Fund Q.* 1966;44:166–206.
6. Paine LA, Baker DR, Rosenstein B, Pronovost PJ. The Johns Hopkins Hospital: identifying and addressing risks and safety issues. *Jt Comm J Qual Saf.* 2004;30:543–550.
7. Rubin H, Pronovost PJ, Diette G. The advantages and disadvantages of process-based measures of health care quality. *Int J Qual Health Care.* 2001;13:469–474.
8. Pronovost PJ, Nolan T, Zeger S, Miller M, Rubin H. How can clinicians measure safety and quality in acute care? *Lancet.* 2004;363:1061–1067.
9. Sexton JB, Helmreich RL, Thomas EJ. Error, stress, and teamwork in medicine and aviation: cross-sectional surveys. *Brit Med J.* 2000;320:745–749.
10. Shortell SM, Marsteller JA, Lin M, et al. The role of perceived team effectiveness in improving chronic illness care. *Medical Care.* 2004;42:1040–1048.
11. Sexton JB. The link between safety attitudes and observed performance in flight operations. Columbus, OH: Ohio State University; 2001.
12. Pronovost P, Weast B, Bishop K, et al. Senior executive adopt-a-work unit: a model for safety improvement. *Jt Commission J Qual Saf.* 2004;30:59–68.
13. Division of Healthcare Quality Promotion, National Center for Infectious Disease, Center for Disease Control. National Nosocomial Infections Surveillance (NNIS) System Report, data summary from January 1992 through June 2003, issued August 2003. *Am J Infect Control.* 2003;31:481–498.
14. Bates D, Leape L, Cullen D, et al. Effect of computerized physician order entry and a team intervention on prevention of serious medication errors. *JAMA.* 1998;280:1311–1316.
15. Flynn E, Barker KN, Pepper GA, Bates DW, Mikeal RL. Comparison of methods for detecting medication errors in 36 hospitals and skilled-nursing facilities. *Am J Health-Sys Pharm.* 2002;59:436–446.
16. Lesar TS, Briceland L, Delcoure K, Parmalee JC, Masta-Gornic V, Pohl H. Medication prescribing errors in a teaching hospital. *JAMA.* 1990;263:2329–2334.
17. Lesar TS, Briceland L, Stein DS. Factors related to errors in medication prescribing. *JAMA.* 1997;277:312–317.

18. Leape L, Cullen D, Clapp M, et al. Pharmacist participation on physician rounds and adverse drug events in the intensive care unit. *JAMA*. 1999;282:267–270.

19. Lilford R, Mohammed MA, Braunholtz D, Hofer TP. The measurement of active errors: methodological issues. *Qual Saf Health Care*. 2004;12(suppl II):ii8–ii12.

20. Hayward R, Hofer TP. Estimating hospital deaths due to medical errors: preventability is in the eye of the reviewer. *JAMA*. 2004;286:415–420.

21. Cook DJ, Montori VM, McMullin JP, Finfer SR, Rocker GM. Improving patients' safety locally: changing clinician behaviour. *Lancet*. 2004;363:1224–1230.

22. Brook R. The RAND/UCLA Appropriateness Method. AHCPR Pub. No. 95–0009. Rockville, MD: Public Health Service; 1994.

23. Lilford R, Mohammed MA, Spiegelhalter D, Thomson R. Use and misuse of process and outcome data in managing performance of acute medical care: avoiding institutional stigma. *Lancet*. 2004;363:1147–1154.

24. Pronovost P, Jenckes M, To M, et al. Reducing failed extubations in the intensive care unit. *Jt Comm J Qual Improv*. 2002;28:595–604.

25. McGlynn EA, Asch SM, Adams J, et al. The quality of health care delivered to adults in the United States. *N Engl J Med*. 2003;348:2635–2645.

26. Berenholtz S, Pronovost PJ, Lipsett PA, et al. Eliminating catheter-related bloodstream infections in the intensive care unit. *Crit Care Med*. 2004;32:2014–2020.

27. Romano PS, Geppert JJ, Davies S, Miller MR, Elixhauser A, McDonald KM. A national profile of patient safety in U.S. hospitals. *Health Aff (Millwood)* 2003;22:154–166.

28. Zhan C, Miller MR. Excess length of stay, charges, and mortality attributable to medical injuries during hospitalization. *JAMA*. 2004;290:1868–1874.

29. Reason J. Combating omission errors through task analysis and good reminders. *Qual Saf Health Care*. 2002;11:40–44.

30. Reason J. *Managing the Risks of Organizational Accidents*. Burlington, VT: Ashgate Publishing Company; 2000.

31. Weick K, Sutcliffe K. *Managing the Unexpected: Assuring High Performance in an Age of Complexity*. San Francisco: Jossey-Bass; 2001.

32. Grol R. Improving the quality of medical care: building bridges among professional pride, payer profit, and patient satisfaction. *JAMA*. 2001;286:2578–2585.

33. Gross PA, Greenfield S, Cretin S, et al. Optimal methods for guideline implementation: conclusions from Leeds Castle meeting. *Med Care*. 2001;39(8 suppl 2):II85–II92.

34. Klein G. *Sources of Power: How People Make Decisions*. Cambridge: Massachusetts Institute of Technology; 1999.

35. Rubin H, Pronovost P, Diette G. From a process of care to a measure: the development and testing of a quality indicator. *Int J Qual Health Care*. 2001;13:489–496.

36. Rubin HR, Pronovost P, Diette GB. The advantages and disadvantages of process-based measures of health care quality. *Int J Qual Health Care*. 2001;13(6):469–474.

2
The Evolution of the Health Care System

KENNETH HILLMAN, JACK CHEN, and LIS YOUNG

Introduction

In the past, hospital administrators have concentrated on meeting their budget and staying out of the newspapers. Over the last 10 years, however, there has been a shift to concentrating on patient safety in hospitals. This chapter will first examine hospital patient safety in a historical context, explaining how the patient safety anomaly is related to a 19th century hospital construct that is no longer appropriate for an increasingly at-risk group of patients. The final section of the chapter will concentrate on the emergence of systems to improve patient safety in acute care hospitals.

Historical Perspective

In many ways acute care hospitals are designed to deliver health care as it was practiced in the 19th century. The technological advances in medicine of the late 20th century are superimposed on a system originally designed to care for patients admitted largely for bed rest and convalescence.

Originally hospitals were charitable institutions established to care for the poor (1). Apart from performing a limited number of operations, hospitals offered little that could not be provided by a doctor in the home. Medical students learned their craft in acute care hospitals, mainly how to make sense of symptoms and signs to reach a diagnosis. Therapeutic options were few. Medical specialists earned their living in their consulting rooms or by visiting patients in their homes. They went to the hospital only once or twice a week to make rounds, accompanied by their assigned team of students and doctors-in-training. They gave freely of their time, and in return maintained a profile as a source of patient referrals and benefited from the prestige and sense of charity associated with a teaching hospital appointment.

The hospital was constructed around the needs of specialist doctors, who in return for giving their time freely had their own wards, operating theaters, recovery areas, nursing staff, and medical teams. They visited the hospital and did rounds at their convenience. Patients were cared for within the limits of what was available. Pain relief was possible, but curative drugs were relatively rare. Diagnostic services were limited to simple x-rays and basic blood tests. Intravenous fluid was rarely used. Operations were limited and not supported by the same sophisticated perioperative care we have today. If one was seriously ill, it was more common to call a doctor to come to the patient, rather than call an ambulance to take the patient to a hospital.

Around the late 1940s, health care delivery changed and has continued to evolve exponentially to the present day. Antibiotics were developed; drugs controlling cardiovascular and respiratory conditions became available; chemotherapy and radiotherapy were increasingly used for cancer; dialysis and other supportive interventions for chronic conditions became widely available; diagnostic procedures enabled us to image and understand much of the body's disease processes previously guessed at by external signs and symptoms; and the number of noninvasive and invasive surgical options expanded.

Hospitalized patients are now admitted for cure or at least control of their diseases. The hospital population is older, usually with multiple co-morbidities, and often further at risk as a result of the procedures and drugs being used. Expectations of hospitalized patients are high—often unrealistically so—and reinforced by widespread and frequent media reports of wonder drugs and miracle operations with little in the way of balance. People still age and become ill with diseases for which medicine has little or nothing to offer.

While the nature of the hospital patient population and its expectations has changed considerably, the system within which they are managed has evolved little since the 19th century. Patients in emergency departments are still processed in the same way. Patients are still "owned" by a single specialist doctor, and most of the day-to-day activities are supported by doctors-in-training. Nursing staff still records vital signs manually, with little or no power to act on abnormalities. Consultant physicians who are ultimately responsible for the patient's care still largely manage from a distance.

What may have worked well in the 19th century does not necessarily guarantee safe management in the 21st century. Specialization may not equip consultants with the skills, knowledge, and experience necessary to care for the complex co-morbidities that patients increasingly have, or for when the patient becomes seriously ill. Junior house doctors are either too inexperienced and lack the skills and knowledge to care for complex at-risk patients, or they tend to become too specialized and fail to receive adequate training in the other areas that are necessary to treat complex patients, especially those who become seriously ill. Silos, or vertical structures within hospitals such as wards, units, and departments, are well developed in acute care hospitals, but there is a paucity of horizontal system integration across the silos.

While the silos adequately manage the specialized component of a patient's condition, they usually prove inadequate for co-existing conditions and for patient complications. The hospital usually does not provide the necessary systems, or horizontal connections, to support the vertical silos.

It is not surprising therefore that there are many potentially preventable deaths and serious adverse events in acute care hospitals (2–4). Moreover, many of these potentially preventable deaths are preceded for many hours by a slow deterioration in vital signs (5). For example, up to 90% of hospital cardiac arrests are preceded by relatively slow and potentially reversible deterioration (6). Admissions of patients to the intensive care unit (ICU) from the general wards are often preceded by the same predictable slow deterioration (7–10). If we are concerned about a seriously ill patient in the community, we call an ambulance. If we have a similar patient in an acute care hospital, it appears we have little in the way of systematic intervention. Nurses record abnormal findings; junior doctors may be informed about the patient in a hierarchical way—the most junior first, with information passed up the line, depending on the level of understanding and awareness of how serious the patient's condition may be. Alternatively, in non-teaching hospitals, the nurse would first contact the patient's primary physician, who might not even be on-site. If unable to attend to the patient, this person may request a consultation by someone more available or expert. Sometimes the patient may be referred to an acute care physician, such as an intensivist. Thus, the response to the crisis is built in an ad-hoc manner, piece by piece. The only systematic and organized approach is often the cardiac arrest team (a predefined and prepared group of responders with specialized resources), called after the patient has "died" (11).

Preemptive Patient Safety Systems

For these reasons, patient safety in hospitals has become a major focus of health care delivery (12–17). How can we provide a safer environment for hospital patients? One way is to train health care workers in health care systems and team-based care (18,19). Adverse event reporting is occurring with increasing frequency (20,21). Information management and communication is improving (22–25). Specifically, more hospitalists are being employed who are trained in acute medicine and in managing the patient's course through the hospital (26).

This book discusses models for delivering acute care, specifically the development of the Medical Emergency Team (MET) (27), a system-based approach to the acutely ill that recognizes the discontinuities in patient care as a result of the vertical silos on which we have constructed hospital care. Potentially avoidable adverse events are caused by suboptimal training and inadequate awareness of at-risk patients, poor supervision, and lack of a timely response at an early stage in the patient's deterioration (8,9,12).

A specialist usually refers to other specialists through a process of formal consultation. For this to occur, the specialist must be aware that the patient has a medical need outside the specialist's own area of expertise. This works well for most referrals. However, the referral system for a patient who is becoming seriously ill offers a set of challenges that is outside the hospital system's ability to address. The deterioration can occur at any time and is often unexpected or unanticipated. The general awareness by medical and nursing staff of what constitutes an at-risk patient is often inadequate, and even if that recognition occurs, response is often not timely and may not result in the right expertise being rapidly provided to the patient when needed.

The patients meeting MET criteria define what constitutes an at-risk patient, and they receive care immediately by staff with appropriate expertise (27–31). The MET concept cuts across the usual silos in health care by providing a team-based, immediate, and appropriate response to at-risk patients.

Recent approaches to improving patient safety are numerous (12,32–35), including a rapidly expanding quality industry; better data analysis; plan-do-study-act (PDSA) cycles (36); and learning lessons from other industries. While these concepts may be intuitively appealing, they have enormous cost implications and until now have not been subject to rigorous evaluation. On the other hand, the MET concept works at the patient–health care deliverer interface, using strict criteria to identify at-risk patients and a nondiscretionary and rapid response by a team with specific skills and knowledge in the care of the seriously ill.

The MET fulfills the criteria for a system approach to patient safety by radically changing the way we respond to patients at risk for developing serious complications. It concentrates on "real-time" adverse event monitoring and response, rather than retrospective data analysis. The World Health Organization has emphasized 3 important features for enhancing patient safety, which mesh with the MET system (37): (1) preventing adverse events irrespective of the cause; (2) making the events visible in terms of data collected on MET responses; and (3) investigating the effects of the adverse event.

Finally, the MET system provides a platform for exploring existing weaknesses in hospital systems and offers knowledge as a basis for improving patient safety.

References

1. Abel-Smith B. *The Hospitals 1800–1948*. London: Heinemann; 1964.
2. Brennan TA, Leape LL, Laird N, et al. Incidence of adverse events and negligence in hospitalized patients: results of the Harvard Medical Practice Study I. *N Engl J Med*. 1991;324:370–376.

3. Leape LL, Brennan TA, Laird N, et al. Nature of adverse events in hospitalized patients: results of the Harvard Medical Practice Study II. *N Engl J Med.* 1991; 324:377–384.
4. Wilson RM, Runciman WB, Gibberd RW, et al. The quality in Australian health care study. *Med J Aust.* 1995;163:458–471.
5. Hillman KM, Bristow PJ, Chey T, et al. Antecedents to hospital deaths. *Intern Med J.* 2001;31:343–348.
6. Schein RMH, Hazday N, Pena M, et al. Clinical antecedents to in-hospital cardiopulmonary arrest. *Chest.* 1990;98:1388–1392.
7. Hillman KM, Bristow PJ, Chey T, et al. Duration of life-threatening antecedents prior to intensive care admission. *Intensive Care Med.* 2002;28:1629–1634.
8. McQuillan P, Pilkington S, Alan A, et al. Confidential inquiry into quality of care before admission to intensive care. *BMJ.* 1998;316:1853–1858.
9. Goldhill DR, White SA, Sumner A. Physiological values and procedures in the 24 hours before ICU admission from the ward. *Anaesthesia.* 1999;54:529–534.
10. McGloin H, Adam SK, Singer M. Unexpected deaths and referrals to intensive care units of patients on general wards: are some cases potentially avoidable? *J Royal Coll Physicians Lond.* 1999;33:255–259.
11. Hillman K, Parr M, Flabouris A, Bishop G, Stewart A. Redefining in-hospital resuscitation: the concept of the medical emergency team. *Resuscitation.* 2001;48: 105–110.
12. Bion JF, Heffner JE. Challenges in the care of the acutely ill. *Lancet.* 2004;363: 970–977.
13. Kohn LT, Corrigan JM, Donaldson MS, eds. *To Err Is Human: Building a Safer Health System.* Washington, DC: National Academies Press; 2000.
14. Vincent C, Neale G, Woloshynowych M. Adverse events in British hospitals: preliminary retrospective record review. *BMJ.* 2001;322:517–519.
15. Shaw C, Coles J. Reporting of adverse clinical incidents: international views and experience. London: CASPE Research; 2001.
16. Baker GR, Norton P. Patient safety and healthcare error in the Canadian healthcare system: a systematic review and analysis of leading practices in Canada with reference to key initiatives elsewhere. Report to Health Canada. 1964. Available at: http://www.hc-sc.gc.ca/english/care/report/index.html. Accessed January 2004.
17. Shojania KG, Duncan BW, McDonald KM, et al. *Making Health Care Safer: A Critical Analysis of Patient Safety Practices.* Rockville, MD: Agency for Healthcare and Research Quality; 2001.
18. Intercollegiate Board for Training in Intensive Care Medicine. Available at: http://www.ics.ac.uk. Accessed January 2004.
19. Estrada CA. Medical errors must be discussed during medical education. *BMJ.* 2000;321:507.
20. Leape L. Reporting of adverse events. *N Engl J Med.* 2002;347:1633–1638.
21. Classen DC, Kilbridge PM. The roles and responsibility of physicians to improve patient safety within health care delivery systems. *Acad Med.* 2002;77:963–972.
22. Leapfrog patient safety standards. Leapfrog Group Web site. Available at: http://www.leapfroggroup.org. Accessed January 2004.
23. Bates DW, Teich JM, Lee J, et al. The impact of computerized physician order entry on medication error prevention. *J Am Med Inform Assoc.* 1999;6: 313–321.

24. Dexter PR, Perkins S, Overhage JM, Maharry K, Kohler RB, McDonald CJ. A computerized reminder system to increase the use of preventive care for hospitalized patients. *N Engl J Med*. 2001;345:965–970.
25. Kilbridge P. Computer crash: lessons from a system failure. *N Engl J Med*. 2003;348:881–882.
26. Wachter RM, Goldman L. The emerging role of "hospitalists" in the American health care system. *N Engl J Med*. 1996;335:514–517.
27. Lee A, Bishop G, Hillman KM, Daffurn K. The Medical Emergency Team. *Anaesth Intensive Care*. 1995;23:183–186.
28. Hourihan F, Bishop G, Hillman KM, Daffurn K, Lee A. The Medical Emergency Team: a new strategy to identify and intervene in high-risk patients. *Clin Intensive Care*. 1995;6:269–272.
29. Hillman KM ed. Redefining resuscitation. *Aust NZ J Med*. 1998;28:759.
30. Hillman KM. Reducing preventable deaths and containing costs: the expanding role of intensive care medicine. *Med J Aust*. 1996;164:308–309.
31. Hillman K. A hospital-wide system for managing the seriously ill. *Minerva Anestesiologica*. 1999;65:346–347.
32. McNutt R, Abrams R, Hasler S. Why blame systems for unsafe care? *Lancet*. 2004;363:913–914.
33. Pande PS, Neuman RP, Cavanagh RR. *The Six Sigma Way: How GE, Motorola, and Other Top Companies Are Honing Their Performance*. New York: McGraw-Hill; 2000.
34. Berwick DM. Errors today and errors tomorrow. *N Engl J Med*. 2003;348: 2570–2572.
35. McNutt RA, Abrams R, Hasler S. Patient safety efforts should focus on medical error. *JAMA*. 2002;287:1997–2001.
36. Cleghorn GD, Headrick LA. The PDSA cycle at the core of learning in health professions' education. *Jt Comm J Qual Improv*. 1996;22:206–212.
37. World Health Organization. World Alliance for Patient Safety: Forward Programme. 2004. Available at: http://www.who.int/patientsafety/en/brochure_final.pdf

3
Process Change in Health Care Institutions: Top-Down or Bottom-Up?

LAKSHMIPATHI CHELLURI

Leadership is powerless without followership—a broad constituency that is ready and willing to be led.

—David Blumenthal

Introduction

Medical errors and quality of medical care have been identified by the Institute of Medicine as issues adversely affecting contemporary medical care (1,2). Since the publication of the report *To Err Is Human*, the focus on decreasing the number of medical errors and improving safety and quality has strengthened. In the past few years, there have been many reports on the inadequacies of and possible interventions to improve the health care system (3–6). The difficulties in changing health care culture and the reluctance of the medical establishment to change have been well documented (3). Donnabedian, a leader in quality improvement, described his personal experience as a patient and the care he received for cancer of the prostate as disappointing and frustrating (4). Similarly, Lawrence, who was chairman and CEO of one of the largest HMOs in the United States, described the chaotic medical care his mother received and concluded that the health care system does not work as well as it could (5). In addition, patients and families of patients who suffered iatrogenic injury are taking an active role in efforts to improve patient safety and quality of care (7,8). Many of these reports discuss the need for a change in culture and the improvement of patient safety and quality of medical care through implementing systems that are available and known to be effective. Change can be brought about either by the leadership or by middle managers and frontline workers. But the elements that lead to successful change, whether initiated by leadership (top-down) or frontline workers (bottom-up), are not well studied in health care.

In the past decade, with an increased focus on medical errors and concern about the poor quality of medical care, many initiatives have sought to improve safety and quality. Some were spearheaded by leadership that set the vision and goals for improvement (9–14), while others were initiated by individuals or groups in nonleadership positions (15–19). This chapter reviews examples of projects in health care initiated either using a top-down or bottom-up approach, and discusses the critical elements for success. First we will look at projects that were led by leadership. These include the Veterans Affairs Quality of Care and Patient Safety programs (9,10); the Pittsburgh Regional Health Care Initiative (11,12); the Quality Institute of the Cleveland Clinic Health System (13); and the Toyota Production System Initiative at the University of Pittsburgh Medical Center (14). We will also review projects led by non-leadership (middle management and direct health care deliverers) that include Medical Emergency Team (MET) responses to identify errors and potential errors (15,16); mortality reviews (17,18); and the initiative to decrease the rate of cesarean sections in Green Bay, WI (19).

Leadership Initiatives

Veterans Affairs Quality of Care and Patient Safety Programs

The Department of Veterans Affairs (VA) initiated a reengineering of health care delivery to improve quality in the mid-1990s, and established the National Center for Patient Safety (NCPS) in 1998. The VA leadership initiated both programs with a major focus on improving quality and safety of care delivered to veterans of the US armed forces. They encouraged an organized approach to measurement and management of quality of care, and built incentives and accountability for performance improvement into the process. The managers were given performance contracts for improvement and were accountable for achieving the goals. These programs resulted in significant improvements in preventive care, outpatient care, and acute inpatient care (9).

It must be noted that patient safety activities at the VA are coordinated by the NCPS. The original VA Patient Safety Improvement program initiated in 1997 was unsuccessful, resulting in the formation of the NCPS with a mandate to lead VA patient safety initiatives. The NCPS identified suspected obstacles including inadequate resources, poor accountability, and less than ideal implementation of patient safety initiatives. This resulted in the establishment of a system for reporting errors, a system to prioritize errors in which the causes of errors are analyzed based on potential for harm and/or frequency, a method to perform analysis of causes, and interventions to minimize recurrence. The program resulted in a 30-fold increase in events reported, and a 900-fold increase in reported "close calls" (10). Analysis of these events led to many changes in practice at individual VA hospitals, in addition to serving as a model for other health care systems.

Pittsburgh Regional Health Care Initiative

Pittsburgh Regional Health Care Initiative (PRHI) is a consortium of businesses, hospitals, insurers, and organizations that provide health care services to people in western Pennsylvania. High costs and poor comparative quality resulted in the formation of the PRHI in 1997. The model is based on identifying and analyzing causes of the problems at the point of care, involvement of frontline workers in identifying solutions, and encouraging change based on shared learning (11,12). PRHI focused on improving clinical outcomes in patients undergoing coronary artery bypass graft surgery, those with depression or diabetes, for maternal and child care, and for hip and knee surgeries. In addition, medication errors and nosocomial infections were addressed. The project created a shared database between the participating health care organizations to collect data on processes of care and link outcomes to them. The information and outcomes of successful processes are then shared with frontline workers, so that they can provide appropriate care. The goal is to develop a system of care with real-time feedback and to connect processes to outcomes for continuous improvement in quality. Significant improvements in nosocomial infections and medication error reporting have been achieved.

Quality Institute of the Cleveland Clinic Health System

The Cleveland Clinic Health System is a consortium of health care institutions led by the Cleveland Clinic that was created between 1996 and 1998. The Quality Institute was established to coordinate system-wide quality improvement activities and "promote evidence-based care within a culture of safety" (13). The institute's staff serves as consultants to the individual hospitals and facilitates communication and the exchange of information leadership. The institute's leadership includes the physician and administrative leaders known as the Medical Operations Council, which identifies and prioritizes quality improvement initiatives based on volume, impact on quality, and potential for improvement, and then allocates resources as needed. Patient care initiatives include the evaluation of clinical processes such as treatment of breast and colorectal cancer, diabetes, stroke, heart failure/myocardial infarction, pediatric asthma and chronic obstructive pulmonary disease. Patient safety initiatives include monitoring medication errors, improving medication safety, and encouraging patients/families to participate in care as well as initiatives to decrease medical errors. These initiatives resulted in improvements in use of angiotensin-converting enzyme inhibitors for heart failure, platelet inhibitors, Beta-blockers for acute myocardial infarction, intravenous thrombolysis for acute stroke, and appropriateness of cesarean sections. The system was awarded the Ernest A. Codman award by the Joint Council on the Accreditation of Health Care Organizations in 2001.

The Toyota Production System Initiative at Presbyterian University Hospital, University of Pittsburgh Medical Center

The Toyota Production System (TPS) is based on involving workers in the building of a defect-free product by specifying responsibilities of individuals and holding them accountable, simplifying processes, and making all changes in processes based on appropriate scientific evidence. The Toyota motor company achieved significant success by following these principles, and TPS has been adopted by other industries, including health care. The leadership at University of Pittsburgh Medical Center introduced TPS to the process of providing medication to patients on the ward by improving communication between patient care wards and the pharmacy (14). A multidisciplinary team of administrative leaders, physicians, pharmacists, and nursing staff on a patient care ward worked together to identify problems and then create and implement solutions. The project resulted in faster delivery of medications and more efficient use of pharmacists' time, and the improvements led to implementation of the process throughout the hospital. The same process was also used to improve physician ordering practices and decrease medication errors.

The preceding examples summarize the quality of care and safety efforts led by the leadership in a large government organization, in a regional organization led by leaders in business and health care, in a large health care system, and at a hospital in a large health care system. The common features of these initiatives include: (1) leadership with vision to improve care and the willingness to commit adequate resources; (2) communication of the vision to the employees and participants; (3) institutional support and appropriate incentives; and (4) involvement of the physicians and staff in identifying solutions and implementation. Kotter describes the key stages in implementing new programs as creating a sense of urgency; building a team that can guide the change; creating a vision that is simple and can be communicated in a short time; obtaining support from all the appropriate staff; empowering people to act as needed; creating short-term wins; and continuing to improve and change the culture for the long-term (20). The programs described above included many of these elements, and emphasize the need for an organized structure for successful implementation of quality improvement and safety projects.

Quality Improvement and Safety Programs Initiated by Individuals in Non-Leadership Positions

Identifying Medical Errors Through Review of the Medical Emergency Team Response

The University of Pittsburgh Medical Center introduced a MET in 1988; however, it was not until 1999 that the institution could reliably initiate the MET response when a patient developed a medical crisis. The keys to effective implementation are described by Foraida et al. (15) and include the creation of objective criteria, posting the criteria in every nursing unit, getting medical executive committee support to allow nursing staff to trigger a MET response without physician approval, and both positive and negative reinforcement through email. The MET quality improvement committee, which includes physicians, nursing staff, and others, reviews all MET responses to identify medical errors and provides this information to the appropriate department for follow-up and suggestions for improvement (16). The team identified errors in patient management in 114 (31.4%) of the total MET responses over an 8-month period, including: patient treatment errors such as hyperkalemia and narcotic overdose; pneumothorax related to insertion of a feeding tube; hypoxia related to an empty oxygen tank; problems with patient-controlled analgesia pumps; and diagnostic errors such as cardiac arrest secondary to delay in diagnosis. There were also prevention errors, or errors resulting from inadequate pre-emptive care in areas such as inadequate respiratory care in patients with tracheostomy, hypoglycemia in a patient receiving long-acting insulin and oral hypoglycemic agents, and injuries related to falls. Identification of the errors resulted in process improvement and minimized the possibility of recurrence.

Mortality Reviews to Identify Quality of Care Issues

Wilson and Soffel (17) and Seward et al. (18) reported on reviewing medical records of patients dying in the hospital to identify quality of care issues. Over the period 1988–1993, Wilson and Soffel found that problems with clinical quality of care issuses were identified in 3% of deaths. Approximately half of the problems identified were related to delays and appropriateness of treatment (17). Seward et al. reviewed 200 consecutive deaths in patients admitted for an emergency at a tertiary care hospital, and reported that 11% of the deaths were unexpected and had some evidence of care management problems that included errors in diagnosis and delays in treatment, particularly at night (18).

Green Bay Wisconsin Cesarean Section Study

Sandmire and DeMott studied the cesarean section practices in Green Bay and reported that the variability in the incidence of cesarean section was related primarily to physician practice and liability risk (19). They also found that higher cesarean rates did not result in better outcomes. They attempted to influence practice by changing their own practice and convincing others that higher cesarean section rates do not result in better outcomes. In addition, information on incidence of cesarean deliveries and outcome was provided to the obstetricians in the area. These efforts resulted in a decrease in incidence of cesarean deliveries from 13.3% to 10.2% over a 6-year period.

Patient safety and quality improvement practices can be designed and implemented by individuals in non-leadership positions. The key elements for success reported by the preceding authors are: identifying a problem that has a significant impact; the commitment and involvement of physicians and staff; effectively communicating the problems and solutions to both leadership and staff; obtaining support from the staff; serving as a role model; and persistence over time.

Change: Top-Down or Bottom-Up

Changes in behavior and culture in organizations can be initiated and successfully implemented by either the leadership or frontline workers, but it is most successful when a leader with vision and excellent communication skills works together with committed and enthusiastic employees. Kenneth Kiser at the Veterans Affairs department made safety and quality the major focus of his organization, and he generated improvements by providing leadership and vision. Although the chances of success may be higher for those programs initiated by leadership, Kotter described many examples in which change was successfully initiated by middle managers and other employees (20). The individual attempting to change behavior and culture in an organization has to be an effective communicator and be able to lead by serving as a role model. The story of Ignac Semmelweis illustrates an unsuccessful attempt to change practice, and the potential for positive impact of the change was monumental (21). Semmelweis was an obstetrician in Vienna in the 19th century, and hypothesized that mortality secondary to puerperal fever (childbed fever) could be improved if physicians washed their hands between patient contacts. He showed that mortality decreased from 20% to less than 2% after the introduction of hand washing. However, he was not able to influence his contemporaries because he believed that the superiority of his practice was obvious and delayed publication of his findings. He also insulted those who did not accept his practice and accused his superiors of causing increased maternal mortality because they disagreed with him. In addition, the manuscript describing his findings was poorly written and difficult to read, so when it was published it was ignored by many physicians at the time. His story shows that the individual who wants to initiate change needs to be able to communicate the ideas to both superiors and coworkers in a nonthreatening manner.

METs are an example of an at-the-bedside change that is particularly effective for several reasons: it employs a methodology to find high-risk patients (those with sudden onset of critical illness, often resulting from errors), and to immediately bring additional resources to bear to prevent harm. Review of cases enables high-yield error identification, which, because of the severity of the adverse outcome (or near-miss), motivates hospital workers to prevent future occurrences of a similar event. METs are likely to become a key component of every hospital's safety net for suddenly critically ill patients, and part of their quality improvement processes. In summary, leadership with a clear vision and employees with commitment are crucial, and both are needed to successfully implement change. It seems MET programs may blend both top-down and bottom-up approaches to great effect.

References

1. Kohn LT, Corrigan JM, Donaldson MS, eds. *To Err Is Human: Building a Safer Health System*. Washington, DC: National Academies Press; 2000.
2. Institute of Medicine. Crossing the Quality Chasm. A New Health System for the 21stCentury. National Academy Press. 2001. Committee on Quality of Health Care in America, Institute of Medicine. *Crossing the Quality Chasm: a New Health System for the 21st Century*. Washington, DC: National Academies Press; 2001.
3. Millenson ML. The silence. Medicine's continued quiet refusal to take quality improvement actions has undermined the moral foundations of medical professionalism. *Health Affairs*. 2003;22:103–111.
4. Mullan F. A founder of quality assessment encounters a troubled system firsthand. *Health Affairs*. 2001;20:137–141.
5. Lawrence DM. My mother and the medical care ad-hoc-racy. *Health Affairs*. 2003;22:238–242.
6. Wachter RM, Shojania KG. *Internal Bleeding: The Truth Behind America's Terrifying Epidemic of Medical Mistakes*. New York: Rugged Land; 2004.
7. Gibson R, Singh JP. *Wall of Silence: The Untold Story of the Medical Mistakes That Kill and Injure Millions of Americans*. Washington, DC: Lifeline Press; 2003.
8. National Patient Safety Foundation Web site. Available at: http://www.npsf.org. Accessed January 10, 2005.
9. Jha AK, Perlin JB, Kizer KW, et al. Effect of the transformation of the Veterans Affairs health care system on the quality of care. *N Engl J Med*. 2003;348:2218–2227.
10. Bagian JP, Lee C, Gosbee J, et al. Developing and deploying a patient safety program in a large health care delivery system: you can't fix what you don't know about. *Jt Comm J Qual Improv*. 2001;27:522–530.

11. Pittsburgh Regional Healthcare Initiative. Central line bloodstream infection rate study. Available at: http://www.prhi.org. Accessed October 12, 2004.
12. Sirio CA, Segel KT, Keyser DJ, et al. Pittsburgh Regional Health Care Initiative: a systems approach for achieving perfect patient care. *Health Affairs*. 2003;22:157–165.
13. Nadzam DM, Waggoner M, Hixon E, et al. Introducing the Quality Institute of the Cleveland Clinic Health System. *Am J Med Qual*. 2003;18:204–213.
14. Thompson DN, Wolf GA, Spear SJ. Driving improvement in patient care: lessons from Toyota. *J Nurs Adm*. 2003;33:585–595.
15. Foraida M, DeVita MA, Braithwaite RS, et al. Improving the utilization of medical crisis teams (Condition C) at an urban tertiary care hospital. *J Crit Care*. 2003;18:87–94.
16. Braithwaite RS, Devita MA, Mahidhara R. Use of medical emergency team responses to detect medical errors. *Qual Saf Health Care*. 2004;13:255–259.
17. Wilson OF, Soffel RA. Quality improvement through review of inpatient deaths. *J Healthc Qual*. 1997;19:12–18.
18. Seward E, Greig E, Preston S, et al. A confidential study of deaths after emergency medical admission: issues relating to quality of care. *Clin Med*. 2003; 3:425–434.
19. Sandmire HF, DeMott RK. The Green Bay cesarean section study. III. Falling cesarean birth rates without a formal curtailment program. *Am J Obstet Gynecol*. 1994;170:1790–1802.
20. Kotter JP, Cohen DS. *The Heart of Change. Real-Life Stories of How People Change Their Organizations*. Boston: Harvard Business School Press; 2002.
21. Nuland SB. *The Doctors' Plague: Germs, Childbed Fever, and the Strange Story of Ignac Semmelweis*. New York: W.W. Norton & Company; 2003.

4
The Challenge of Predicting In-Hospital Iatrogenic Deaths

MICHAEL BUIST and DONALD CAMPBELL

Introduction

In this chapter, we first explore the similarities and differences between the current hospital crisis of iatrogenic patient deaths—which is now the fourth most common cause of death in the United Kingdom (1), and the sixth most common in the United States (2)—and the theories that have been used to explain and manage organizational crises that occur in other industries. We then critically examine the studies to date that attempt to predict in-hospital patient management crises. Finally, we conclude that in the short term patients need more "hard defenses" to protect them from the health care system. In the long term, there needs to be a significant and fundamental change to the "soft defenses," such as the training of frontline health care workers, so that potential patient crises are predicted and managed earlier to prevent iatrogenic morbidity and mortality.

Organizational Crisis Theory: Hazards, Defenses, and Latent Conditions

In his book *Managing the Risks of Organizational Accidents*, Reason states that organizational accidents, as opposed to individual accidents, are predictable events (3). An individual accident is one in which a person or group of people make an individual slip, lapse, or error of judgment with the net result being an adverse outcome either to the person or the people who erred, or to those in the immediate vicinity. There is usually a relatively tight, simple explanation for cause and effect in an individual accident. For example, if a person makes the error of judgment to drive a car on the wrong side of the road, there is a high likelihood of an accident, which will involve the person who made the error along with any bystanders. Organizational accidents have "multiple causes involving many people at different levels of an organization" (4). While usually infrequent, these events are often catastrophic. Analyses of such organizational accidents often reveal that the defenses an organization has to prevent such catastrophes are breached by a unique series of sequential hazards that play out in an environment of latent conditions.

There is always a tension within an organization to balance resource allocation for production and profit generation against the implementation, maintenance, and updating of defenses to protect the organization from crisis. Resource allocation for production of profit is a core tenant of a commercial organization; it is a process that has easily measured endpoints with relatively simple relationships between resource allocation and production. On the other hand, resource allocation for organizational defenses has no such relationship, and the benefits of such defenses are difficult to measure. If an organization has little exposure to hazards that may cause a crisis, it can be difficult to allocate resource to defenses in the face of societal or financial drivers to maximize production. This tension thus creates the landscape, or latent conditions, that may predispose an organization to crisis (4). An organization's defenses can be simply categorized into either "hard" or "soft." Hard defenses are physical barriers where no human discretion applies. Soft defenses relate to laws, rules, policies, procedures, guidelines, and, often as a last resort, common sense. Because these soft defenses are human constructs, their implementation, utilization, analysis, improvement, and even avoidance can occur at an individual operator level. Furthermore, operator interpretation and implementation, or lack thereof, inevitably becomes an organizational issue that is often dependent on where in a particular organization the tension between production and protection sits (4).

Iatrogenic Patient Death: Individual or Organizational Accident?

Thus we turn to the crisis in the safety of health care. Up to this point, the terms "crisis," "catastrophe," and "accident" have been used to mean the same thing: a sudden, overwhelming event with considerable damage to those involved. For the purposes of the remainder of this chapter, we shall confine ourselves to a definition of crisis as an unexpected, iatrogenic in-hospital death (Box 4.1 and 4.2). That these deaths constitute a crisis in an epidemiological, societal, political, and medico-legal sense will be made in other chapters.

A patient entering a hospital enters a system where they will be exposed to a variety of hazards, which in turn have numerous defenses in place to prevent an adverse patient outcome. Operations, anesthesia, medical interventions and procedures, drugs and fluids, and even oxygen therapy constitute the hazards. Some hard defenses exist in anesthesia, whereby the administration of hypoxic gas mixtures is physically prevented; otherwise, most other defenses in the general hospital ward environment are soft. These soft defenses include treatment policies and procedures, manual

Box 4.1

A 47-year-old, previously healthy male underwent a semi-elective thoracotomy for an empyema. The surgical procedure and anesthesia were uneventful. The patient returned to the ward at 3 pm with a heart rate of 130 beats per minute. Otherwise his observations were unremarkable. The surgical registrar was concerned about the heart rate and the patient's inability to pass urine post-operatively. She instructed the intern to insert a urinary catheter if the patient failed to pass urine by 6 pm. At 6 pm there was no urine output, and the heart rate was 140 beats per minute. Despite the intern's insistence, the patient refused to have a urinary catheter inserted. Otherwise the patient's condition was stable. At the end of the shift, the day intern presented a verbal report to the night resident medical officer on the patient at 10 pm.

The night resident medical officer was summoned urgently to see the patient at 11:30 pm when the patient's blood pressure dropped to 85/60mmHg. The heart rate was now 150 beats per minute. The medical officer assessed that the patient was hypovolemic and administered 2 liters of intravenous fluid, and ordered a blood transfusion. With this intervention, the blood pressure improved and the medical officer went about his other tasks. There were no further observations on the patient until 2:30 am, when the blood pressure was observed to be 75/55mmHg. The medical officer again responded promptly and commenced further fluid resuscitation. Again there was a transient improvement in the patient's condition. At about 4 am, the medical officer was concerned enough about the patient to telephone the on-call surgical registrar (offsite, on-call due to financial restraints) and explained the patient's condition. The surgical registrar was concerned and stated that he would come in early at 7 am to review the patient prior to the commencement of his operating list. At 5:30 am, the patient lost consciousness, and the nursing staff put out a cardiac arrest call. Despite the best efforts of the anesthetic registrar and the ICU registrar, the patient could not be resuscitated and died at 6 am.

Box 4.2.

It was the case of Mike Hurewitz, a journalist who decided to donate part of his liver to his ailing brother 2 years ago, which framed the new "legend" of American health care. Mr. Hurewitz is no longer alive to tell his story, but it has become a morality tale for much that is wrong.

His brother, Adam, 54, suffered from hepatitis C and his liver was rapidly failing. The elder brother, 57, resolved to save the younger and they both checked into the legendary Mount Sinai Hospital, a hospital specializing in living-donor liver transplants.

Charles Miller, who performed New York's first liver transplant over 15 years ago, ran the transplant unit. He removed 60% of Mike's liver on January 10, 2002. Mike was a healthy patient whose main anxiety was saving his brother.

Adam was transferred to intensive care, but Mike was sent to an ordinary ward. This ward—filled with 34 transplant patients—was overseen by a first-year resident. Mike soon developed a rapid heart rate. Doctors were unaware of this, however, as his vital signs were not checked by nursing staff, and the surgeon, Miller, did not visit Mike after the operation.

When Mike then developed an infection and his condition worsened, Miller was paged by concerned nursing staff. But according to reports, the doctor lingered in a bookshop, taking his time. When he returned to the hospital, he did not visit Mike, but instead went to see another patient due for surgery. Mike died after choking on his own blood in the ward, 3 days after giving Adam the gift of life.

alarm systems, and ad hoc hierarchical and lateral human check systems. Soft defenses are very reliant on the training and education that health care workers receive. Superimposed on these layers of hazards and defenses with which the patient is confronted are the latent conditions that exist, most obviously within the patient but more insidiously within the hospital as an organization. A patient's past medical history, family history, social history, associated co-morbidities, drug regimen, and allergies largely constitute their latent conditions. These conditions and their relation to the current presenting complaint that brings the patient into the hospital system comprise territory that individual health care workers are usually extremely well trained in and familiar with. Hospital latent conditions are not so explicit, particularly to the patient or the frontline health care worker. They include a complex matrix of production imperatives such as the financial operating environment, political and societal imperatives, medico-legal and insurance concerns, compliance issues imposed by various regulatory bodies (often with associated financial incentives or disincentives), and workforce and work-practice issues.

In the acute care hospital the distinction between individual and organizational accidents is blurred. First, the crisis of iatrogenic patient death is insidious. Epidemiologically, this crisis may constitute an epidemic; however, to the individual practitioner, or even hospital, it may not appear as such, largely because at an individual level these events occur relatively infrequently, over a long time frame. For example, the Quality in Australian Healthcare Study (QAHS) looked at a random sample of 14 179 admissions to 28 hospitals in 2 states of Australia in 1992 and documented 112 deaths (0.79%) and 109 cases where the adverse event caused greater than 50% disability (0.77%) (5). Nearly 70% of the deaths and 58% of the cases of significant disability were considered to have a high degree of preventability. For the individual clinicians, treating departments, and units, and even the study hospitals themselves, their actual experience of these outcomes over the year would be minimal (1 or 2 cases).

Secondly, the defenses that hospitals have to protect patients have not been changed significantly in the past few decades. In particular there are few, if any, "hard" defenses, and the "soft" defenses are overly reliant on the skills and abilities of frontline health care workers, principally the junior doctor and nurse. In Australia and the United Kingdom, several studies indicate that their medical undergraduate syllabuses do not provide graduates with the basic knowledge, skills, and judgment to manage acute life-threatening emergencies (6–9). These studies identified deficiencies in cognitive abilities, procedural skills, and communication. Further analysis of the causative factors associated with the adverse events in the QAHS found that cognitive failure was a factor in 57% of these adverse events (10). In this analysis, cognitive failure included such errors as: failure to synthesize, decide, and act on available information; failure to request or arrange an investigation, procedure, or consultation; lack of care or attention; failure to attend; misapplication of or failure to apply a rule, or use of a bad or inadequate rule (10). In a 2-hospital study from the United Kingdom that looked at 100 sequential admissions to the intensive care unit (ICU) from wards, it was found that 54 had suboptimal care on the ward prior to transfer (11). This group of patients had a mortality rate of 56%. Some of the suboptimal treatment factors included: failure to seek advice, lack of knowledge, failure to appreciate clinical urgency, and lack of supervision. Undergraduate and postgraduate curricula have been slow to embrace a culture of patient safety (12,13). The hospital organizational response to the issue of adverse events and iatrogenic deaths has generally been to attempt to document and audit incidence, reinforce the traditional hierarchal referral model of care, and to incorporate a plethora of written policies and procedures into the clinical environment with few sustained organizational attempts to "close the loop." In the acute hospital setting, the frequent turnover of workers through frontline care delivery positions and the expectation that the hospital is a training setting may reduce the organizational ability to "see" such events and retain corporate memory of them—let alone to have the sophisticated procedures in place to undertake root-cause analysis and organizational learning.

Finally, the hospital environment is a complex and dynamic matrix of political, administrative, financial, workplace and workforce variables that interact to provide patient care (14). This effect overwhelms the fact that one could probably argue that the hazards a patient may encounter at worst have changed little, and at best have diminished somewhat thanks to better operative and perioperative techniques and safer drugs.

Attempts to Predict Hospital Iatrogenic Death

Implicit in the prediction of iatrogenic hospital death is the need to have a number of easily identifiable, simple clinical markers or factors that predict death. There have been 3 study types used to look for such markers. First, the large, retrospective, epidemiological case note review studies to determine incidence and outcome from hospital adverse events have shed some light on factors that may predispose a patient to iatrogenic hospital death (1,5,10,15–18). The Harvard Medical Practice Study (HMPS) and the QAHS both performed a separate analysis of the documented adverse events, by an iterative process with expert reviewers, to look for causative factors, degrees of preventability, and, with HMPS, associated negligence. The HMPS found that age, operative status, and negligence were associated with poor outcomes (death and permanent disability) from adverse events, with associated high degrees of preventability. The HMPS documented that patients over 65 years had double the risk of an adverse event than patients aged 16 to 44 years (15,16). It also estimated that 51.3% of the deaths from adverse events were caused by negligence. In a re-examination of the 2351 adverse events from the QAHS, 34.6% of the adverse events were categorized as "a complication of, or the failure in the technical performance of an indicated procedure or operation" (10). However, more significantly, 81.8% of events were associated with human error and cognitive failure as discussed above (10). The QAHS also found that delay both in diagnosis and in treatment was associated with 20% of adverse events, and that 86% to 90% of these events were assessed to be highly preventable (10).

A second methodology employed has been the retrospective case note review, which has considered the features of care received by patients who had an unexpected in-hospital death or a high-risk event (in-hospital cardiac arrest or unplanned ICU admission), including an examination of the observation charts prior to the index event. A New South Wales (NSW) study of 50 942 acute care admissions to 3 hospitals performed over a 6-month period in 1996 documented the antecedents of 778 deaths (19). Of these only 66 were classified as unexpected in that they did not have a do-not-resuscitate order or were preceded by a cardiac arrest or intensive care unit admission. In the 8 hours prior to the deaths of these patients, 50% had severe abnormalities documented in the observation charts or concerns noted in the nursing or medical record. Furthermore, 33% of these patients had abnormal observations or concerns noted up to 48 hours prior to their death. The most common abnormal observations were hypotension (systolic blood pressure <90 mmHg) and tachypnea (respiratory rate >36 per minute). Several studies have examined cardiac arrest calls or unplanned intensive care unit admissions from within hospitals on the assumption that these events were "unexpected," in that there were no do-not-resuscitate orders in place or that whatever process was happening could have been reversed with intensive care interventions. Although only 15% to 30% of patients survive to hospital discharge following in-hospital cardiac arrest (20–27), there is good evidence that the majority of these arrests are not unexpected. In common with the findings from the NSW study (19), retrospective analysis of simple bedside observations prior to inpatient cardiac arrest call or referral for intensive care unit admission has demonstrated prolonged periods of documented clinical instability in a significant number of patients. A retrospective case note review at the Jackson Memorial Medical Center, Florida over a 4-month period in 1987 documented 64 consecutive in-hospital cardiac arrests in the general ward areas (28). Of these, 54 (84%) had documented observations of clinical deterioration or new complaints within 8 hours of the arrest. In a similar study performed at the Cook County Hospital, Illinois, 150 cardiac arrests were observed in the medical wards over a 20-month period from 1990 to 1991 (29). In 99 of these (64%), a nurse or physician documented deterioration in the patient's condition within 6 hours of the cardiac arrest; the hospital mortality rate of the 150 cardiac arrests was 91%. In addition, in a 28-week period reported in 1999 at the Manchester Royal Infirmary in England, 47 cardiac arrest calls in the general ward areas were analyzed (30), and 24 (51%) had premonitory signs prior to the cardiac arrest call. Similarly, in a study in a tertiary care hospital in metropolitan Melbourne over the calendar year 1997, there was a median period of documented clinical instability of 6.5 hours (range 0 to 432 hours) prior to either cardiac arrest call or intensive care unit referral among 122 in-hospital patients (31). This was despite that over the period of instability on average these patients were reviewed twice by junior medical staff (31).

In a case control study performed at Selly Oak Hospital in Birmingham, England, of 118 consecutive cardiac arrests in 1999, multivariate analysis identified abnormal breathing, abnormal pulse, and abnormal systolic blood pressure in the hours prior to the cardiac arrest as being positively associated with the event (32). More simply, Goldhill and Sumner made the observation across a group of UK hospitals that admission to the intensive care unit from the general ward areas, as compared to ICU admission from surgery or the emergency department resulted in significantly higher mortality (33). Furthermore, in a study of 7190 ICU admissions across 24 UK hospitals, the actual length of stay in a general hospital ward was an independent predictor of hospital mortality (34). This study documented a hospital mortality rate of 67.2% for patients who were on the ward for greater than 15 days.

The major limitation of the studies cited above is that they primarily examined the numerator (unplanned ICU admission, cardiac arrest, and in-hospital unexpected death) without reference to denominator data (number of persons or person-days at risk). As such the clinical value of this knowledge is limited, and estimates of relative risk for the risk factors that have been identified cannot be estimated. Four prospective cohort studies have attempted to overcome this problem (35–38). In the first,

Bellomo et al. followed 1125 patients admitted for greater than 48 hours (to exclude day case surgical admissions) to the surgical units at the Austin Hospital over a 6-month period in 1999 (35). They documented 414 serious adverse events including 80 patient deaths (7.1%). This study also identified increased age as a risk factor for death from adverse events. The mortality rate for patients aged more than 75 years who underwent unscheduled surgery was 20%. The major limitation of this study was that the definition of serious adverse events included postoperative complications such as sepsis, pulmonary edema, and acute myocardial infarction, events that although serious and adverse, may not have been preventable.

In a second prospective study, a daily review of the bedside observation charts in the 165 acute general surgical and general medical beds (5 wards) was undertaken at Dandenong Hospital in Melbourne over a 33-week period in 1999 (36). During the study, 6303 patients were admitted, and of these 564 (8.9%) experienced a total of 1598 abnormal observations. The 2 most common abnormal observations were desaturation to less than 90% (51% of all events) and hypotension (17.3%). During the study, 146 patients died. When the abnormal observations were considered simultaneously in a multiple linear logistic regression model, the following events were found to be significant predictors of mortality: decrease of consciousness, loss of consciousness, hypotension, respiratory rate < 6/min, oxygen saturation >90%, and tachypnea <30/min. The presence of any 1 of the 6 events was associated with a 6.8-fold (95% CI: 2.7–17.1) increase in the risk of mortality. A cross-sectional survey undertaken at the Royal London Hospital came to a similar conclusion (37). On a single day, the following data was collected from 433 adult nonobstetric inpatients: respiratory rate, heart rate, systolic blood pressure, temperature, oxygen saturation, level of consciousness, and urine output for catheterized patients. Mortality status at hospital discharge was then determined. Logistic regression modeling identified level of consciousness, heart rate, age, systolic blood pressure, and respiratory rate as important variables in predicting outcome. Patients receiving a lower level of care than desirable also had an increased mortality rate ($P < 0.01$).

A potentially major shortcoming of these studies that may limit our ability to generalize from the findings is that they were all undertaken in a single institution. The only prospective multi-center study is the ACADEMIA study, undertaken jointly by the UK Intensive Care Society and the Australia and New Zealand Intensive Care Society clinical trials group (38). In this study, data was collected on the incidence of serious physiological abnormalities that were preceded in hospital death, cardiac arrest, or unanticipated ICU admission over 3 consecutive days in 90 hospitals in the 3 study countries. There were 638 such events, of which 60% had a total of 1032 serious physiological abnormalities prior to the index event.

These studies to identify factors that may predict unexpected iatrogenic hospital death (Table 4.1) have major limitations, which hamper the ability

TABLE 4.1. Risk factors for patient crisis

Adverse event epidemiological studies
Increased age
Negligence
Operative procedure
Human error and cognitive failure
Diagnostic and treatment delay
Retrospective case control studies
Hypotension
Tachypnea
Documentation of concern
Abnormal pulse
Level of Consciousness
Prospective studies
Hypotension
Bradypnea
Tachypnea
Oxygen desaturation
Level of consciousness
Receiving a lower level of care for illness state

to generalize the findings. All of the data in these studies has been collected manually from existing (paper) records; if variables of interest are not documented, they are not included in the analysis. Furthermore, all of the studies have collected data at one point in time or, at best, over a limited time, thus allowing for observation bias and Hawthorne effect (39). The time delay from data collection and publication in most of the studies mentioned is years, during which time the hospital latent conditions and patient case mix may have altered significantly. There is presently no capacity to collect this data in a usable format in "real time." Finally there is the issue of patient resuscitation status, or do-not-resuscitate orders, that may complicate the interpretation of what is, or is not, an unexpected iatrogenic hospital death. None of the above studies have a consistent methodology that documents the frequency and application of such orders on the study populations.

Prevention of Futile Clinical Cycles With Hard Defenses

Given the data concerning the incidence and risk factors for unexpected hospital deaths, a wide range of interventions has been proposed to prevent them. These include the Medical Emergency Team (MET) (40–43), outreach teams (44–46), the "intensive care unit without walls" (47,48), the hospitalist (49,50), the British Early Warning System (51–53), and various education systems for both undergraduates and postgraduates (54,55).

However, all of these strategies constitute soft defenses. As such, success or otherwise is dependent on human cognitive processes and abilities.

An alternative methodology to address the issue of the patient crisis is to examine the processes surrounding and leading up to such an event. This is sometimes described as a clinical audit and may be reported as a root-cause analysis when it examines both circumstances and latent conditions. In the case report of an in-hospital death presented in Box 4.1, there was no Medical Emergency Team call, consultation with the treating surgeon, or on-call intensive care specialist during the period of the patient's post-operative course. This death occurred in a hospital where the MET had been in operation for over 4 years and where a full-time nurse educator was employed to ensure optimal compliance, education, and MET utilization. The issues that this death raised were crystallized in the letter of complaint that the family wrote to the state coroner that asked among other things:

- *"Why didn't the resident doctor contact the surgeon who operated on ..., during the night if there were signs of distress, complications, or a deterioration in his condition?"*
- *"Why didn't the resident doctor contact the registrar? Was there a registrar on duty during the night?"*
- *"Why wasn't a MET call put into place after 11 PM when ... blood pressure fell and remained low? What criteria or symptoms presented by a patient instigates the MET process. ... ?"*

The expert witness appointed by the coroner made the obvious conclusion:

"Another important observation is that the patient fulfilled the criteria for activation of the MET for at least 14 hours. I understand that XXXX Hospital had a MET at the time of the patient's death and that these MET criteria were widely advertised and known throughout the hospital. I also understand that these criteria were attached to the back of the hospital medical officer's ID card and thus easily available in case of doubt when faced with a sick patient. The timely activation of the hospital MET might have saved the patient's life."

However, the real question remained: why didn't the extremely competent and experienced medical and nursing staff involved with this man's care call for some sort of help, even if it was not the MET? Why did the soft defenses fail? Some answers came from the detailed debriefing that took place with the involved staff. First, because the patient was discharged from recovery with a heart rate of 130 beats per minute, the junior medical staff assumed that the patient was "okay" from both the consultant surgeon and anesthetist's point of view. They assumed that if the operating team were in any way unhappy with the patient's condition, the patient would have been transferred to the intensive care unit postoperatively. However, both the surgeon and anesthetist were unaware that the patient was discharged from recovery with an elevated heart rate that mandated a MET call. Second, despite the patient's heart rate, he "looked okay"; in particular, the patient was sitting up, having a cup of tea, and talking to relatives early that evening. Third, members of the nursing staff were reassured that the junior medical staff attended promptly to their concerns about the patient and seemed to be managing the situation appropriately. Finally, it was a very busy night for all concerned. With the benefit of hindsight, everyone involved would have put out a MET call. The traditional hierarchal referral model of care is the manner in which most Western hospitals manage these and other acute medical scenarios in the general ward setting. In this model, when a patient deteriorates, the bedside nurse invariably documents the deterioration and then has to decide whether or not to communicate this information, and to whom. If this communication occurs it is usually to the most junior member of the treating medical team—often a junior doctor with less than 12 months of experience. To receive this communication, this doctor needs to be available and not distracted by other tasks, and then read an alphanumeric pager and call the nurse back (assuming that the line is not busy). The degree to which this vital, first information-transfer step succeeds is very much dependent on the communication skills of the nurse and the junior doctor. Based on this information and a large number of hospital latent conditions, the junior doctor will turn up and make an assessment of the patient. In most instances the junior doctor will lack the skills, confidence, and experience to manage the situation (6–9). As such, the communication step and associated processes will be repeated with the medical team's next most senior doctor, generally a specialty trainee registrar or fellow. This person, because of their position in the hospital hierarchy, generally cannot stop what they are doing to attend to the patient—this type of "medical middle manager" in the hospital hierarchy is usually busy in surgery, the emergency department, doing ward rounds, outpatients, or attending to their education. Although generally more experienced, particularly in their chosen specialization, even at this level the registrar/fellow may suffer from the same inadequacies as the junior doctor (56). However, at this level some actions (often telephone orders) are undertaken at the behest of the registrar/fellow. Some of these actions include patient case assessment, investigation, and management. In some instances, there are further referrals to subspecialty units and transfer of patient care to different teams of on-call doctors. The consultant is usually contacted about the patient's situation. This traditional hierarchal referral model of care, while arguably appropriate for more chronic outpatient medical conditions, is not well suited for the acutely ill patient in the general ward setting. For it to be successful in this setting, all of the following steps need to occur:

1. Timely response of all staff in a well-coordinated sequence
2. Correct diagnosis
3. Correct assessment of the severity of the patient's condition is appropriately communicated

4. Appropriate actions are taken
5. The actions taken are documented
6. Response is documented

In a previously reported study, the median duration of these processes prior to cardiac arrest and/or ICU admission in 112 patients was 6.5 hours, ranging up to 432 hours (31). When one considers these "clinical futile cycles" (41) and the complexities in which all of these "soft defenses" must operate, it is little wonder that there are not more unexpected iatrogenic inpatient deaths. Often the only factors that prevent greater mortality are patient physiological resilience and the hypervigilance of a junior medical or nursing staff member, which has been shown to be an inadequate defense against organizational accidents.

MET and MET Calling Criteria

The concept behind a MET is based on 2 premises: first that there is a significant mortality rate among those patients that have an in-hospital cardiac arrest (57,58), and second that it would seem logical to treat the patients before the cardiac arrest occurs. As such, there is a requirement for calling criteria to activate the MET. To date, most of the MET calling criteria implemented (Table 4.3) have been developed on the basis of clinical intuition and without rigorous validation. For example, it would seem reasonable that a patient with a systolic blood pressure of less than 90 mmHg at least be assessed by a trained resuscitation expert. However, in most hospitals we have no idea of the true incidence of this degree of hypotension and its natural history without MET intervention. This highlights the requirement that if MET criteria are to be useful to general ward staff, they need to have a high degree of face validity. It would seem from the limited number of observational studies that have attempted to validate MET criteria (36,37) that abnormal neurological and respiratory observations have the greatest

TABLE 4.2. Automated, escalated alert interventions for Box 4.1

Time	Abnormal observation	Alert status	Alert recipient	Action required
3 PM	1. Heart Rate: 130 bpm	2	1. Receiving surgical ward	Patient reviewed within 3 hours
			2. Junior Medical Officer	?return to operating room
6 PM	1. Heart Rate: 140 bpm	3	1. Surgical Registrar	Urgent patient review within 1 hour
11:30 PM	1. Heart Rate: 150 bpm	4	1. MET	Urgent resuscitation
	2. SBP: <90 mmHg		2. Treating surgeon and ICU specialist	

TABLE 4.3. MET Calling Criteria (PR = pulse rate, RR = respiratory rate, SBP = systolic blood pressure)

	Dandenong Hospital (41)	Austin Hospital (42)	Merit Study (43)	UPMC Presbyterian Hospital (59)
Airway	Threatened airway, respiratory distress		Threatened	Difficulty breathing
Breathing	RR < 6/min RR > 30/min O2 Sat < 90% (despite O2)	RR < 8/min RR > 30/min O2 Sat < 90% (despite O2)	All respiratory arrests RR < 5/min RR > 36/min	RR < 8 RR > 36 O2 Sat < 8
Circulation	PR > 130/min SBP < 90 mmHg (despite treatment)	PR > 130/min PR < 40/min SBP < 90 mmHg	All cardiac arrests PR < 40/min PR > 140/min SBP < 90 mmHg	PR < 40 PR > 140 with symptoms Any PR > 160 SBP < 80 SBP > 200 DBP > 110
Neurology	Fitting Decreased LOC	Acute change in conscious state	Sudden fall in level of consciousness (Fall in GCS of > 2 points) Repeated or prolonged seizures	Acute loss of consciousness New lethargy or difficulty waking Collapse Seizure Sudden loss of limb or facial movement
Other	Concerned Need of treatment Prompt help	Staff member is worried about the patient	Any patient that you are seriously worried about that does not fit the above criteria	Chest pain unresponsive to nitroglycerine Color change Uncontrolled bleeding Bleeding into airway Naloxone use without response

TABLE 4.4. Risk of Mortality: Independent Predictors

Event	Odds ratio and 95% CI
Decrease of consciousness	6.4 (2.6–15.7)
Hypotension	2.5 (1.6–4.1)
Loss of consciousness	6.4 (2.9–13.6)
Bradypnea	14.4 (2.6–80.0)
SaO₂ < 90%	2.4 (1.6–4.1)
Tachypnea	7.2 (3.9–13.2)

positive predictive value for valid MET activation. As discussed previously, from our own work in this area we found that loss of consciousness, decreased consciousness, respiratory rate of less than 6 per minute and greater than 30 per minute, had far greater significant predictive value for in-hospital death than cardiovascular instability and oxygen desaturation (Table 4.4) (36). The creation of MET criteria has at least some documented, objective parameters, which should aid in the identification of the potential patient crisis, and once it is recognized, there is an improved likelihood that the appropriate response will occur (e.g. calling a MET). Having MET criteria has other benefits: it helps identify the onset of the crisis objectively and enables those reviewing the case in retrospect to identify whether a delay in care occurred and the consequent impact of the delay.

Communication Technology as a Hard Defense

With the advances in communication technology and given that there are easily identifiable risk factors for unexpected iatrogenic patient demise (Table 4.1), there is a need for a patient-centric system that communicates accurate patient abnormal physiological data to the most appropriate personnel in a timely fashion. Such a system would require electronic entry of simple bedside observational data, which could then be processed to determine appropriate severity and communication of this to the most appropriate doctors and nurses. This would remove many of the subjective, human cognitive factors that so often either fail or simply do not occur in the acute hospital setting when patients become acutely ill. Considering the case history in Box 4.1, such a system could function with the treating clinical staff as outlined in Table 4.2. The alerts are graded according to the severity of the clinical observations and allow for escalation if the appropriate management does not occur. Alert escalation can be configured individually, to alert other, more senior staff of "failed alerts," or to automatically page the MET/cardiac arrest teams when appropriate. Theoretically such a system should significantly reduce important errors of cognition and delays in diagnosis and treatment, and thus reduce morbidity and mortality from adverse events, in particular cardiac arrest.

References

1. Adam D. The counting house. *Nature.* 2002;417:898.
2. Kohn LT, Corrigan JM, Donaldson MS, eds. *To Err Is Human: Building a Safer Health System.* Washington, DC: National Academies Press; 2000.
3. Reason J. *Managing the Risks of Organizational Accidents.* Aldershot, England: Ashgate Publishing Limited; 1998.
4. Reason J. *Hazards, Defence, and Losses in Managing the Risks of Organizational Accidents.* Ashgate Publishing Limited, Aldershot, 1998.
5. Wilson RM, Runciman WB, Gibberd RW, et al. The quality in Australian health care study. *Med J Aust.* 1995;163:458–471.
6. Harrison GA, Hillman KM, Fulde GWO, Jacques TC. The need for undergraduate education in critical care. *Anaesth Intensive Care.* 1999;27:53–58.
7. Taylor D. Undergraduate procedural skills training in Victoria: is it adequate? *Med J Aust.* 1997;171:22–25.
8. Buist M, Jarmolovski E, Burton P, McGrath B, Waxman B, Meek R. Can interns manage clinical instability in hospital patients? A survey of recent graduates. *Focus Health Prof Edu.* 2001;3:20–28.
9. Cooper N. Medicine did not teach me what I really needed to know. *BMJ.* 2003;327(suppl):S190.
10. Wilson R, Harrison B, Gibberd R, Hamilton J. An analysis of the causes of adverse events from the quality in Australian health care study. *Med J Aust.* 1999;170:411–415.
11. McQuillan P, Pilkington S, Allan A. Confidential enquiry into the quality of care before intensive care unit admission. *BMJ.* 1998;316:1853–1858.
12. McDonald R. New initiative to improve undergraduate teaching in acute care. *Student BMJ.* 2004;12:68.
13. Stevens DP. Finding safety in medical education. *Qual Saf Health Care.* 2002; 11:109–110.
14. Buist M, Bellomo R. MET: The medical emergency team or the medical education team? *Crit Care Resuscitation.* 2004;6;83–91.
15. Brennan TA, Leape LL, Laird N, et al. Incidence of adverse events and negligence in hospitalized patients: results of the Harvard Medical Practice Study I. *N Engl J Med.* 1991;324:370–376.
16. Leape LL, Brennan TA, Laird N, et al. The nature of adverse events in hospitalized patients: results of the Harvard Medical Practice Study II. *N Engl J Med.* 1991;324:377–384.
17. Thomas EJ, Studdert DM, Burstin HR, et al. Incidence and types of adverse events and negligent care in Utah and Colorado. *Med Care.* 2000;38:261–271.
18. Davis P, Lay-Yee R, Briant R, Wasan A, Scott A, Schug S. Adverse events in New Zealand public hospitals: occurrence and impact. *NZ Med J.* 2002;115: 203–205.
19. Hillman KM, Bristow PJ, Chey T, et al. Antecedents to hospital deaths. *Intern Med J.* 2001;31:343–348.
20. Berger R, Kelley M. Survival after in-hospital cardiopulmonary arrest of non-critically ill patients: a prospective study. *Chest.* 1994;106:872–879.
21. McGrath RB. In-house cardiopulmonary resuscitation—after a quarter of a century. *Ann Emerg Med.* 1987;16:1365–1368.

22. Ebell MH, Becker LA, Barry HC, Hagen M. Survival after in-hospital cardiopulmonary resuscitation. A meta-analysis. *J Gen Intern Med.* 1998; 13: 805–816.
23. Bedell SE, Delbanco TL, Cook EF, Epstein FH. Survival after cardiopulmonary resuscitation in the hospital. *N Engl J Med.* 1983;309:569–576.
24. Debard ML. Cardiopulmonary resuscitation: analysis of six years' experience and review of the literature. *Ann Emerg Med.* 1981;10:408–415.
25. George AL, Folk BP, Crecelius PL, Campbell WB. Pre-arrest morbidity and other correlates of survival after in-hospital cardiopulmonary arrest. *Am J Med.* 1989;87:28–34.
26. Bedell SE, Deitz DC, Leeman D, Delbanco TL. Incidence and characteristics of preventable iatrogenic cardiac arrests. *JAMA* 1991;265:2815–2820.
27. Tortolani AJ, Risucci DA, Rosati RJ, Dixon R. In-hospital cardiopulmonary resuscitation: patient and resuscitation factors associated with survival. *Resuscitation.* 1990;20:115–128.
28. Schein RM, Hazdat N, Pena M, et al. Clinical antecedents to in-hospital cardiopulmonary arrest. *Chest.* 1990;98(6):1388–1392.
29. Franklin C, Mathew J. Developing strategies to prevent in-hospital cardiac arrest: analyzing responses of physicians and nurses in the hours before the event. *Crit Care Med.* 1994; 22:244–247.
30. Smith AF, Wood J. Can some in-hospital cardio-respiratory arrests be prevented? A prospective survey. *Resuscitation.* 1998;37:133–137.
31. Buist MD, Jarmolowski E, Burton PR, Bernard SA, Waxman BP, Anderson J. Recognising clinical instability in hospital patients before cardiac arrest or unplanned admission to intensive care. A pilot study in a tertiary-care hospital. *Med J Aust.* 1999;171:22–25.
32. Hodgetts T, Kenward G, Ioannis V, Payne S, Castle N. The identification of risk factors for cardiac arrest and formulation of activation criteria to alert a medical emergency team. *Resuscitation.* 2002;54:125–131.
33. Goldhill DR, Sumner A. Outcome of intensive care patients in a group of British intensive care units. *Crit Care Med* 1998;28:1337–1345.
34. Goldhill DR, McNarry AF, Hadjianastassiou VG, Tekkis PP. The longer patients are in hospital before intensive care admission the higher their mortality. *Intensive Care Med.* 2004;30:1908–1913.
35. Bellomo R, Goldsmith D, Russell S, Uchino S. Postoperative serious adverse events in a teaching hospital: a prospective study. *Med J Aust.* 2002;176:216–218.
36. Buist M, Nguyen T, Moore G, Bernard S, Anderson J. Association between clinically abnormal bedside observations and subsequent in-hospital mortality: a prospective study. *Resuscitation.* 2004;62:137–141.
37. Goldhill DR, McNarry AF. Physiological abnormalities in early warning scores are related to mortality in adult inpatients. *Br J Anaesth.* 2004;92:882–884.
38. Kause J, Smith G, Prytherch D, Parr M, Flabouris A, Hillman K. A comparison of antecedents to cardiac arrests, deaths, and emergency intensive care admissions in Australia and New Zealand, and the United Kingdom—the ACADEMIA study. *Resuscitation.* 2004;62:275–282.
39. Campbell JP, Maxey UA. The Hawthorne effect: implications for pre-hospital research. *Ann Emerg Med.* 1995;26:590–594.

40. Bristow PJ, Hillman KM, Chey T, et al. Rates of in-hospital arrests, deaths, and intensive care admissions: the effect of a medical emergency team. *Med J Aust.* 2000;173:236–240.
41. Buist MD, Moore GE, Bernard SA, Waxman BP, Anderson JN, Nguyen TV. Effects of a medical emergency team on reduction of incidence of and mortality from unexpected cardiac arrests in hospital: preliminary study. *BMJ.* 2002; 324:1–6.
42. Bellomo R, Goldsmith D, Uchino S, et al. A prospective before and after trial of a medical emergency team. *Med J Aust.* 2003;179:283–287.
43. MERIT study investigators. A cluster randomized controlled trial of the medical emergency team. Abstract from the ANZICS ASM, Melbourne, Australia, October 2004.
44. Goldhill D, McGinley A. Outreach critical care. *Anaesthesia.* 2002;57:183.
45. Goldhill DR. Preventing surgical deaths: critical care and intensive care outreach services in the postoperative period. *Br J Anaesth.* 2005 Jul;95(1):88–94.
46. Garcea G, Thomasset S, McClelland L, Leslie A, Berry D. Impact of a critical care outreach team on critical care readmissions and mortality. *Acta Anaesthesiol Scand.* 2004;48:1096–1100.
47. Hillman K. Critical care without walls. *Curr Opin Crit Care.* 2002;8:594–599.
48. Hillman K. Expanding intensive care medicine beyond the intensive care unit. *Crit Care.* 2004;8:9–10.
49. Hillman K. Hospitals and hospitalists: an alternative view. *Med J Aust.* 2000;172: 299.
50. Hillman K. The hospitalist: A US model ripe for importing? *Med J Aust.* 2003; 178:54–55.
51. Goldhill DR. The critically ill: following your MEWS. *QJM.* 2001;94:507–510.
52. Subbe CP, Davies RG, Williams E, Rutherford P, Gemmell L. Effect of introducing the Modified Early Warning Score on clinical outcomes, cardiopulmonary arrests and intensive care utilization in acute medical admissions. *Anaesthesia.* 2003;58:797–802.
53. Cuthbertson BH. Outreach critical care—cash for no questions? *Br J Anaesth.* 2003;90:4–6.
54. Anderson ID, ed. *Care of the Critically Ill Surgical Patient.* London: Arnold, 2003.
55. Harrison J, Buist M, Flanagan B. A simulation-based MET training course for physician trainees at Southernhealth. Abstract book, the 9th national forum for pre-vocational medical education. Melbourne, October 24–26th 2004.
56. Harrison J, Flanagan B. What are PGY3's worried about? Exploration of physician trainees concerns regarding their resuscitation skills. Abstract book, the Ninth National Forum for Pre-vocational Medical Education; October 24–26, 2004; Melbourne.
57. Peatfield RC, Taylor D, Sillett RW, McNicol MW. Survival after cardiac arrest in hospital. *Lancet.* 1977; I:1223–1225.
58. Redell SL, Delbanco TL, Cook EF, Epstein FH. Survival after cardiopulmonary resuscitation in the hospital. *N Engl J Med.* 1983;309(10):569–576.
59. DeVita MA, Braithwaite RS, et al. Condition C. . .Quality and Safety in Health Care 2004.

5
Overview of Hospital Medicine

DAVID J. MCADAMS

History of the Hospitalist Movement

Traditionally the primary care physician (PCP), usually an internist or family practice physician, has been responsible for outpatient and inpatient care. Many forces in health care have pushed toward a separation of care provided to patients in these separate locations. Changes in hospital management systems, hospital size, the increasing severity of patient illness, and out-of-control health care costs have been integral in the push toward an inpatient physician care model (1). Within the context of these changes, there has been a growing sense of dissatisfaction among PCPs regarding the ability to provide timely and efficient care to both their outpatient and inpatient populations. This has given rise to the hospital medicine "specialist," an emerging specialty that is defined, much like critical care and emergency medicine, by the site of care rather than a disease, patient population, or organ system.

While physicians with inpatient care duties have existed both in North America and Europe for some time, the appearance of the hospital physician, or "hospitalist," is a newer phenomenon. Certainly, the ever-present house officer has had a place in history as the physician who essentially lives in the hospital. However, this role has been mainly restricted to the medical trainee with little experience and much responsibility, serving as a rite of passage toward becoming the more senior and less-present attending physician. In contrast, the hospital physician is a more experienced physician, not under the same training and hierarchical constraints as the house-officer, who is available at almost all times to care for the needs of patients in the hospital setting.

It has been almost 10 years since the coining of the term "hospitalist" by Wachter and Goldman (1). Definitions have been reworked and adapted, but currently the Society of Hospital Medicine defines hospitalists as: "physicians whose primary professional focus is the general medical care of hospitalized patients. Their activities include patient care, teaching, research, and leadership related to hospital medicine" (2). The drive and

49

expansion of this field of medicine has been felt throughout the United States and abroad, and its popularity continues to grow. During the past decade this new specialty has formed its own professional society, created dedicated journals, and inundated well-respected, traditionally general medicine journals with abundant evidence-based literature. Society of Hospital Medicine estimates indicate that there were about 2000 hospitalists in 1998 and 8000 in 2003, with that number expected to rise as high as 25 000 by 2010 (2). Indeed, this is one of the only fields of medicine where there is a vast surplus of jobs comparative to physicians to fill them.

Most hospitalists have been trained in internal medicine, mostly general internal medicine, although there is a large subset that has subspecialty training, usually in critical care medicine. The remainder are mainly family practice physicians, pediatricians, and others who specialize in infectious diseases and cardiology. Currently, no formal training is required to become a hospitalist—indeed, a significant amount of training in internal medicine is geared toward care of the hospitalized patient. However, there are 6 hospitalist fellowships currently with more being planned for the future. In many ways they are designed like general internal medicine fellowships, gearing the physician toward further experience in education and clinical research while providing continued exposure to inpatients and their medical problems.

Models of Hospitalist Care

Wachter has described 4 stages of hospital care that help to illustrate the driving forces behind hospitalist models (3). These stages help us to understand inpatient care structure, but they are not meant to be hierarchical, nor do hospital systems pass through them sequentially. Rather, this is a tool that helps us to understand that many external forces predicate how hospital care is provided.

The first stage is the PCP model, in which PCPs care for their own patients admitted to the hospital. This has been the classic model of care in medicine. The second stage involves rotating coverage of hospitalized patients between members in a private practice, where each physician takes turns caring for those patients admitted. This model became popular as physician groups got larger and the number of patients in their practices increased. In the third stage, we see the emergence of a dedicated hospital physician who cares for inpatients; PCPs may pass on care of patients to the hospital physician, but are not required to do so. In the fourth stage, in contrast to the voluntary hospitalist stage, PCPs are required to hand over care of patients to the inpatient physician. Every stage has its own associated advantages and disadvantages. For example, in stages 3 and 4, the inpatient physician can provide continuous care to admitted patients while the PCP is free to spend more time in the office. However, this may lead to discontinuity of care due to multiple providers, or dissatisfaction in not being able to see one's own doctor. Given the forces of health care today, many if not most hospital systems are relying at least in part on a voluntary hospitalist system of care, as described in stage 3.

Numerous hospitalist models of care are in place today. In many ways, the models continually redefine themselves based on changes in the hospitals and in physician training. For example, recent restrictions in housestaff work hours have necessitated that hospitals find alternative ways to cover patients.

One type of model includes a private practice group employing a hospitalist to admit and care for patients. A much more popular model involves a private practice group of inpatient physicians providing care to patients admitted to the hospital; typically such hospitalist groups contract out to private practices or hospitals to care for their patients. These models are popular with community facilities. Other models include those in which hospitals and health maintenance organizations hire their own inpatient physicians. Finally, many academic centers now have divisions or sections of hospital medicine. Academic hospitalists generally do less direct work with direct patients than private hospitalists—usually between 1 and 6 months per year—but their time is usually supplemented by activities such as housestaff training, academic research, and administrative duties.

Benefits of Hospitalist Systems

There are several benefits inherent in having a dedicated physician caring for patients requiring hospitalization. The hospitalist is not limited or constrained by the problems that come with an office practice. As such, the hospitalist is available throughout the day or night to see patients immediately, to meet with patient family members and loved ones, and to respond to emergency situations. The hospitalist is also in a prime position to foster a culture of patient safety, primarily by participating in multidisciplinary teams (4). Additionally, since this doctor practices only in the hospital, over time the hospitalist becomes more attuned to developing and maintaining the necessary skills to manage acute inpatient medical issues.

Hospital medicine is a relatively young field, but the body of evidence in literature showing the benefits of this new system is growing rapidly. Published data demonstrates that utilizing hospitalists decreases total costs per case and patient's length of stay (5); preserves patient satisfaction despite no direct PCP involvement in care (5); helps lower short-term mortality (6); provides benefit in end-of-life care (7); and improves resident education (8). Data also suggests that some of these changes, particularly length of stay and cost per case, are derived only when experienced hospitalists are present in a program or after a program has been established for some time (6). This should be noted with concern, since the recent explosion in this position's popularity in hospital medicine has left many slots open for inexperienced hospitalists, and since some programs are designed to be transient and are filled by recent residency graduates. Nonetheless, the benefits derived from hospitalist use are evident, and certainly this concern will diminish over the next decade as the number of providers begins to equilibrate with the number of available employable positions.

A large number of hospitalist journals now exist. Interestingly, nearly every one has a section focusing on quality improvement or patient safety. Again, because these physicians are working within the hospital most of the time they are afforded the unique ability to police the system, recognize areas of improper or inefficient care management, and formulate and carry out care plans that have been proven to enhance inpatient care.

Hospitalists as Acute Providers

Compared to past decades, sicker patients are being admitted to the hospital, and they are staying longer. Most patients are no longer simply staying in facilities awaiting tests—they have serious, volatile problems, with conditions that can change at any time. One can argue that 24/7 care of patients by an in-house physician is much more beneficial than traditional, outside, overnight call coverage (9).

By virtue of focused training in hospital medicine and advanced cardiac life-support techniques, the hospitalist is in a prime position to care for the inpatient in urgent and emergent situations. In general, adverse events follow a gradual clinical patient deterioration, and often the signs go unrecognized or are even ignored (10). While there is not much direct data yet to suggest a link between hospitalists and early recognition of deterioration, there is some suggestion that the omnipresence of the hospitalist allows for more prompt recognition of acute problems with patients and implementation of appropriate and directed care to prevent adverse outcomes (6,8).

The hospitalist can work alone in this venue, but more commonly he or she works as part of either a multidisciplinary team or a Medical Emergency Team (MET). The concept of a "code team" is not new, and certainly many facilities rely on intensivists and intensive care unit (ICU) teams to provide emergency care. The newer trend is an attempt to make these teams more universal and more rapid to respond. The use of a hospitalist system does not preclude the need for a MET—the hospitalist, both intensivist and non-intensivist, can be a part of this response team. Physicians trained in internal medicine (who do not then do subspecialty training) often do not have major instruction beyond basic life support and advanced cardiac life-support techniques, particularly complex airway management. More often the non-intensivist hospitalist is the first responder to urgent or emergent situation, calls the MET to the bedside, and can certainly be involved as an integral member of the MET as the "code leader." However, the more challenging aspects of code management are usually reserved for the intensivist. Again, the major benefit of the hospitalist to the hospital system is being in a position to foster a more astute recognition of the clinical deterioration of patients, and then set into motion the necessary elements to call the MET to the patient's aid.

Many clinical trials now are underway to examine the usefulness of METs. At least 2 studies (both were non-randomized and non-blinded) have shown some benefit to having a MET—namely a decreased incidence of unanticipated ICU transfers, lower incidence of death without a do-not-resuscitate order, a deceased incidence of and mortality for in-hospital cardiac arrests, and a reduction in overall hospital mortality (11,12). There certainly appears to be some advantage from in-house METs, but the extent of it remains to be seen.

Thoughts for the Future

The wave of the future in hospital care will almost universally involve the hospitalist. Yet given the rapid nature with which this is occurring, steps need to be taken to ensure that hospitalists are prepared for the situations they will encounter on a daily basis.

Instituting steps to improve retention (incentive programs, reasonable shifts, and work hours, etc.) will likely improve performance and care delivery in programs that employ hospitalists. Changes may also be made in residency training programs to allow candidates interested in a career in hospital medicine the opportunity to obtain more experience in the care of the inpatient and in managing inpatient emergencies. While more fellowships for hospital medicine may continue to emerge, it remains to be seen if completing a fellowship will be required for those wishing to pursue a hospital-based position.

It may become necessary to define the specific types of training required for hospital medicine, and almost certainly this will evolve around management of acute scenarios. Hospitalists need to be fully trained to deal with emergent events, particularly non-intensivists. In academic centers, residents receive less and less exposure to urgent or emergent events and procedures. Interestingly, they are getting more controlled experience in the lab setting, but much less bedside emergency situation experience. And since no formal training is required in hospital medicine, much of these duties are falling onto the shoulders of already busy and short-staffed intensivists.

Focused training for hospitalists participating in multidisciplinary teams or METs may prove to be extremely beneficial for every aspect of patient care. While the former will almost certainly allow for better management of quality issues and patient safety, the latter will be the basis for provision of care during acute hospital emergencies.

References

1. Wachter RM, Goldman L. The emerging role of "hospitalists" in the American health care system. *N Engl J Med*. 1996;335:514–517.
2. Society of Hospital Medicine. Available at: http://www.hospitalmedicine.org. Accessed January 2005.
3. Wachter RM. An introduction to the hospitalist model. *Ann Intern Med*. 1999; 130:338–342.
4. Shojania KG, Wald H, Gross R. Understanding medical error and improving patient safety in the inpatient setting. *Med Clin North Am*. 2002;86:847—867.
5. Wachter RM, Goldman L. The hospitalist movement 5 years later. *JAMA*. 2002; 287:487–494.
6. Meltzer D, Manning WG, Morrison J, et al. Effects of physician experience on costs and outcomes on an academic general medicine service: results of a trial of hospitalists. *Ann Intern Med*. 2002;137:866–875.
7. Auerbach AD, Pantilat SZ. End-of-life care in a voluntary hospitalist model: effects on communication, processes of care, and patient systems. *Am J Med*. 2004;116:669–675.
8. Kulaga ME, Charney P, O'Mahony SP, et al. The positive impact of initiation of hospitalist clinician educators: resource utilization and medical resident education. *J Gen Intern Med*. 2004;19:293–301.
9. SHM Benchmarks Committee. Value added by hospitalists: hospital medicine programs add value through extraordinary availability (24/7). *Hospitalist*. 2004; 8:19–22.
10. Buist M, Bernard S, Anderson J. Epidemiology and prevention of unexpected hospital deaths. *Surgeon*. 2003;1:265–268.
11. Bristow PJ, Hillman KM, Chey T, et al. Rates of in-hospital arrests, deaths, and intensive care admissions: the effect of a medical emergency team. *Med J Aust*. 2000;173:236–240.
12. Buist MD, Moore GE, Bernard SA, Waxman BP, Anderson JN, Nguyen TV. Effects of a medical emergency team on reduction of incidence of and mortality from unexpected cardiac arrests in hospital: preliminary study. *BMJ*. 2002; 324:1–6.

6
Medical Trainees and Patient Safety

STEPHEN W. LAM and ARTHAS FLABOURIS

Health Care, Health Care Facilities, and Medical Trainees

Medical trainees form an important part of the medical profession. They are vital health care resources, contributing both to the delivery of health care to patients as well as advancements in research and academic medicine. Their contribution is profoundly influenced by their prior undergraduate academic education and supervised clinical experience. Progression through the postgraduate years is associated with a diminishing level of clinical supervision as clinical expertise is accumulated. Assessment is typically a combination of formative and summative assessment, until the trainee is considered safe to practice without further supervision.

Postgraduate clinical training generally occurs in large health care facilities. The patient profiles and illness types (or "case mix") found in these facilities influence the health care provision that is required from medical trainees. These factors, in addition to others such as level and quality of supervision, available resources, and working conditions, determine a trainee's learning environment. Together, this creates a "shared dependence," where patients depend on a trainee capable of providing them with safe care, while the trainee relies on patients to be part of a learning environment from which to gain quality training and experience.

The hospital inpatient population is becoming increasingly complex. The population is aging (1,2), with increasing co-morbidities, changing disease demographics (3–5), increasing complexity of health care technology (6), and patients with chronic and often terminal conditions in acute care facilities due to the lack of available chronic and aged care facilities. Meanwhile hospitals seek to achieve cost efficiency through reducing acute hospital beds, streamlining inpatient care, staff reductions, and greater emphasis on home care. The changing needs of patients is also reflected by an increase in demand for a new specialist in hospital medicine, or "hospitalist," capable of providing competent institutional care in a team environment and handling both acute medical events (7) and palliative care issues (6,8).

The rapid growth in technological and scientific advances resulting from better understanding of complex disease processes and how to deal with them has fueled the growth of medical specialization. The number of American Medical Association–accredited specialties and subspecialties increased from 14 in 1927 to 41 by 1985, after which growth was exponential, reaching 124 by the year 2000 (9). Highly technical proceduralists and specialists are now limiting their practices to specific diseases, organs, or parts of the body. Because of the associated technical complexity and cost of such procedures, many of these services are restricted to academic and acute care medical facilities. As a result, there has been a decline in the number of medical practitioners devoted to comprehensive and whole individual care. Medical specialization has been criticized as being unnecessarily fragmented (10) and confusing to patients and general practitioners alike, with risk to the perception of medicine as an integrated profession (11).

Undergraduate Years

The primary role of medical schools is the education of medical students—preparing them with the necessary knowledge and skills for structured, supervised practice in acute care facilities. Increasingly this role has had to compete with research and other non-teaching activities. In the 1990s, the medical curriculum was criticized for being too rigid, overuse of didactic teaching methods, and too much emphasis on rote memorization (12). Since then the emphasis of undergraduate training and examination has shifted away from the didactic acquisition of academic knowledge and toward a focus on patient-oriented knowledge and problem-based learning (6,13,14). The adoption of patient-based learning methods has been undertaken with a view to improving the link between undergraduate training and postgraduate provision of patient care (6,13–15). It also allows undergraduate training to evolve with changing patient needs on the wards.

Recognition of the importance of practical skills assessment has lead to the use of such examination techniques as the Observed Structured Clinical Examination (OSCE). For the assessment for competency in critical care skills, a teaching methodology that incorporates structured clinical, objective, multidisciplinary, problem-based instruction (16) with that of OSCE and/or computer simulation–based assessment have been shown to be effective (17).

Medical Trainees and Patient Safety—The First Few Years

Despite lacking a strong base of medical experience, postgraduate medical education in acute care facilities is tailored toward clinical expertise in select medical domains through a specialized, structured curriculum, which deviates from a more whole-patient approach. Medical trainees often lack sufficient skills to meet patient needs (14,18–20): training in the basic aspects of recognizing and caring for the critically ill patient is often lacking not only in the undergraduate years (21,22) but often in postgraduate studies as well (23,24), and may remain in a poor state after completion of the chosen medical specialty and among specialty supervisors (25).

Because of the frequent and routine nature of many aspects of general ward care, such as handling minor complaints and prescribing intravenous fluids, at many health care institutions the most junior member of the health care team are the first point of contact when an issue arises. Such issues are often nonspecific and undifferentiated complaints, or requests made by patients, nursing/paramedical, or medical staff. Under such circumstances, most junior trainees remain unsupervised and receive little feedback, unless an adverse event is the result.

The high frequency of minor medical issues arising in ward care has also created the need for 24-hour "on-call" medical officers to deal with them. On such shifts, medical trainees often are given a wide range of smaller, less focused tasks. Several tasks for multiple patients may be allocated to the individual simultaneously from different areas of the hospital. Such tasks may be of varying priority, and for reasons ranging from the urgency of the patient's clinical condition to time frames and deadlines (e.g. awaiting transfer to the operating room).

As such, medical trainees often are faced with the need to triage priorities and handle important tasks with multiple distracting issues under significant time pressures. "On-call" shifts are typically long and extend outside normal working hours.

Frequently the mode of presentation of medical emergencies is subtle or nonspecific; and their early recognition and correct management is crucial to patient safety and outcome (7,26–30). Subtle indicators of a more severe underlying process can be easily overlooked among the burden of routine tasks. A recent survey of patients who suffered cardiac arrests, death, or unanticipated intensive care unit admission in hospitals in 3 countries revealed that significant physiological abnormal findings were present in many patients prior to those events. For some patients there was documentation of review by medical staff, thus highlighting the possible preventability of such adverse events (31). Similarly other studies have documented patients with abnormal and/or inadequately attended clinical findings who subsequently experience potentially preventable adverse events (30,32). Inappropriate working conditions can hinder a trainee's ability to correctly identify and separate warning signs of impending disaster from more minor complaints and issues, and provide appropriate care in a timely manner where required (33–37).

Improving Patient Safety in Institutions with Medical Trainees

The delivery of health care can be separated into 2 types:

* predictable by the presenting illness (e.g. provision of elective surgical procedure or drug treatment for a known problem), or
* an unanticipated acute medical problem or complication (e.g. undiagnosed illnesses, idiosyncratic drug reactions, iatrogenic and nosocomial complications)

The supervision of postgraduate trainees in their provision of patient care that is predictable by the presenting illness should be adjusted according to the trainees' level of experience and assessed competency. Predictable illness clinical pathways can be used to oversee clinical performance, but the value of senior clinical oversight should not be ignored (26). Such oversight can be useful in detecting missed diagnoses as well as providing educational feedback upon performance.

Responses to acute medical emergencies should be immediate, organized, predetermined and involve of a team of appropriately trained and resourced clinical staff. A good example is a trauma team response (38,39). The organization of trauma management has resulted in a significant reduction in preventable deaths (40,41). However, for inpatients with acute medical emergencies, often the most junior doctors are left to manage such emergencies on their own. Not only may they lack the required critical care skills, but they also lack the crucial skills of being able to communicate, coordinate, and organize a team response. Often monitoring and procedural equipment are not available, and senior assistance may be remote or not provided in a timely fashion. This is especially so in acute care facilities, where response to acute ward medical emergencies may be limited to a team that responds only to cardiac arrests.

As demonstrated in this book, a team that responds to acute medical emergencies other than cardiac arrest for hospital inpatients is a concept that is becoming increasingly popular (42–45). Ideally medical trainees should be trained in basic and advanced resuscitation skills, no matter what their primary specialty training. However, the expectation that all such trainees would be able to regularly perform or practice those skills is hard to sustain. It is more important that trainees be instructed in the early recognition of at-risk patients, and/or patients that may go on to experience an acute medical illness (7,26–30), and possess the skills to integrate themselves within any available hospital medical emergency response team.

Postgraduate Training and Specialization

Complicated patients need practitioners who are able to manage undifferentiated illnesses, often along with multiple specialist teams and/or other generalists. Focus on one area of practice with specialist training invariably leads to a lack of knowledge and experience in other areas.

The multifactorial causes of adverse events in the Quality in Australian Health Care Study shows that technical competency, problem-solving ability, communication, performance, and system design all contribute to the quality of medical care and thus should be considered integral components to postgraduate education curricula (46).

Thus, in this age of increasing specialization it is crucial that postgraduate training maintains a more balanced approach to acute care for the whole of the patient. At the very least medical trainees should be taught to distinguish warning signs that may herald a greater emergency requiring need of further attention, recognize their limitations, and be empowered to refer as appropriate or seek other critical care involvement during times of medical crises.

Support for the concept of the hospitalist has grown as a result of issues of patient safety and a drive for lower inpatient costs (47,48). The rise of the hospitalist mirrors that of the critical care domains of intensive care and emergency medicine, which pioneered and continues to promote coordinated, whole-patient acute care for inpatients. Hospitalists have become the preferred providers of postgraduate medical education among medical trainees in some countries (49).

Training and retention of basic and advanced life-support skills requires a multidisciplinary, coordinated, and integrated team approach, one that is far removed from the current situation of a junior doctor acting in isolation within a hospital ward. Such training is best served through clinical exposure within dedicated critical care units, simulation technology, and skills laboratories (50). Training that also involves instruction in triage, emergency planning and preparation, team leadership, teamwork, and team organization during emergency response should be included. Consideration for such training should begin in the undergraduate years. A system of regular reaccreditation is an essential component.

Summary

With changing hospital patient demographics and rapidly advancing health care technology, it is becoming increasingly important for health care systems to evolve to meet their new challenges. Medical trainees, as a vital health care resource, provide both elective and emergency medical care within acute health care facilities. Postgraduate training and medical team structure often place junior trainees at the forefront of identifying and responding to inpatient acute medical needs. This requires them to deal with issues ranging from the trivial to the more complicated and often subtle presentations of acute medical emergencies. Their ability to recognize these signs and alert and participate in the response to acute medical events with hospital medical emergency teams is crucial to minimizing serious adverse events for such patients.

For medical trainees to safely and efficiently fulfill their roles in emergent and elective patient care, undergraduate and postgraduate training will need to provide them with the appropriate skills, environment, balance between specialization and general medicine, and appropriate supervision.

References

1. Population Division, Department of Economic and Social Affairs, United Nations Secretariat (2003). World Population Prospects: The 2002 Revision. Highlights, New York: United Nations. Available at: http://www.un.org/esa/population/publications/wwp2002/wpp2002.highlightsrev1.pdf.
2. World Health Organization. The World Health Report 1998: life in the 21st century—a vision for all. Geneva: WHO;May 1998.
3. van Weel C. Chronic diseases in general practice: the longitudinal dimension. *Eur J Gen Pract.* 1996;2:17–21.
4. van Weel C, Michels J. Dying, not old age, to blame for costs of health care. *Lancet.* 1997;350:1159–1160.
5. Resnick NM, Marcantonio ER. How should clinical care of the aged differ? *Lancet.* 1997;350:1157–1158.
6. Chantler C. National Health Service: the role and education of doctors in the delivery of health care. *Lancet.* 1999;353:1178–1181.
7. McQuillan P, Pilkington S, Allan A, et al., Confidential inquiry into quality of care before admission to intensive care. *BMJ.* 1998;316:1853–1858.
8. McCahill, Dunn GP, Mosenthal AC, Milch RA, Krouse RS. Palliation as a core surgical principle: part 1. *J Am Coll Surg.* 2004;199:149–160.
9. Donini-Lenhoff FG, Hedrick HL. Growth of specialization in graduate medical education. *JAMA.* 2000;284:1284–1289.
10. Grumbach K. Primary care in the United States—the best of times, the worst of times. *N Engl J Med.* 1999;341:2008–2010.
11. Martini CJ. Graduate medical education in the changing environment of medicine. *JAMA.* 1992;268:1097–1105.
12. Christakis NA. The similarity and frequency of proposals to reform US medical education: constant concerns. *JAMA.* 1995;274:706–711.
13. Howe A, Campion P, Searle J, Smith H. New perspectives—approaches to medical education at four new UK medical schools. *BMJ* 2004;329:327–331.
14. Jones R, Higgs R, Angelis C, Prideaux D. Changing face of medical curricula. *Lancet.* 2001;357;699–704.
15. Dornan T, Bundy C. What can experience add to early medical education? Consensus survey. *BMJ.* 2004;329:834–840.
16. Hill D, Stalley P, Pennington D, Besser M, McCarthy W. Competency-based learning in traumatology. *Am J Surg.* 1997;173:136–140.
17. Rogers PL, Jacob H, Rashwan AS, Pinsky MR. Quantifying learning in medical students during a critical care medicine elective: a comparison of three evaluation instruments. *Crit Care Med.* 2001;29:1268–1273.

18. Smith GB, Poplett N. Knowledge of aspects of acute care in trainee doctors. *Postgrad Med J*. 2002;78:335–338.
19. Meek T. New house officers' knowledge of resuscitation, fluid balance, and analgesia. *Anaesthesia*. 2000;55:1128.
20. Goldacre MJ, Lambert T, Evans J, Turner G. Preregistration house officers' views on whether their experience at medical school prepared them well for their jobs: national questionnaire survey. *BMJ*. 2003;326:1011–1012.
21. Harrison GA, Hillman KM, Fulde GW, Jacques TC. The need for undergraduate education in critical care (results of a questionnaire to year 6 medical undergraduates, University of New South Wales and recommendations on a curriculum in critical care.) *Anaesth Intensive Care*. 1999;27:53–58.
22. Buchman TG, Dellinger RP, Raphaely RC, Todres ID. Undergraduate education in critical care medicine. *Crit Care Med*. 1992;20:1595–1603.
23. Gillard JH, Dent TH, Jolly BC, Wallis DA, Hicks BH. CPR and the RCP. Training of students and doctors in UK medical schools. *J R Coll Physicians Lond*. 1993;27:412–417.
24. Redmond AD. Training in resuscitation. *Arch Emerg Med*. 1987;4:205–206.
25. Thwaites BC, Shankar S, Niblett D, Saunders J. Can consultants resuscitate? *J Roy Coll Physicians Lond*. 1992;26:265–267.
26. Reilly BM. Physical examination in the care of medical inpatients: an observational study. *Lancet*. 2003;362:1100.
27. Hillman K, Bristow PJ, Chey T, et al. Antecedents to hospital deaths. *Intern Med J*. 2001;31:343–348.
28. Franklin C, Mathew J. Developing strategies to prevent inhospital cardiac arrest analyzing responses of physicians and nurses in the hours before the event. *Crit Care Med*. 1994;22:244–247.
29. Bedell SE, Deitz DC, Leeman D, Delbanco TL. Incidence and characteristics of preventable iatrogenic cardiac arrest. *JAMA*. 1991;265:2815–2820.
30. Schein RM, Hazday N, Pena M, Ruben BH, Sprung CL. Clinical antecedents to in-hospital cardiopulmonary arrest. *Chest*. 1990;98:1388–1392.
31. Kause J, Smith G, Prytherch D, Parr M, Flabouris A, Hillman K; Intensive Care Society (UK); Australian and New Zealand Intensive Care Society Clinical Trials Group. A comparison of antecedents to cardiac arrests, deaths, and emergency intensive care admissions in Australia and New Zealand, and the United Kingdom—the ACADEMIA study. *Resuscitation*. 2004;62:275–282.
32. Garrad C, Young D. Suboptimal care of patients before admission to intensive care is caused by a failure to appreciate or apply the ABCs of life support. *BMJ*. 1998;316:1841–1842.
33. Homes G. Junior doctors' working hours: an unhealthy tradition? [editorial]. *Med J Aust*. 1998; 68:587–588.
34. Olson L, Ambrogetti A. Working harder—working dangerously? *Med J Aust*. 1998;168:614–616.
35. Sexton JB. Error, stress, and teamwork in medicine and aviation: cross sectional surveys. *BMJ*. 2000;320:745–749.
36. Lockley SW, Cronin JW, Evans EE, et al. Effect of reducing interns' weekly work hours on sleep and attentional failures. *N Engl J Med*. 2004:351:1829–1837.
37. Landrigan CP, Rothschild JM, Cronin JW, et al. Effect of reducing interns' work hours on serious medical errors in intensive care units. *N Engl J Med*. 2004: 351:1838–1848.

38. West JG, Williams MJ, Trunkey DD, Wolferth CC. Trauma systems. Current status—future challenges. *JAMA*. 1988;259:3597–3600.
39. Pagliarello G, Dempster A, Wesson D. The integrated trauma program: a model for cooperative trauma triage. *J Trauma*. 1992;33:198–204.
40. Shackford SR, Hollingworth-Fridlund P, Cooper GF, et al. The effect of regionalization upon the quality of trauma care as assessed by concurrent audit before and after institution of a trauma system. *J Trauma*. 1986;26:812–820.
41. Draaisma JM, de Haan AF, Goris RJ. Preventable trauma deaths in the Netherlands—a prospective multicenter study. *J Trauma*. 1989;29:1552–1557.
42. Lee A, Bishop G, Hillman KM, Daffurn K. The medical emergency team. *Anaesth Intensive Care*. 1995;23:183–186.
43. Stenhouse C, Coates S, Tivey M, Allsop P, Parker T. Prospective evaluation of a Modified Early Warning Score to aid detection of patients developing critical illness on a surgical ward. *Br J Anaesth*. 2000;179(6):663P.
44. Kerridge RK, Saul WP. The medical emergency team, evidence-based medicine and ethics. *Med J Aust*. 2003;179:313–315.
45. Goldhill OR, Worthing L, Mulcahy A, Tarling M, Sumner A. The patient-at-risk team: identifying and managing seriously ill ward patients. *Anaesthesia*. 1999;54:853–860.
46. Wilson RM, Runciman WB, Gibberd RW, et al. The quality in Australian health care study. *Med J Aust*. 1995;163:458–471.
47. Wachter RM, Goldman L. The emerging role of hospitalists in the American health care system. *N Engl J Med*. 1996;335:514–517.
48. Wachter RM. Hospitalists in the United States—mission accomplished or work in progress? *N Engl J Med*. 2004;350:1935–1936.
49. Hauer KE, Wachter RM, McCulloch CE, Woo GA, Auerbach AD. Effects of hospitalist attending physicians on trainee satisfaction with teaching and with internal medicine rotations. *Arch Intern Med*. 2004;164:1866–1871.
50. Riley RH, Grauze AM, Chinnery C, Horley RA, Trewhella NH. Three years of "CASMS:" the world's busiest medical simulation centre. *Med J Aust*. 2003; 179:626–630.

7
Matching Levels of Care with Levels of Illness

GARY B. SMITH and JULIANE KAUSE

My ward was now divided into three rooms; and, under favor of the matron, had managed to sort out the patients in such a way that I had what I called my "duty room," my "pleasure room," and my "pathetic room," and worked for each in a different way. One, I visited with a dressing tray full of rollers, plasters, and pins; another, with books, flowers, games, and gossip; a third, with teapots, lullabies, consolation and sometimes, a shroud.

—Louisa May Alcott (1)

Matching the level of care to the severity of a patient's illness seems fundamental to the provision of quality health care. However, until recently admission to the hospital has generally been an unplanned process, with patients being admitted directly from home, an outpatient clinic, or the emergency department (ED) to a general ward. A few very sick patients were admitted directly from the emergency department to a high dependency unit (HDU) or an intensive care unit (ICU) for higher levels of monitoring or care, but the majority were placed in general, poorly monitored environments. In times of high HDU/ICU occupancy, even sick patients are triaged to lower care areas (2).

The placement of patients on general wards has often been based on the type of disease, rather than their care needs or severity of illness. As a result, patients of different illness severity have been treated together. Medical and nursing care was usually specialty-based, with most urgent clinical care being provided by trainee staff working in hierarchical structures. Patients were admitted under specialists who were experts in their field but often lacked the ability to detect and manage critical illness arising from conditions outside their specialty. There was often little planning of the patients' in-hospital stay, and patient flow through hospital areas often bore little relation to their level of acuity. While these systems served some patients well, others were disadvantaged and often received suboptimal care (3–10).

Today reduced hospital beds and increased reliance on outpatient surgery mean that only the sickest patients are now hospitalized. In general, patients are older and more dependent than in previous decades; the incidence of co-existing morbidity is higher, and patient management has become more complex, placing greater pressure on health care staff. Developments in nursing, medical, surgical, and anaesthetic care mean that complex therapies and investigations that were previously unavailable or deemed too risky are now commonplace. In effect, the hospital has become the "intensive care unit of the community."

Evidence of Incorrect Placement of Patients

In an ideal world, the sickest patients should be admitted to an area that can provide the greatest supervision and the highest level of organ support and nursing care. While this is often so, it is clear that many patients are incorrectly placed for their level of acuity (11–17). For example, in a 2-week survey of medical and surgical wards in a UK hospital, Leeson-Payne et al. recorded 111 "HDU days," representing 57 patients (11). Similarly, Crosby and Rees showed that 6.8% of patients in surgical ward beds and 50.8% of patients in ICU beds would have been more appropriately cared for in an HDU (12). Over 60% of patients in a group of Welsh HDUs were also incorrectly placed; the majority of them were well enough to be cared for on a general ward (13). Similarly, a study of 8040 ICU admissions in the United States demonstrated that 76.8% of patients admitted simply for monitoring were reported to have a 10% chance of receiving active ICU treatment during their stay; only 4.4% actually received it (14). These data suggest that, although ICU and HDU beds are scarce, low acuity patients are often placed there. This is important, as inability to admit sick patients to an ICU when they require intensive care leads to poor outcomes (18–20). Improvements in these processes have occurred, due to the introduction of recommendations for admission and discharge criteria for critical care units and the associated levels of care (21–27).

The mismatch of patient needs and the care capabilities is not limited to those who are sufficiently sick to warrant an HDU or ICU bed. For instance, surgical patients "lodged" on medical wards may also receive care that is not matched appropriately to their disease or level of acuity if ward staff are unfamiliar with the disease process or its treatment; the same is true for patients who are in ICU but should be on the medical ward.

Definitions of Levels of Care

The disparity between patient severity of illness and the location of their care has encouraged the UK health service to define levels of care for hospitalized patients (25). Using this system, patients are allocated to a level of care according to their clinical need; location and prevailing nurse-to-patient ratio are not considered (25). The system uses 4 levels of care:

Level 0: Patients whose needs can be met through normal ward care in an acute hospital. Such patients would usually only require oral or bolus intravenous medication, patient-controlled analgesia, and vital sign observations performed once every 4 hours.

Level 1: Patients at risk of their condition deteriorating, or those recently relocated from higher levels of care whose needs can be met on an acute care ward with additional support from the critical care team. Such patients might require vital sign monitoring on a more frequent basis than Level 0 patients, regular physiotherapy, airway suction every 2 to 6 hours, or advanced techniques such as epidural analgesia.

Level 2: Patients requiring more detailed observation or intervention, including support for a single failing organ system or postoperative care, and those stepping down from higher levels of care.

Level 3: Patients requiring advanced respiratory support alone or basic respiratory support together with support of at least 2 organ systems. This level includes all complex patients requiring support for multi-organ failure.

Unfortunately, the UK classification system shares some terminology with the Society of Critical Care Medicine's recommendations for categorizing intensive care units (23). Nevertheless it does provide a starting point from which levels of care can be matched to patient severity of illness. Patient movement between these levels of care has been portrayed as linear (28), but the speed of physiological deterioration can be dramatic and sudden as compensatory mechanisms fail. Occasionally, patients will suffer acute deterioration and a "false arrest;" 33% of these patients subsequently die in the hospital (29). When in doubt, it is probably wise to opt for a higher level of care, as it is much easier to step down care if the patient is later found to be stable or improving.

Identifying the Patient's Level of Illness

Signs of illness reflect the interaction between the patient's physiological reserve (i.e., age, prior health), physiological deterioration (particularly respiratory rate, heart rate, S_aO_2, and level of consciousness), and the underlying clinical condition. The level of treatment being received by the patient should also be considered, as this will influence physiological values; for example, consider the impact of supplementary oxygen on S_aO_2.

In general, clinical signs of acute illness are similar whatever the underlying process, as they reflect failing cardiovascular, respiratory, and neurological systems. Consequently, sensitive methods of identifying those patients at risk of deterioration are difficult to develop, and current practice depends upon the use of systems incorporating measures of vital sign deterioration (30–34). These systems are intuitive; however, their sensitivity, specificity, and accuracy in predicting certain clinical outcomes have yet to be widely validated (33,35–37). Indeed, although numerous studies have identified heart rate, blood pressure, respiratory rate, and conscious level abnormalities to be markers of impending critical events (38–42), suggestions that their incidence have predictive value must be questioned, as not all important vital signs are, or can be, recorded continuously in general ward areas. Several studies confirm that the charting of vital signs is often poor, with resultant gaps in data (41–45). While the use of physiological systems can increase the frequency of vital sign monitoring (46), they will only truly be useful for outcome prediction if widespread monitoring of hospitalized patients becomes available.

It is rare for a single symptom, clinical sign, vital sign measurement, or laboratory investigation to be pathognomonic of a specific clinical condition. Consequently, clinical decisions are usually based upon more than one piece of information, each of which is weighted for its significance in the context under consideration. While the use of a warning score based on common physiological abnormalities is appealing, it is possible that a more subjective approach, based loosely on staff experience and expertise may also be effective (47–49). Future research needs to consider how the performance of physiologically based scoring systems can be enhanced by the inclusion of factors such as the results of routine investigations (50,51), symptoms, diagnosis, and therapy (52). If such scoring systems can be incorporated into computerized monitoring systems that include so-called "smart alarms" and decision-support and neural network technology, they may prove useful in detecting subtle trends sufficiently early for critical illness to be averted.

Response to Acute Illness

Even when medical staff is alerted to a patient's abnormal physiology, there is often delay in attending to the patient or in referral for higher levels of care (3,41,42,53,54). The use of algorithms that dictate specific actions and response times are helpful but not perfect (53,54). Delayed treatment on wards can result in poor outcomes (55).

Knowledge and Experience of Ward Staff

Patients should expect to be treated in areas where the knowledge and clinical expertise of doctors, nurses, and physiotherapists is appropriate for their condition. However, at a time when hospitalized patients' acuity is increasing, deficiencies in the acute care knowledge and skills of medical staff have been identified in numerous studies (56–69). For example, recent research papers suggest that junior trainee doctors may have knowledge gaps concerning resuscitation (57), fluid and electrolyte balance (57,58), analgesia (59), issues of consent (60,61), pulse oximetry (62,63) and drug dosages

(64,65). Similar deficiencies in skills and ability have been documented, with trainee doctors unable to perform simple clinical procedures such as drug calculations (66), nasogastric tube placement, bladder catheterization (67,68), and electrocardiogram interpretation (69). Often medical trainees had not observed common or essential procedures (70), and this is supported by the documented diminishing exposure to clinical cases (71–74), which reflects condensed training and shorter hours of work (75,76). The acute care knowledge and skills of senior ward doctors has not yet been assessed, but there is little to suggest that their performance is likely to be better (77,78).

"Deskilling" of ward nurses seems to have been one of the adverse outcomes of the opening of ICUs and HDUs. Previously, when overall hospital acuity levels were low, patients with complex medical problems and invasive monitoring could easily be admitted to these new, high-care areas. However, over time, hospital activity levels have risen, patients have become sicker, and ICUs and HDUs have become full. Ill patients are now discharged earlier to the general wards, where some clinical skills have not been maintained (79,80) (since patients of the highest acuity have been removed to the ICUs) and as a result staff often lack confidence when dealing with acute care problems (81). Ward staff rarely use a systematic approach to the assessment of critically ill patients (81). Consequently, courses in acute care are being developed that are suitable for ward nurses (82,83).

The discovery that trainee doctors and ward nurses often lack the skills necessary to detect critical illness and manage sick patients is worrying, as they are usually the first to assess and treat patients. Of particular concern are reports that medical school training provides poor preparation for doctors' early careers in clinical medicine and fails to teach essential aspects of applied physiology and acute care (84–89). Furthermore, the common textbooks used by medical students and trainee doctors to learn how to examine patients rarely offer advice on how to assess the acutely ill patient (90). In the UK, these shortfalls have led to the development of postgraduate courses to teach doctors, nurses, and physiotherapists how to recognize and manage critical illness on general wards (82,91,92). The Society of Critical Care Medicine has also introduced a course, directed at non-intensivists, which focuses on managing sick patients in the first 24 hours of critical illness when more direct critical care expertise is unavailable (93). Similarly, an advanced resuscitation course forms part of the Medical Emergency Team (MET) programs established in Australia (94).

It is recognized that training in acute and critical care should commence early on, and many countries have established curricula for inclusion in undergraduate medical education programs (89, 95–97). New educational techniques are often used, including simulation and computer-assisted learning (98–100). Training opportunities in critical care are now available for large numbers of medical school graduates in the UK (101). There are also attempts to standardize training and education for medical and nursing staff who are interested in careers in critical (102–105) and acute medicine (106). Increasingly, these require the trainee to demonstrate acquisition of certain core competencies.

Potential Impact of Staffing Levels and Patient Flow on Outcomes

Hospital staffing tends to be at its lowest during night-time hours and on weekends, potentially making it difficult to match levels of care to patient acuity. Admission to a general medical ward after 5 PM (107) or to the hospital on weekends (108) is associated with increased mortality. Patients who are discharged from ICUs to general wards at night have an increased risk of in-hospital death compared to those discharged during the day and to those discharged to HDUs (109,110). If hospitals were well staffed at all times, the temporal variation might be eliminated. Often those who need to be readmitted to ICU are shown to have residual organ failure at the time of ICU discharge (111). Ward nurses are often uncertain about the dependency of patients received from ICU; better communication from ICU staff might improve this (112).

In US hospitals, greater registered nurse staffing was associated with a reduction in rates of pneumonia, shock, cardiac arrest, and death (113). Mortality in the ICU is also increased at times of lower staffing levels (114), perhaps suggesting poor matching of care with demand.

New Approaches to Matching Care with Patient Severity of Illness

Many of the reported deficiencies in acute care relate to inadequate management of the patient's airway, breathing, and circulation, or aspects of patient monitoring (3–5, 38–42). These areas of practice are extremely familiar to specialists working in critical care, anaesthesia, and emergency medicine, but less so to the clinicians under whom patients are traditionally admitted. Consequently, many new models of care delivery attempt to support the primary admitting team with the skills of resuscitation specialists (115,116). These advances can be categorized into new patient admission processes, early emergency department treatment, new general medicine specialists, rapid response teams, and better decisions about limitation of care and resuscitation.

New Patient Admission Processes

In many UK hospitals, emergency patients are now rarely admitted directly to a general ward without a degree of in-hospital triage. As before, some of this occurs from the emergency department; however, new admission wards—medical and surgical assessment units—have been created for the rapid triage for patients referred by primary physicians (117). These units perform 2 major functions; they monitor and observe patients for up to 72 hours, and act as a single location for all acute admissions until their required level of care is evaluated. The single location provides rapid access to senior medical staff, diagnostics, and urgent treatment, acting as a central focus for on-call medical, nursing, and physiotherapy staff, in contrast to the traditional system in which staff and patients were dispersed throughout the hospital. In some centers, the opening of assessment units has been accompanied by the appointment of senior clinicians in acute medicine (118). Other developments that have accompanied the introduction of medical assessment units and surgical assessment units are the concepts of post-admission ward rounds and, perhaps more appropriately, multiple ward rounds during a single day (119).

Early Treatment of Patients in the Emergency Department

Many acutely ill patients enter the hospital via the emergency department and are obviously in need of immediate ICU-type interventions. It makes little sense to defer these interventions until ICU admission, which may be delayed by organizational factors. Emergency departments usually have the resources to intervene with techniques, such as invasive cardiovascular monitoring, non-invasive cardiac output measurement, and oximetry, which facilitate the use of early goal-directed therapy (120). Early therapy in the emergency department reverses physiological deterioration (121), and although several publications demonstrate that late application of goal-directed therapy in critically ill patients is not beneficial (122,123), early therapy appears capable of improving patient survival (120).

New General Medicine Specialists

In the United States, cost pressures, increased patient acuity, shortened hospital stays, and time pressures on primary physicians led to the development of the hospitalist, a new type of generalist physician who cares for patients with a wide range of organ dysfunction (124). In this book, the role of the hospitalist is described in detail in Chapter 5. The hospitalist provides the immediate, cross-specialty, clinical care that has so often been lacking in the hospital from community-based, primary care physicians. The majority of hospitalists are specialists in general internal medicine (125). While their primary professional focus is general inpatient care, 80% of hospitalists also care for these patients when they are admitted to critical care units (126). Hospitalists also have teaching, research, and administrative responsibilities, and where they have been introduced they seem to have been beneficial (124,127).

In the UK, many hospital physicians have specialized to the point where their involvement with the "on-call" admission of unselected, acutely ill medical patients has become intermittent and a minor part of their work. Many also state that they would never participate in hands-on emergency care (119). In response, some hospitals have appointed acute care physicians who often work within medical assessment units (118). Others have introduced systems in which the on-call physician is relieved of all conflicting duties while on call (119), or have adopted the concept of "physician of the week," in which a senior clinician's schedule for the week is dedicated exclusively to the care of medical emergencies (119,128).

Rapid Response Teams

In most hospitals, the only nonspecific acute care team in existence is the cardiac arrest team. Although such teams appear to improve the rates of survival for patients after cardiac arrest in circumstances where no team had previously existed (129,130), there is evidence that most victims survive due to the actions of staff before the team arrives (131). Cardiac arrest also has appallingly low rates of survival (132,133). Consequently, some hospitals in Australia and the United States have introduced Medical Emergency Teams whose role is much broader than, but includes, care of the patient in cardiac arrest (134–142). The early involvement of the MET, which usually comprises medical and nursing staff from intensive care and general medicine responding to specific calling criteria (34), seems to reduce cardiac arrests, deaths, and unanticipated intensive care unit admissions (42, 137–139); they may also detect medical error, improve treatment limitation decisions, and reduce postoperative deaths (94,140–142).

In the UK, the Department of Health supported the development of a similar system of preemptive ward care, based predominantly on individual members or teams of nursing staff (143). Models of outreach services are, perhaps, less prescriptive than that described for the MET. For instance, they may range from a single critical care consultant nurse (144) to a 24-hour, 7-day-per-week multi-professional team. Some are based upon existing acute pain relief teams (145) while others may manage only postoperative patients (146,147). Evidence suggests that the effects of outreach teams or systems are beneficial (148–151). A disadvantage of nurse-based outreach teams is that, although they may use patient group directives to enable them to administer fluids and oxygen without consultation with doctors, their pharmacological interventional armamentarium is limited.

Better Decisions About Limitation of Care and Resuscitation

If a hospital patient is not expected to live, alterations are often made in the level of care required. Although a do-not-resuscitate decision does not exclude other active care, for some patients the focus of care will shift to palliation of symptoms. However, there is evidence that the resuscitation status of many patients referred for active therapy has often not been considered, or that the decision made was inappropriate (94). Even when patients have clear evidence of severe physiological deterioration, which could be anticipated to lead to cardiac arrest or death, decisions about resuscitation status are uncommon (42). This may be due to a reluctance of staff to engage in difficult do-not-resuscitate discussions with patients or their relatives, or because their knowledge of such policies is poor (152). Internationally, there are varying attitudes with regard to the training and practice of ethical aspects of resuscitation (153,154). For example, many European countries have no formal policy for recording –do-not-resuscitate decisions, and the practice of consulting patients about the decision is variable (153). Improved treatment limitation decision-making is likely to improve patient care, reduce unnecessary and futile cardiopulmonary resuscitation attempts, and make resource utilization more rational.

Summary

Existing models of acute care do not match care provision with patient severity of illness and may lead to substandard care and medical error. New methods of care delivery, in which the work of primary clinicians is supported by the skills of resuscitation specialists, provide opportunities to improve this situation. These advances involve medical and surgical assessment units, hospitalists, consultants in acute care, early emergency department treatment, medical emergency and outreach teams, and better decisions about limitation of care and resuscitation.

References

1. Alcott LM. *Hospital Sketches*. Boston: James Redpath Publishers; 1863.
2. Strauss MJ, LoGerfo JP, Yeltatzie JA, Temkin N, Hudson LD. Rationing of intensive care unit services. An everyday occurrence. *JAMA*. 1986;255:1143–1146.
3. McQuillan PJ, Pilkington S, Allan A, et al. Confidential inquiry into quality of care before admission to intensive care. *BMJ*. 1998;316:1853–1858.
4. Neale G. Risk management in the care of medical emergencies after referral to hospital. *J Roy Coll Physicians Lond*. 1998;32:125–129.
5. McGloin H, Adam S, Singer M. Unexpected deaths and referrals to intensive care of patients on general wards. Are some cases potentially avoidable? *J Roy Coll Physicians Lond*. 1999;33:255–259.

6. Vincent C, Neale G, Woloshynowych M. Adverse events in British hospitals: preliminary retrospective record review. *BMJ*. 2001;322:517–519.
7. Brennan TA, Leape LL, Laird NM, et al. Incidence of adverse events and negligence in hospitalized patients: results of the Harvard Medical Practice Study I. *N Engl J Med*. 1991;324:370–376.
8. Kohn LT, Corrigan JM, Donaldson MS, eds. *To Err Is Human: Building a Safer Health System*. Washington, DC, National Academies Press; 2000.
9. Wilson RMcL, Runciman WB, Gibberd RW, Harrison BT, Newby L, Hamilton JD. The quality in Australian health care study. *Med J Aust*. 1995;163:458–471.
10. Seward E, Greig E, Preston S, et al. Confidential study of deaths after emergency medical admission: issues relating to quality of care. *Clin Med*. 2003; 3:425–434.
11. Leeson-Payne CG, Aitkenhead AR. A prospective study to assess the demand for a high dependency unit. *Anaesthesia*. 1995;50:383–387.
12. Crosby DL, Rees GA. Provision of postoperative care in UK hospitals. *Ann R Coll Surg Engl* 1994;76:14–18.
13. Donnelly P, Sandifer QD, O'Brien D, Thomas EA. A pilot study of the use of clinical guidelines to determine appropriateness of patient placement on intensive and high dependency care units. *J Public Health Med*. 1995;17:305–310.
14. Zimmerman JE, Wagner DP, Knaus WA, Williams JF, Kolakowski D, Draper EA. The use of risk predictions to identify candidates for intermediate care units. Implications for intensive care utilization and cost. *JAMA*. 1995;108: 490–499.
15. Bodenham AR, Knappett P, Cohen A, Bensley D, Fryers P. Facilities and usage of general intensive care in Yorkshire. A need for high-dependency units. *Clin Intensive Care*. 1995;6:260–265.
16. Ryan DW, Bayly PJ, Weldon OG, Jingree M. A prospective two-month audit of the lack of provision of a high-dependency unit and its impact on intensive care. *Anaesthesia*. 1997;52:265–270.
17. Kilpatrick A, Ridley S, Plenderleith L. A changing role for intensive therapy: is there a case for high dependency care? *Anaesthesia*. 1994;49:666–670.
18. Frisho-Lima P, Gurman G, Schapira A, Porath A. Rationing critical care —what happens to patients who are not admitted? *Theor Surg*. 1994;9:208–211.
19. Simchen E, Sprung CL, Galai N, et al. Survival of critically ill patients hospitalized in and out of intensive care units under paucity of intensive care unit beds. *Crit Care Med*. 2004;32:1654–1661.
20. Metcalfe A, Slogget A, McPherson K. Mortality among appropriately referred patients refused admission to intensive care units. *Lancet*. 1997;350:7–12.
21. Society of Critical Care Medicine Task Force of the American College of Critical Care Medicine, Society of Critical Care Medicine. Guidelines on intensive care unit admission, discharge, and triage. *Crit Care Med*. 1999;27:633–638.
22. Nasraway S, Cohen IL, Dennis RC, et al. Guidelines on admission and discharge for adult intermediate care units. *Crit Care Med*. 1998;26:607–610.
23. Haupt, MT, Bekes CE, Brilli RJ, et al. Guidelines on critical care services and personnel: recommendations based on a system of categorization of three levels of care. *Crit Care Med*. 2003;31:2677–2683.
24. Department of Health. Guidelines on admission to and discharge from intensive care and high dependency units. HMSO, London: March 1996.

25. Intensive Care Society. Levels of critical care for adult patients. London: Intensive Care Society; 2002.
26. Smith G, Nielsen M. ABC of intensive care: criteria for admission. *BMJ*. 1999; 318:1544–1547.
27. European Society of Intensive Care Task Force. Guidelines for utilisation of intensive care units. *Intensive Care Med*. 1994;20:163–164
28. Intensive Care Society. Guidelines for the introduction of outreach services. London: Intensive Care Society; 2002.
29. Cashman JN. In-hospital cardiac arrest: what happens to the false arrests? *Resuscitation*. 2002;53:271–276.
30. Morgan RJ, Williams F, Wright MM. An early warning scoring system for detecting developing critical illness. *Clin Intensive Care*. 1997;8:100.
31. Stenhouse C, Coates S, Tivey M, Allsop P, Parker T. Prospective evaluation of a modified Early Warning Score to aid earlier detection of patients developing critical illness on a surgical ward. *Br J Anaesth*. 2000;84:663.
32. Goldhill DR, Worthington L, Mulcahy A, Tarling M, Sumner A. The patient-at-risk team: identifying and managing seriously ill ward patients. *Anaesthesia*. 1999;54:853–860.
33. Subbe CP, Hibbs R, Williams E, Rutherford P, Gemmel L. ASSIST: a screening tool for the critically ill patients on general medical wards. *Intensive Care Med*. 2002;28:S21.
34. Houlihan F, Bishop G, Hillman K, Daffurn K, Lee A. The Medical Emergency Team: a new strategy to identify and intervene in high-risk patients. *Clin Intensive Care*. 1995;6:269–272.
35. Smith G. To M.E.T. or not to M.E.T.—that is the question. *Care Critically Ill*. 2000;16:198–199.
36. Cuthbertson BH. Outreach critical care—cash for no questions? *BJA*. 2003; 90:5–6.
37. Subbe CP, Kruger M, Rutherford P, Gemmel L. Validation of a modified Early Warning Score in medical admissions. *QJM* 2001;94:521–526.
38. Franklin C, Mathew J. Developing strategies to prevent in-hospital cardiac arrest: analyzing responses of physicians and nurses in the hours before the event. *Crit Care Med*. 1994;22:244–247.
39. Schein RM, Hazday N, Pena M, Ruben BH, Sprung CL. Clinical antecedents to in-hospital cardiopulmonary arrest. *Chest*. 1990;98:1388–1392.
40. Hodgetts TJ, Kenward G, Vlachonikolis IG, Payne S, Castle N. The identification of risk factors for cardiac arrest and formulation of activation criteria to alert a medical emergency team. *Resuscitation*. 2002;54:125–131.
41. Hillman K, Bristow PJ, Chey T, et al. Duration of life-threatening antecedents prior to intensive care admission. *Intensive Care Med*. 2002;28:1629–1634.
42. Kause J, Smith GB, Hillman K, Prytherch D, Parr M, Flabouras A. A comparison of antecedents to cardiac arrests, deaths and emergency intensive care admissions in Australia and New Zealand, and the United Kingdom—the ACADEMIA study. *Resuscitation*. 2004;62:275–282.
43. Chellel A, Fraser J, Fender V, et al. Nursing observations on ward patients at risk of critical illness. *Nurs Times*. 2002;98:36–39.
44. Kenward G, Hodgetts T, Castle N. Time to put the R back in TPR. *Nurs Times*. 2001;97:32–33.

45. Subbe CP, Williams EM, Gemmell LW. Are medical emergency teams picking up enough patients with increased respiratory rate? *Crit Care Med.* 2004; 32:1983–1984.
46. McBride J, Knight D, Piper J, Smith GB. Long-term effect of introducing an early warning score on respiratory rate charting on general wards. *Resuscitation.* In press.
47. Cioffi J. Recognition of patients who require emergency assistance: a descriptive study. *Heart Lung.* 2000;29:262–268.
48. Cioffi J. Nurses' experiences of making decisions to call emergency assistance to their patients. *J Adv Nurs.* 2000;2:108–114.
49. Boockvar K, Brodie HD, Lachs M. Nursing assistants detect behavior changes in nursing home residents that precede acute illness: development and validation of an illness warning instrument. *J Am Geriatr Soc.* 2000;48:1086–1091.
50. Prytherch DR, Sirl JS, Weaver PC, et al. Towards a national clinical minimum data set for general surgery. *Br J Surg.* 2003;90:1300–1305.
51. Prytherch DR, Sirl JS, Schmidt P, Featherstone PI, Weaver PC, Smith GB. The use of routine laboratory data to predict in-hospital death in medical admissions. *Rescusitation.* 2005;66:203–207.
52. Cullen DJ, Nemeskal AR, Zaslavsky AM. Intermediate TISS: a new Therapeutic Intervention Scoring System for non-ICU patients. *Crit Care Med.* 1994;22:1406–1411.
53. Day BA. Early warning system scores and response times: an audit. *Nurs Crit Care.* 2003;8:156–164.
54. Carberry M. Implementing the modified early warning system: our experiences. *Nurs Crit Care.* 2002;7:220–226.
55. Lundberg JS, Perl TM, Wiblin T, et al. Septic shock: an analysis of outcomes for patients with onset on hospital wards versus intensive care units. *Crit Care Med.* 1998;26:1020–1024.
56. Smith GB, Poplett N. Knowledge of aspects of acute care in trainee doctors. *Postgrad Med J.* 2002;78:335–358.
57. Meek T. New house officers' knowledge of resuscitation, fluid balance and analgesia. *Anaesthesia.* 2000;55:1127–1143.
58. Somasekar K, Somasekar A, Hayat G, Haray PN. Fluid and electrolyte balance: how do junior doctors measure up? *Hosp Med.* 2003;64:369–370.
59. Gould TH, Upton PM, Collins P. A survey of the intended management of acute postoperative pain by newly qualified doctors in the South West region of England in August 1992. *Anaesthesia.* 1994;49:807–810.
60. Jackson E, Warner J. How much do doctors know about consent and capacity? *J R Soc Med.* 2002;95:601–603.
61. Arumugam PJ, Harikrishnan AB, Carr ND, Morgan AR, Beynon J. A study on surgical knowledge of house officers and their role in consent. *Hosp Med.* 2003; 64:108–109.
62. Kruger PS, Longden PJ. A study of a hospital staff's knowledge of pulse oximetry. *Anaesth Intensive Care.* 1997;25:38–41.
63. Stoneham MD, Saville GM, Wilson IH. Knowledge about pulse oximetry among medical and nursing staff. *Lancet.* 1994;344:1339–1342.
64. Gompels LL, Bethune C, Johnston SL, Gompels MM. Proposed use of adrenaline (epinephrine) in anaphylaxis and related conditions: a study of senior

house officers starting accident and emergency posts. *Postgrad Med J.* 2002; 78: 416–418.

65. Wheeler DW, Remoundos D, Whittlestone KD, et al. Doctors' confusion over ratios and percentages in drug solutions: the case for standard labelling. *J R Soc Med.* 2004;97:380–383.

66. Rolfe S, Harper NJ. Ability of hospital doctors to calculate drug doses. *BMJ.* 1995;310:1173–1174.

67. Board P, Mercer M. A survey of the basic practical skills of final-year medical students in one UK medical school. *Med Teacher.* 1998;20:104–108.

68. Goodfellow PB, Claydon P. Students sitting medical finals—ready to be house officers? *J R Soc Med.* 2001;94:516–520.

69. Montgomery H, Hunter S, Morris S, et al. Interpretation of electrocardiograms by doctors. *BMJ.* 1994;309:1551–1552.

70. Moercke AM, Eika B. What are the clinical skills levels of newly graduated physicians? Self-assessment study of an intended curriculum identified by a Delphi process. *Med Educ.* 2002;36:472–478.

71. McManus IC, Richards P, Winder BC. Clinical experience of UK medical students. *Lancet.* 1998;351:802–803.

72. McManus IC, Richards P, Winder BC, Sproston KA, Vincent CA. The changing clinical experience of British medical students. *Lancet.* 1993;341: 941–944.

73. Dickson L, Heymann TD, Culling W. What the SHO saw. *J R Coll Physicians Lond.* 1994;28:523–526.

74. Pearse RM, Mitra AV, Heymann TD. What the SHO really does. *J R Coll Physicians Lond.* 1999;33:553–556.

75. MacDonald R. Implementing the European working time directive. *BMJ.* [Career Focus] 2003;327:s9–s11.

76. Philibert I, Friedmann P, Williams WT, for the members of the ACGME Work Group on Resident Duty Hours. New requirements for resident duty hours. *JAMA.* 2002;288:1112–1114.

77. Mather HM, Elkeles RS. Attitudes of consultant physicians to the Calman proposals: a questionnaire survey. North West Thames Diabetes and Endocrinology Specialist Group. *BMJ.* 1995;311:1060–1062.

78. Thwaites BC, Shankar S, Niblett D, Saunders J. Can consultants resuscitate? *J R Coll Physicians Lond.* 1992;26:265–267.

79. Ingelby S, Eddleston J, Naylor S. Evaluating knowledge in acute illness: Critical Care Educational Project. *Crit Care.* 2003;7:S119.

80. Quniton S, Higgins Y. Critical care training needs analysis for ward staff. *Crit Care.* 2003;7:S119–120.

81. Featherstone P, Smith GB, Linnell M, Easton S, Osgood VM. Impact of a one-day inter-professional course (ALERT™) on attitudes and confidence in managing critically ill adult patients. *Resuscitation.* 2005;65:329–336.

82. Smith GB, Osgood VM, Crane S. ALERT™—a multiprofessional training course in the care of the acutely ill adult patient. *Resuscitation.* 2002;52:281–286.

83. O'Riordan B, Gray K, McArthur-Rouse F. Implementing a critical care course for ward nurses. *Nurs Stand.* 2003;17:41–44.

84. Cooper N. Medical training did not teach me what I really needed to know. *BMJ.* [Career Focus] 2003;327:190s.

85. Goldacre MJ, Lambert T, Evans J, Turner G. Preregistration house officers' views on whether their experience at medical school prepared them well for their jobs: national questionnaire survey. *BMJ*. 2003;326:1011–1012.
86. Frankel HL, Rogers PL, Gandhi RR, Freid EB, Kirton OC, Murray MJ. What is taught, what is tested: findings and competency-based recommendations of the Undergraduate Medical Education Committee of the Society of Critical Care Medicine. *Crit Care Med*. 2004;32:1949–1956.
87. Shen J, Joynt GM, Critchley LA, Tan IK, Lee A. Survey of current status of intensive care teaching in English-speaking medical schools. *Crit Care Med*. 2003;31:293–298.
88. Phillips PS, Nolan JP. Training in basic and advanced life support in UK medical schools: questionnaire survey. *BMJ*. 2001;323:22–23.
89. Harrison GA, Hillman KM, Fulde GW, Jacques TC. The need for undergraduate education in critical care. (Results of a questionnaire to year 6 medical undergraduates, University of New South Wales and recommendations on a curriculum in critical care). *Anaesth Intensive Care*. 1999;27:53–58.
90. Cook CJ, Smith GB. Do textbooks of clinical examination contain information regarding the assessment of critically ill patients? *Resuscitation*. 2004;60: 129–136.
91. Anderson ID. Care of the Critically Ill Surgical Patient courses at the Royal College of Surgeons. *Br J Hosp Med*. 1997;57:274–275.
92. White RJ, Garrioch MA. Time to train all doctors to look after seriously ill patients—CCrISP and IMPACT. *Scott Med J*. 2002;47:127.
93. Dellinger RP. Fundamental critical care support: another merit badge or more? *Crit Care Med*. 1996;24:556.
94. Parr MJ, Hadfield JH, Flabouris A, Bishop G, Hillman K. The Medical Emergency Team: 12-month analysis of reasons for activation, immediate outcome, and not-for-resuscitation orders. *Resuscitation*. 2001;50:39–44.
95. Mørcke AM, Wichmann-Hansen G, Guldbrand-Nielsen D, Tønnesen E, Eika B. Searching the core of emergency medicine. *Acta Anaesthesiol Scand*. 2004; 48:243–248.
96. Garcia-Barbero M, Such JC. Teaching critical care in Europe: analysis of a survey. *Crit Care Med*. 1996;24:696–704.
97. Buchman TG, Dellinger RP, Raphaely RC, Todres ID. Undergraduate education in critical care medicine. *Crit Care Med*. 1992;20:1595–1603.
98. Boulet JR, Murray D, Kras J, Woodhouse J, McAllister J, Ziv A. Reliability and validity of a simulation-based acute care skills assessment for medical students and residents. *Anesthesiology*. 2003;99:1270–1280.
99. Rogers PL. Simulation in medical students' critical thinking. *Crit Care Med*. 2004;32:S70–1.
100. Wheeler DW, Whittlestone KD, Smith HL, Gupta AK, Menon DK; East Anglian Peri-Operative Medicine Undergraduate Teaching Forum. A web-based system for teaching, assessment, and examination of the undergraduate peri-operative medicine curriculum. *Anaesthesia*. 2003;58:1079–1086.
101. MacDonald R. New initiative to improve undergraduate teaching in acute care. *BMJ*. [Career Focus] 2004;328:s29.
102. Dorman T, Angood PB, Angus DC, et al. Guidelines for critical care medicine training and continuing medical education. *Crit Care Med*. 2004;32:263–272.

103. Baktoft B, Drigo E, Hohl ML, Klancar S, Tseroni M, Putzai P. A survey of critical care nursing education in Europe. *Connect: World Crit Care Nurs.* 2003;3:85–87.
104. The Intercollegiate Board for Training in Intensive Care Medicine. Available at: http://www.rcoa.ac.uk/ibticm/index.asp?InterPageID=6
105. European Society of Intensive Care Medicine. The ESICM educational project "competency-based training programme." Available at: http://www.esicm.org/PAGE_cobatrice/?1gsl. Accessed August 19, 2005.
106. Available at: http://www.jchmt.org.uk/acute/curr_acute.pdf. Accessed August 19, 2005.
107. Hillson SD, Rich EC, Dowd B, Luxenberg MG. Call nights and patient care: effects on inpatients at one teaching hospital. *J Gen Intern Med.* 1992;7:645.
108. Bell CM, Redelmeier DA. Mortality among patients admitted to hospitals on weekends as compared with weekdays. *N Engl J Med.* 2001;345:663–668.
109. Beck DH, McQuillan PJ, Smith GB. Waiting for the break of dawn? The effects of discharge time, discharge scores, and discharge facility on hospital mortality after intensive care. *Intensive Care Med.* 2002;28:1287–1293.
110. Goldfrad C, Rowan K. Consequences of discharges from intensive care at night. *Lancet.* 2000;355:1138–1142.
111. Moreno R, Miranda DR, Matos R, Fevereiro T. Mortality after discharge from intensive care: the impact of organ system failure and nursing workload use at discharge. *Intensive Care Med.* 2001; 27: 999–1004.
112. Whittaker J, Ball C. Discharge from intensive care: a view from the ward. *Intensive Crit Care Nurs.* 2000;16:135–143.
113. Needleman J, Buerhaus P, Mattke S, Stewart M, Zelevinsky K. Nurse-staffing levels and the quality of care in hospitals. *N Engl J Med.* 2002;346:1715–1722.
114. Tarnow-Mordi WO, Hau C, Warden A, Shearer AJ. Hospital mortality in relation to staff workload: a 4-year study in an adult intensive-care unit. *Lancet.* 2000;356:185–189.
115. Szalados JE. Critical care teams managing floor patients: the continuing evolution of hospitals into intensive care units? *Crit Care Med.* 2004;32:1071–1072.
116. Department of Health. Comprehensive critical care. A review of adult critical care services. London; 2000.
117. Cooke MW, Higgins J, Kidd P. Use of emergency observation and assessment wards: a systematic literature review. *Emerg Med J.* 2003;20:138–142.
118. Armitage M, Raza T. A consultant physician in acute medicine: the Bournemouth Model for managing increasing numbers of medical emergency admissions. *Clin Med.* 2002;2:331–333.
119. Mather HM, Connor H. Coping with pressures in acute medicine—the second RCP consultant questionnaire survey. *J R Coll Physicians Lond.* 2000;34:371–373.
120. Rivers E, Nguyen B, Havstad S, et al.; Early Goal-Directed Therapy Collaborative Group: Early goal-directed therapy in the treatment of severe sepsis and septic shock. *N Engl J Med.* 2001;345:1368–1377.
121. Nguyen HB, Rivers EP, Havstad S, et al. Critical care in the emergency department: a physiologic assessment and outcome evaluation. *Acad Emerg Med.* 2000;7:1354–1361.

122. Hayes MA, Timmins AC, Yau EHS, Palazzo M, Hinds CJ, Watson D. Elevation of systemic oxygen delivery in the treatment of critically ill patients. *N Engl J Med.* 1994;330:1717–1722.
123. Gattinoni L, Brazzi L, Pelosi P, et al. A trial of goal-oriented hemodynamic therapy in critically ill patients. SvO2 Collaborative Group. *N Engl J Med.* 1995;333:1025–1032.
124. Wachter RM, Goldman L. The hospitalist movement 5 years later. *JAMA.* 2002;287:487–494.
125. Hoff TH, Whitcomb WF, Williams K, Nelson JR, Cheesman RA. Characteristics and work experiences of hospitalists in the United States. *Arch Intern Med.* 2001;161:851–858.
126. Lindenauer PK, Pantilat SZ, Katz PP, Wachter RM. Hospitalists and the practice of inpatient medicine: results of a survey of the National Association of Inpatient Physicians. *Ann Intern Med.* 1999;130:343–349.
127. Baudendistel TE, Wachter RM. The evolution of the hospitalist movement in the USA. *Clin Med.* 2002;2:327–330.
128. Worth R, Youngs G. Consultant physician of the week: a solution to the bed crisis. *J R Coll Physicians Lond.* 1996;30:211–212.
129. Sandroni C, Ferro G, Santangelo S, et al. In-hospital cardiac arrest: survival depends mainly on the effectiveness of the emergency response. *Resuscitation.* 2004;62:291–297.
130. Henderson SO, Ballesteros D. Evaluation of a hospital-wide resuscitation team: does it increase survival for in-hospital cardiopulmonary arrest? *Resuscitation.* 2001;48:111–116.
131. Soar J, McKay U. A revised role for the hospital cardiac arrest team? Resuscitation 1998; 38: 145–149.
132. Tunstall-Pedoe H, Bailey L, Chamberlain DA, Marsden AK, Ward ME, Zideman DA. Survey of 3765 cardiopulmonary resuscitations in British hospitals (the BRESUS study): methods and overall results. *BMJ.* 1992;304: 1347–1351.
133. Gwinnutt CL, Columb M, Harris R. Outcome after cardiac arrest in adults in UK hospitals: effect of the 1997 guidelines. *Resuscitation.* 2000;47:125–135.
134. Hillman K, Bishop G, Lee A, et al. Identifying the general ward patient at high risk of cardiac arrest. *Clin Intensive Care.* 1996;7:242–243.
135. Hourihan F, Bishop G, Hillman KM, Daffurn K, Lee A. The medical emergency team: a new strategy to identify and intervene in high-risk patients. *Clin Intensive Care.* 1995;6:269–272.
136. Lee A, Bishop G, Hillman KM, Daffurn K. The medical emergency team. *Anaesth Intensive Care.* 1995;23:183–186.
137. Buist MD, Moore GE, Bernard SA, Waxman BP, Anderson JN, Nguyen TV. Effects of a medical emergency team on reduction of incidence of and mortality from unexpected cardiac arrests in hospital: preliminary study. *BMJ.* 2002;324:1–6.
138. DeVita MA, Braithwaite RS, Mahidhara R, Stuart S, Foraida M, Simmons RL. Medical Emergency Response Improvement Team (MERIT). Use of medical emergency team responses to reduce hospital cardiopulmonary arrests. *Qual Saf Health Care.* 2004;13:251–254.
139. Bellomo R, Goldsmith D, Uchino S, et al. A prospective before-and-after trial of a medical emergency team. *Med J Aust.* 2003;179:283–287.

140. Braithwaite RS, DeVita MA, Mahidhara R, Simmons RL, Stuart S, Foraida M. Medical Emergency Response Improvement Team (MERIT). Use of medical emergency team (MET) responses to detect medical errors. *Qual Saf Health Care.* 2004;13:255–259.

141. Bristow PJ, Hillman KM, Chey T, et al. Rates of in-hospital arrests, deaths, and intensive care admissions: the effect of a medical emergency team. *Med J Aust.* 2000;173:236–240.

142. Bellomo R, Goldsmith D, Uchino S, et al. Prospective controlled trial of effect of medical emergency team on postoperative morbidity and mortality rates. *Crit Care Med.* 2004;32:916–921.

143. Anderson K, Atkinson D, McBride J, Moorse S, Smith S. Setting up an outreach team in the UK. *Crit Care Nurs Eur.* 2002:2:8–12.

144. Jones P. Consultant nurses and their potential impact upon health care delivery. *Clin Med.* 2002;2:39–40.

145. Counsell DJ. The acute pain service: a model for outreach critical care. *Anaesthesia.* 2001;56:925–926.

146. Bamgbade OA. The peri-operative care team: a model for outreach critical care. *Anaesthesia.* 2002;57:1028–1044.

147. Goldhill D. Introducing the postoperative care team. *BMJ.* 1997;314:389.

148. Ball C, Kirkby M, Williams S. Effect of the critical care outreach team on patient survival to discharge from hospital and readmission to critical care: non-randomised population based study. *BMJ.* 2003;327:1014–1016.

149. Garcea G, Thomasset S, McClelland L, Leslie A, Berry DP. Impact of a critical care outreach team on critical care readmissions and mortality. *Acta Anaesthesiol Scand.* 2004;48:1096–1100.

150. Pittard AJ. Out of our reach? Assessing the impact of introducing a critical care outreach service. *Anaesthesia.* 2003;58:882–885.

151. Story DA, Shelton AC, Poustie SJ, Colin-Thome NJ, McNicol PL. The effect of critical care outreach on postoperative serious adverse events. *Anaesthesia.* 2004;59:762–766.

152. Smith GB, Poplett N, Williams D. Staff awareness of a 'do not attempt resuscitation' policy in a district general hospital. *Resuscitation.* In press.

153. Mohr M, Bahr J, Kettler D, Andres J. Ethics and law in resuscitation. *Resuscitation.* 2002;54:99–102.

154. Baskett PJ, Lim A. The varying ethical attitudes towards resuscitation in Europe. *Resuscitation.* 2004;62:267–273.

8
General Principles of Medical Emergency Teams

DARYL JONES, RINALDO BELLOMO, and DONNA GOLDSMITH

There is nothing more difficult to take in hand, more perilous in its conduct or more uncertain in its success, than to take the lead in the introduction of a new order of things; because the innovator has for enemies all those who have done well under the old conditions and lukewarm defenders in those who may do well under the new.

—Niccolo Machiavelli

The hospital system of developed countries is highly imperfect. It delivers extraordinarily variable outcomes for a given medical condition or surgical procedure. While some of this difference is due to the inherent biological variability of patients and disease states, much of it is attributable to the variability of the performance of health care providers and of the systems within which they work. Positive variability (excellence) is obviously not a problem; negative variability (error or substandard practice), on the other hand, is a major problem.

From well conducted studies in the United States and Australia (1–3) and assuming that other Western health care systems are similar, somewhere between 200 000 and 400 000 patients in developed countries' hospitals may die needlessly because of such errors every year (4).

Many agree that something must be done to make hospital patients safer and improve systems of care. Few, however, are able to suggest a change that can be implemented reasonably rapidly and shown to decrease morbidity and mortality relatively quickly. Nonetheless, one such system change has been recently proposed: the Medical Emergency Team (MET) (5–10). This chapter will focus on the general principles underlying this approach.

Physiological Principles

The MET as a Logical Approach for Preventing Serious Adverse Events in Hospitalized Patients

Most hospitals have hundreds of patients at any given time. They are receiving care in different wards, with different levels of monitoring, and have a variable intensity of disease and medical intervention. While many of them have a hospital stay without incident, some are at risk of serious adverse events, including cardiac arrest. The care that these patients receive is dependent on the diligence, knowledge, skills, and experience of the doctors and nurses attending them, as well as the hospital infrastructure and resources. While care of hospital patients could be improved by massive and costly changes in the daily allocation of care and resources (such as 1 nurse for 1 patient, or electrocardiogram, oximetry, and other electronic monitors at all beds), it is illogical and unpractical to apply such interventions to all patients in a hospital setting. As most hospital patients are low-risk, thousands would be needed in any given study to show the positive effects of such approaches on reducing the incidence of adverse events or mortality.

However, approximately 15% to 20% of all hospitalized patients will develop serious adverse events including cardiac arrest (1–4,11). These *clinical adverse events* are rarely sudden or unpredictable, and are frequently preceded by 1 or more signs of *physiological and biochemical deterioration* that occur over hours and sometimes days (12–14). This is the first of a number of important factors underlying the notion that the MET is a logical approach for the prevention of serious adverse events (Table 8.1) (15–17).

Using preset criteria of *physiological* instability, any member of the ward staff can activate the MET to rapidly mobilize intensive care staff to deliver prompt and definitive treatment in the early phase of clinical deterioration. The MET system aims to reduce cardiac arrests, morbidity, and mortality. To achieve this goal, the hospital must develop the capability to deliver intensive care services promptly to critically ill patients, regardless of the patient's location. Just as an ambulance goes to the patient within the community, so the MET must go to the patient within the hospital.

And just as lay people cannot be expected to deal with acute illness in the community, junior and inexperienced doctors cannot be expected to reliably deal with life-threatening critical illness in the hospital. Thus, objective, reproducible, and easily measured criteria must be developed to trigger intervention by the MET (Table 8.2). Preset criteria increase the reliability of MET calls, and allow auditing of the appropriateness of the calls and any delays. In addition to being objective and reproducible, the criteria are noninvasive, and thus provide potential benefit with minimal risk of harm. They include familiar and routine nursing vital signs as well as a "worried" criterion (caregiver "worried" about patient and wants help) to allow flexibil-

TABLE 8.1. Physiological rationale for the MET as approach for preventing serious adverse events in hospitalized patients

Principle 1: There is time for intervention (12–14).
• The evolution of clinical and physiological deterioration is relatively slow.

Principle 2: There are warning signs (12–14).
• Clinical deterioration is preceded by physiological deterioration in commonly measured **vital signs.**
• These observations are easy to measure, inexpensive, and non-invasive (measuring them does not hurt the patient).

Principle 3: There are effective treatments if dangerous conditions are recognized.
• Examples include beta-blockers for myocardial ischemia, fluid therapy for hypovolemia, non-invasive ventilation and oxygen for respiratory failure, and anticoagulation for thrombo-embolic disease.
• The majority of MET interventions are inexpensive, relatively simple, and non-invasive (7).

Principle 4: Any member of staff can activate the MET.

Principle 5: Early intervention improves outcome.
• The assumption that early intervention saves lives has been shown for the treatment of trauma (15) as well as septic shock (16).
• The hospital survival for cardiac arrest is at best 14% (17).
• It is intuitive that sick people are easier to treat than dead people.

Principle 6: The expertise exists and can be deployed.
• Intensive care doctors and nurses are experts in the delivery of advanced resuscitation.
• The review of the critically ill patient is prompt.

ity in dealing with any possible emergency situation. Although the "worried" criterion is impossible to validate, it is the most common reason for MET activation in Austin Health in Melbourne.

This observation highlights another principle of the MET system: *calling criteria must be simple, objective, and real to the typical caller (nurses).* These calling criteria are based on clinical experience. It would be unethical to construct a trial in which the control group is left untreated following the discovery of such signs of instability, and it would be impossible to gain

TABLE 8.2. MET calling criteria at Austin Hospital

If 1 of the following is present, call 7777 and ask for the MET.
• Staff member is worried about the patient
• Acute change in heart rate   <40 or >130 bpm
• Acute change in systolic blood pressure   <90 mmHg
• Acute change in respiratory rate   <8 or >30 bpm
• Acute change in saturation   <90% despite oxygen
• Acute change in conscious state
• Acute change in urine output to   <50 ml in 4 hours.

consent and randomize patients rapidly after developing a medical crisis. For these reasons, retrospective and before-and-after trials are important to consider, and retrospective studies have demonstrated that the presence and number of such warning signs are related to mortality (18,19).

Sociological and Cultural Principles

The MET Is a Sociological Process

Those who think that the physiological rationale presented above should be enough to prompt action and a change in systems are not appreciating the sociological aspects of hospitals and medicine.

For the MET to be effective, the first sociological change that needs to occur within the hospital relates to safety. Safety must move up the ladder of priorities for all health care providers. Currently organizations typically focus on "efficacy" and productivity as their priority and pride. Safety must move to an equally important position within the institution.

A second sociological principle is that nurses must be empowered to do more for their patients and call for help outside of the regimented framework created by the history of Western medicine. If a patient is critically ill and needs prompt review, it is unreasonable, illogical, and dangerous to ask the nurse to page junior doctors who may be unavailable (e.g. in the operating room) and/or lack the skills to manage patients in crisis (12,17,20,21). Similarly, the attending specialist or consultant may not even be in the hospital. While a plan to have senior consultants train inexperienced individuals on how to intervene in a medical crisis may make sense, in practice it is difficult to deliver in today's hospitals because of competing responsibilities. Therefore, a new plan like the MET is needed.

Nurses are highly trained professionals; they care about their patients and must be empowered to call for competent and promptly delivered help (the MET). This is a major paradigm shift, but a necessary one for the MET to work. It might meet resistance from physicians used to a hierarchical model of care from the last century, but such resistance must be dealt with politically by the organization. The organization must make it clear that it is hospital policy to enable any member of the staff to seek help via the MET at any time and for any reason they believe appropriate. These issues are covered in more detail in Chapter 9.

If a nurse makes a call for the MET and is criticized later by the attending consultant for following "hospital policy," the attending consultant must be made aware of and asked to work within the new system. These sociological changes are vital.

Hospital staff tends to train and work in discrete care areas or specialties that we call "silos." For example, cardiologists treat patients with heart problems, endocrinologists treat patients with hormonal disorders, and

TABLE 8.3. Aims and potential benefits of the MET

Aim	Potential benefits
•Assist ward doctors and nurses in the management of acutely unwell and complicated patients	•Reduction of cardiac arrests and unplanned ICU admissions •Reduction in morbidity and hospital length of stay
•To educate and supervise junior medical staff in the advanced recuscitation of acutely unwell patients	•Increased use of hospital beds for management of primary surgical diagnosis rather than complications following surgery
•Improve awareness and ability of doctors and nurses to identify and manage acutely unwell patients	•Increased confidence of staff in the management of acutely unwell patients
•Provision of objective calling criteria for activation of the MET	•Empowering of nursing staff and doctors to seek help by a system which is supported by hospital policy
•Early identification and treatment of patients requiring ICU therapies	•Reduced ICU length of stay and disease-related morbidity and mortality
•Assist in advanced treatment directive decision making	•Avoiding unnecessarily invasive therapies and cardiopulmonary resuscitation in patients for whom it is inappropriate, futile, and undignified

orthopedic surgeons treat patients with bone diseases. These divisions must break down in acute situations, when it is clear that expertise from another silo is needed (for example, if an orthopedic patient develops chest pain). Such need for a second opinion is entrenched in chronic (or at least less-acute) hospital medicine. A plan for rapid assistance must also become entrenched in acute medicine, and the response must happen within minutes, not days. The MET, in a sense, is a rapid second opinion—the appropriate expertise gets to the patient promptly.

Of course, an endocrinologist would never be asked to fix a broken neck. Similarly, why should we let a trainee not skilled in lung diseases try to treat a patient with hypoxemic respiratory failure? It is profoundly illogical. The appropriate doctors for such a patient should be those who most frequently treat hypoxemic respiratory failure. Antediluvian concepts like "patient ownership" are unacceptable in an emergency. A model similar to the team approach to managing severe trauma must be adopted for managing the acutely ill ward patient.

In Austin Health, it is no longer acceptable for junior doctors to attempt to treat acutely unwell ward patients in an unsupervised manner at the expense of patient safety. One of the aims and potential benefits of the MET is the provision of appropriate support and supervision of junior doctors in acute resuscitation situations (Table 8.3). The adage in modern medicine of "see one, do one, teach one" must be replaced by a practical plan to always have the best person available to meet the patient's needs, at the patient's bedside. This plan requires a cultural change. These sociological principles are as important to the success of the MET as the physiological principles outlined above.

The MET Is About Organizational Culture

The MET system can only be successful and thrive in the right culture. An organization's culture must be committed to the "Cs" of good patient care: competence in treatment delivery; compassion in the reaction to a patient's problems; communication in dealing with the patient, the family, and members of the health care team and other colleagues; collegiality in dealing with other care groups within the hospital; caring in ensuring that the right outcomes are delivered; and credibility in the eyes of the patient, the family, the health care team, and colleagues.

If organizations do not encourage and reward these values, the MET cannot be successfully implemented and/or remain effective. In particular, if the MET is not viewed as embracing the above values and does not have professional credibility within the organization, it will fail.

The precise personnel composition of the MET varies from model to model. Most often, the MET contains an intensive care fellow and nurse, as well as the receiving medical fellow of the day (Table 8.4), and in some settings, a respiratory care practitioner. Each member of this team has designated roles that may also vary between models. The advantage of the MET system is that the expertise of the team members can be brought together in a timely manner to formulate and deliver a definitive manage-

TABLE 8.4. Structure and roles of MET personnel

Staff member	Role/responsibility
Intensive care fellow	• Thorough understanding of interplay between clinical medicine, mechanism of disease, and therapies for reversal of acute physiological deterioration (advanced resuscitation techniques) • Skills in airway management and advanced cardiac life support • Facilitation of advanced treatment directives • Documentation of issues surrounding MET for ongoing audit and quality control
Intensive care nurse	• Advanced knowledge in the application of therapies required in advanced resuscitation • Provision of ongoing information and advice to ward nurses for patients remaining on the ward following MET-call • Liaising with intensive care unit regarding potential for patient admission
Medical fellow	• Skills in diagnosis and management of underlying etiology of medical condition • Follow-up and ongoing management of patients remaining on ward following MET call
Ward nurse	• Knowledge of patients' nursing issues since admission and leading up to MET call
Respiratory care practitioner (US)	• Assistance with respiratory-related therapies

ment plan. To a varying degree, all members of the hospital community are members of the MET.

Political Principles

The MET Requires Political Support

Any change in an organization's structure will always require an amount of political support, and the MET system is no different. For political support to be obtained, there first must be leadership. This means that opinion leaders, administrative leaders, and academic leaders must be seen to support and promote the MET system. These individuals set the tone of the institution's response to the MET. Their support is vital to its success and must be sought from the start.

The second vital political step is to ensure the support of the stakeholders. Stakeholders include nurses, attending physicians, residents and interns, and training program directors. They should all appreciate the aims of the MET, as well as the potential benefits for them if they support the MET (Table 8.3). Nurses must be made to appreciate that the MET will increase their ability to obtain help immediately. Attending physicians must be made to realize the MET will ensure their patients' safety when they are not in the hospital, and, more importantly, they must also accept that METs do not "take patients away from their care." Residents need to appreciate that the MET is there to support them, or substitute for them if they cannot attend, and interns must be made to understand that the MET is there to teach them, support them, and keep them from having to deal with overwhelming situations alone. In addition staff must realize that reduced length of hospital stay may improve the efficiency of bed use. It is important that the users of the system appreciate that all major decisions will be made only following communication with them.

Our experience is that if these political processes are dealt with carefully and systematically, all stakeholders will support the new approach. Of course, each stakeholder may come to this realization in his or her own time. Nurturing those wary of the MET response must continue long after other caregivers may have given it strong endorsement.

Other political processes need to be put in motion to ensure the success of the MET. They include paving the way by educating nurses, residents, interns, other staff and announcing the imminent introduction of a new system. The system change must be supported with accounts of when and how the current system has failed and continues to fail patients, and these should be related to the stakeholders. Such accounts must come with a vision of how they can be fixed through a MET system, and a sense of urgency that too many patients have already suffered unnecessarily and the time to make the change is now.

This process must not single out units or individuals—it must be made clear that it is the system that must change. There is also a clear political (and scientific) need to define short-term goals that can be achieved and outcomes that can be used to test whether the system is working. If it can be shown that outcomes improved with the MET, the MET will become entrenched in the culture of the organization.

Finally it is absolutely necessary to offer regular feedback to users once the MET is implemented. This is one of the most important means of achieving and maintaining political support for the change. MET callers must always be thanked, and occasionally they must be told they saved a patient's life by calling in a timely fashion. Such immediate and case-relevant feedback is extremely powerful in generating positive emotions and strong support for the MET.

Logistics: Introducing MET into a Hospital System

The system change required for successful introduction of the MET model must occur in a number of phases (Table 8.5), and involves the participation of multiple members of the hospital staff (Figure 8.1). These processes are discussed in detail elsewhere in this book.

The most important aspect of the preparation phase is to collect regional and site-specific data on the qualitative and quantitative aspects of adverse events in the hospital. This data serves as a baseline for historical comparison and acts as a "call to arms" to motivate cultural and social change. Throughout the implementation process, an individual or group of individ-

TABLE 8.5. The phases of introducing a MET service into a hospital setting

Preparation phase
- Accurate collection of baseline levels of serious adverse events and cardiac arrests
- Presentation of preliminary findings and MET model to hospital administration
- Education sessions for medical and nursing staff
- Preparation of members of the MET
- Formulation of MET-resuscitation trolley and instruments for ongoing documentation of MET data

Implementation phase
- Consider initial implementation in high-risk area
- Provide positive feedback to staff after successes
- Follow-up for patients receiving multiple MET calls
- Availability of adequate MET resources on a 24-hour basis
- Evaluation of need for increased HDU/ICU beds

Maintenance phase
- Ongoing audit of cardiac arrests and MET calls
- Continued education of new medical and nursing staff entering the system
- Ongoing feedback of MET effectiveness to hospital community

uals must champion the MET cause. If the culture, politics, and sociological aspects of the hospital are not attended to, all else will fail.

Once administrative and financial support has been secured, the next task is to win over the doctors and nurses who will use the MET system. Information and education sessions should be given on a repeated basis and should be tailored to the audience.

The MET service must be adequately staffed by trained personnel to guarantee a rapid, expert, and effective response. Activation of the MET system should be an easy process (and significantly easier than pre-MET processes for managing a crisis). Accordingly, effort should be made to minimize logistic barriers to triggering and summoning the MET: specifically, calling criteria and the emergency call number should be readily displayed on telephones, large wall posters, and/or on pocket cards for caregivers. In addition, the system should ensure 1-ring operator pick up of calls and a coordinated method of notifying the MET members as to the location of the call. Response time should be measured with "mock MET responses" to prove that responses meet speed and reliability criteria. If these measures are undertaken, then the MET will become embedded in local hospital culture. The experience at Austin Health has been that there is a progressive increase in call rates over time (Figure 8.2).

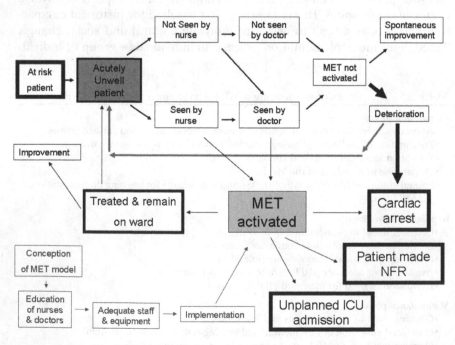

FIGURE 8.1. The plight of the unwell patient in the environment of the MET.

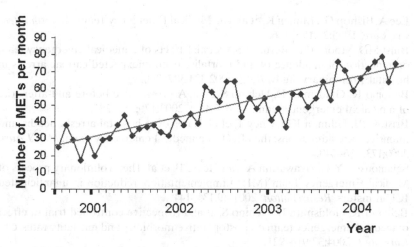

FIGURE 8.2. Progressive increase over time in the number of MET calls at the Austin Hospital from August 2000 to July 2004.

Summary: From Intuition to MET Implementation

The theory behind the MET system and the principle that early intervention improves outcome is intuitive. It is considerably easier to resuscitate a patient who is alive rather than one who is dead. Successful implementation of a MET system relies on support from hospital administrators and participation of staff members at all levels and of all disciplines. Introduction of the MET requires careful planning and information sessions that must be repeated on numerous occasions. An ongoing audit of the impact of the system on adverse outcomes, as well as the experiences of the users of the system, must be maintained.

Above all, it should never be forgotten that the goal of the MET system is to improve the quality of patient care by reducing avoidable morbidity and mortality.

References

1. McGlynn EA, Asch SM, Adams J, et al. The quality of health care delivery to adults in the United States. *N Engl J Med.* 2003;348:2635–2645.
2. Brennan TA, Leape LL, Laird N, et al. Incidence of adverse events and negligence in hospitalized patients: results of the Harvard Medical Practice Study I. *N Engl J Med.* 1991;324:370–376.
3. Wilson RMcL, Runciman WB, Gibberd RW, et al. The quality in Australian health care study. *Med J Aust.* 1995;163:458–471.
4. Lee TH. A broader concept of medical errors. *N Engl J Med.* 2002; 347:1965–1967.

5. Lee A, Bishop G, Hillman K, et al. The Medical Emergency Team. *Anaesth Intensive Care.* 1995;23:183–186.
6. Buist MD, Moore GE, Bernard SA, et al. Effects of a medical emergency team on reduction of incidence of and mortality from unexpected cardiac arrests in hospital: preliminary study. *BMJ.* 2002;324:387–390.
7. Bellomo R, Goldsmith D, Uchino S, et al. A prospective before-and-after trial of a medical emergency team. *Med J Aust.* 2003;179:283–287.
8. Bristow PJ, Hillman KM, Chey T, et al. Rates of in-hospital arrests, deaths, and intensive care admissions: the effect of a medical emergency team. *Med J Aust.* 2000;173:236–240.
9. Salamonson Y, Kariyawasam A, van Heere B, et al. The evolutionary process of Medical Emergency Team (MET) implementation: reduction in unanticipated ICU transfers. *Resuscitation.* 2001;49:135–141.
10. Bellomo R, Goldsmith D, Uchino S, et al. Prospective controlled trial of effect of medical emergency team on postoperative morbidity and mortality rates. *Crit Care Med.* 2004;32:916–921.
11. Bellomo R, Goldsmith D, Russell S, Uchino S. Postoperative serious adverse events in a teaching hospital: a prospective study. *Med J Aust.* 2002;176:216–218.
12. Buist MD, Jarmolowski E, Burton PR, Bernard SA, Waxman BP, Anderson J. Recognizing clinical instability in hospital patients before cardiac arrest or unplanned admission to intensive care. *Med J Aust.* 1999;171:22–25.
13. Franklin C, Mathew J. Developing strategies to prevent in-hospital cardiac arrest: analyzing responses of physicians and nurses in the hours before the event. *Crit Care Med.* 1994;22:244–247.
14. Shein RM, Hazday N, Pena M, Ruben BH, Sprung CL. Clinical antecedents to in-hospital cardiopulmonary arrest. *Chest.* 1990;98:1388–1392.
15. Blow O, Magliore L, Claridge JA, et al. the golden hour and the silver day: detection and correction of occult hypoperfusion within 24 hours improves outcome from major trauma. *J Trauma.* 1999;47:964–969.
16. Rivers E, Nguyen B, Havstad S, et al. Early goal-directed therapy in the treatment of severe sepsis and septic shock. *N Engl J Med.* 2001;345:1368–1377.
17. Hillman K, Parr, M, Flabouris A, Bishop G, Stewart A. Redefining in-hospital resuscitation: the concept of the medical emergency team. *Resuscitation.* 2001; 48:105–110.
18. Goldhill DR, McNarry AF. Physiological abnormalities in early warning scores are related to mortality in adult patients. *Brit J Anaesth.* 2004;92:882–884.
19. Hillman KH, Bristow PJ, Chey T, et al. Duration of life-threatening antecedents prior to intensive care admission. *Intensive Care Med.* 2002;28:1629–1634.
20. Reilly BM. Physical examination in the care of medical patients: an observational study. *Lancet.* 2003;362:1100–1105.
21. Hodgetts TJ, Kenward G, Vlackonikolis, et al. Incidence, location, and reasons for avoidable in-hospital cardiac arrest in a district general hospital. *Resuscitation.* 2002;54:115–123.

9
Potential Sociological and Political Barriers to Medical Emergency Team Implementation

MICHAEL A. DEVITA and KENNETH HILLMAN

Introduction

While there is an abundance of literature on the success or otherwise of simple medical interventions such as a new drug or procedure, there is little in the way of evaluating system implementation. The Medical Emergency Team (MET) system requires implementation across an organization involving clinicians and administration (1). This chapter will discuss potential obstacles to as well as possible enhancement strategies for the implementation of a MET system across an organization. The major barriers and strategies for overcoming them are noted in Table 9.1.

Sources of Obstacles and Inertia

The MET system was first described in 1994 (1), but investigators are still attempting to quantify the types and magnitude of the benefits. A cohort comparison study involving 3 hospitals demonstrated a reduction in case-mix-adjusted rates of unanticipated admissions to the intensive care unit (ICU) (2). Another MET evaluation study demonstrated a significant reduction in the incidence of, and mortality from, unexpected hospital cardiac arrests (3). A further prospective before-and-after trial demonstrated an impressive reduction of in-hospital cardiac arrests, death following cardiac arrest, and overall in-hospital mortality after the introduction of a MET system (4). Although these and other studies are preliminary in the sense that they are not randomized prospective placebo-controlled clinical trials, they nevertheless provide considerable support for the concept of a planned system response to crises that would reliable rescue patients as they deteriorate. Yet few hospitals to date utilize such a system—why is this?

The barriers to the introduction of METs have a number of background and cultural sources that are difficult to discern and to overcome, and they have not been well studied or described. The first barrier is viewing all

TABLE 9.1. Barriers to MET implementation and methods to overcome them

Barrier	Suggested approach
Failure to view errors as products of the system rather than individual mistakes	Multidisciplinary event reviews of care antecedent to a crisis
Lack of data that METs are life-saving	Review current data; run focused trial; multidisciplinary crisis event reviews
Professional silos	Multidisciplinary event reviews; teach "system" of care
Professional control	Emphasize METs to support, not supplant primary team's coverage; return patients to primary team immediately after event
Educational system	Emphasize benefit of better supervision of trainees by crisis team responders; track outcomes, delays in current system
Financial	Utilize current resources to staff MET response; identify frequency of avoiding ICU admission identify mortality benefit to offset cost

errors as a predictable result of the system of care that permits them to occur. While health care delivery may work well in providing individual patient clinical care, few systems cross existing health care "silos"—the professional groupings such as nursing or internal medicine physicians, or geographic groupings like an intensive care unit. Quality work within silos tends to be relatively easy to foster because members of a group tend to have common incentives and disincentives. Hospital-wide systems, however, are more difficult to effectively introduce and maintain in part because the framework for interdisciplinary systems improvement is relatively new to health care organizations and also because the members of diverse groups may have conflicting incentives. This perspective fosters the blaming of an individual or of chance for an error or adverse event, and a system that lacks adequate quality checks (such as double-checking blood prior to transfusion), continuous patient monitoring (such as pulse oximetry), and a rapid recovery system to reliably intercept the consequences of errors and prevent harm is one that will be unsafe. Overcoming the perception that errors are not systematic is essential to creating an effective crisis response system.

The MET system is a hospital-wide patient safety system. It assumes errors will be made, and provides an important (and potentially life-saving) mechanism for the system to recover from a failure and prevent the deterioration of a patient's condition, irrespective of whether the deterioration was due to an error of omission or commission. The MET system requires interdisciplinary resources and teamwork. It presupposes that the system views these events as relatively common and preventable, as well as worth preventing and worth the associated costs. In other words, the hospital system of care must prioritize patient safety and view errors as a problem with the system, instead of an individual error.

A second barrier is the lack of incontrovertible data regarding the benefit of a MET system. The culture of medicine tends to be scientifically based; thus, behavioral changes tend to require evidence that change will have value. Such a study is underway in 23 Australian hospitals involving three-quarters of a million patients, using a cluster control methodology. The study should shed light not only on the effectiveness of a MET system, but also on factors that may affect its degree effectiveness. These factors may include the incidence of vital sign abnormalities that a MET system could respond to, the rate of response once predefined MET criteria have been reached, and the response's effectiveness. Because the study does not focus on the sociological and psychological barriers to creating an effective response, it may not have the full impact one might expect. Further study will be needed to create the cultural change required to support a MET system.

Some might argue that a placebo-controlled trial for METs is impossible because the intervention is performed in a setting that is so large and complex that comparisons are difficult, and because the participating hospitals are sure to demonstrate "contamination" as the people within the study move from hospital to hospital in the normal course of career changes. Thus no trial will truly be controlled or be a "pure placebo." The impediments to research extend to the types of data elucidated, because they are fundamentally different from the data one obtains from, for example, a placebo-controlled drug trial. Endpoints are less discrete and not as easy to measure as patients' clinical data. This difference may lead scientifically scrutinizing readers to devalue the current and perhaps future data regarding the MET system. However, no one can argue against early intervention in serious illness. The effectiveness of the system depends on factors such as the appropriateness of the calling criteria, systematic implementation strategies, and suitable maintenance strategies to ensure ideal functioning of the system over time.

A third barrier is the existence of professional silos. Most hospital professionals were trained in a system in which only their profession is taught. Teaching the various health professionals exclusively their own profession creates a tendency toward cultural and intellectual isolation. Workers also practice their profession within their own silo, and become knowledgeable about the data within their silo, but remain relatively ignorant of data outside their silo or of interactions between the professional silos. The intellectual and role isolationism sets up a system of ownership, competition, and egocentrism, and is perhaps the foundation for blame when things go wrong. Similarly, the "health care team" is often deficient because they are rarely trained together and sometimes do not cooperate in system improvement activities; it is no team at all. Better models for teamwork exist in sports or in the military. For example, the aviation industry sees itself as a global team continually striving to improve effectiveness and reduce error. A team learns and practices together before working together; a prime example is in sports, where there is a long history of effective training to improve effectiveness and reduce error among those competing together as part of a team. In contrast, members of the health care professions tend to view themselves first as a physician, or nurse, rather than a team member. This cognitive "set" can prevent individuals from taking actions that are within their capability but outside the traditional boundaries of their profession.

Another fundamental problem is that health care education is deficient in teaching the "system" of care. Instead it focuses on diseases—diagnostics and therapeutics— and concentrates on procedural skills, such as setting up a ventilator, inserting a central line, or performing a dressing change. Training programs traditionally do not emphasize the "health care system": how a hospital works, including the hospital hierarchy; the roles and responsibilities of various staff; the interactions within the system; and the informatics infrastructure. Implementing systematic change is often left to health graduates to learn while on-the-job. This sets up a system "blindness," where members of the health care professions may not trust the environment within which they are working, which leads them to set up their own methods for "getting around the system to get things done right." In this mindset, the system is the problem, not the solution.

Medicine is relatively resistant to change. For example, it took trauma systems 10 years before they demonstrated a decrease in mortality (5–7). But there is also little acknowledgment or understanding of the complexity of health care and therefore little understanding of implementation strategies for any new process. The identification of facilitators and impeders is for the most part through personal experience, and only for those "trying to get something done" (8–11).

Foundations for System Change

Some recent social changes are laying the foundation for in-hospital transformations. First, recent publications and scandals over potentially preventable deaths in the health care system have highlighted the frequency of errors and the harm that they cause (12). *To Err Is Human*, a book published by the Institute of Medicine in the United States, previously highlighted the under-publicized poor safety record of the US health care system. As a result, society now expects and is demanding more safety from the health care system.

Federal policy is beginning to shift, as constituencies demand safer care and greater accountability. This change is occurring globally. National safety bodies oversee strict standards for drugs and devices, but currently there is little in the way of evaluating and imposing standards around health systems. In the past decade the Joint Council on Accreditation of Health-care Organizations (JCAHO) in the United States has introduced tough new safety system audits (13). Their initiatives coincided with a tragic death in a hospital that had very recently been audited and accredited by the orga-nization, which led some to conclude that the auditing system itself needed repair (14,15). The US Food and Drug Administration has altered its report-ing mechanism and its methodology for notification of important drug error concerns. They now observe for sources of medication error and put pres-sure on manufacturers to alter packaging, labeling claims, and marketing approaches to prevent systematic sources of clinical errors and harm.

Health care marketing strategies have also changed. Health care buyers are working together to get the best value instead of the best cost. For example, the Leapfrog group in the United States has defined system stan-dards and care goals that have prompted providers to alter their approach to care delivery, marketing, and data collection (16–18). Thus, senior health care officials are now attentive to safety as an important indicator of quality of care within a hospital, and a number of agencies in the United States, Australia, and Europe now are showing interest in METs. For example, the Institute for Healthcare Improvement is providing courses on METs, and JCAHO has included information on METs at its national meeting. Both the federal and state governments in Australia are currently sponsoring an evaluation of the MET system. Because safety is a goal for all caregiver organizations, these forces are leading administrators and caregivers to recognize the possible benefit of the MET for their institution and their patients. It would also demonstrate that they are practicing according to newly emerging practice patterns and safety initiatives.

Impediments Within the Hospital

There are a number of impediments within the hospital that my challenge the implementation of a MET system. The first is cost. For at least the last decade in the United States, there has been a huge focus on cutting costs. However, as noted above, there is now a shifting focus to safety. While cost is and will always remain an issue, the balance is changing from favoring cost considerations to a new obsession with quality.

The MET seems to increase cost because MET systems appear to require new equipment and staffing. When a MET system is undertaken, one should expect a 3- to 5-fold rise in the frequency of calls to seriously ill patients (19), although the majority will not be cardiac arrest events (1,20). Based on those numbers, it is easy to predict the staffing required for emergency stabilization. Medical Emergency Teams often include 1 or more intensive care or emergency medicine physicians and nurses, an anesthesiologist or nurse anesthetist, and 1 or more respiratory therapists. In addition, other members of the staff who are not part of the team will respond and attempt to help manage the crisis; this activity is usually in addition to the other responsibilities they have. This perception of added work is a barrier to implementation and may stop discussion before accurate estimates of cost and benefit can be analyzed. It is estimated that training every staff member of a hospital to deal with cardiac arrests would cost over $500 000 per survivor (21). On the other hand, a MET system aims to concentrate a small number of experts who respond to all hospital emergencies, rather than universal training for all staff in basic cardiopulmonary resuscitation. In this sense, METs will save training costs and also decrease the work of those who would otherwise respond to cardiac arrest events.

A second impediment is that crisis teams intervene for patients who are usually being cared for by other individuals. This raises 2 issues. The first is power—who is in "control" of the patient's care. If one group is already treating the patient, calling in a second group sets up a conflict regarding who is in charge, with the implied question of who is better. The second issue is based on historical perceptions that each team should give "total" care to its patients. In this model, calling for help may be perceived as a sign of weakness, perhaps both emotional and intellectual, implying that the caller is somehow not equipped to deal with the situation. These attitudes promoting barriers between clinical services need to be removed and working across traditional silos is required for successful implementation of MET responses.

Because METs require cultural as well as behavioral change, hospital nursing, physician, and administration leadership is required to make the system work. These leaders are needed for political support and for the added funding needed for the program. Without hospital leadership forcefully advocating for improved care of patients in crisis, and finding the resources needed to demonstrate both the need for and benefit of this service, the project is unlikely to succeed.

Senior colleagues in the allied health professions are key allies in culture change, in particular senior nurses and physician leaders. Staff nurses and doctors working in the hospital will not participate fully in the project without support from their leadership. The work occurring at the crisis response requires a significant influx of nursing and physician support; often the support arrives from other areas of the hospital. This shift of work responsibilities will be in addition to other responsibilities and so may be resisted. The leadership has to view the larger hospital perspective and be able to allocate resources that can both handle the added workload and have the skills necessary for the management of hospital crises. To protect these resources from added work, the leaders may balk at lending their support. Opting for the status quo—especially when it seems that individuals rather that systems are the cause of crisis events—is often the politically easier course to take.

We have observed that role perception of caregivers is a barrier to implementation and successful use of METs. Professional differences may create unanticipated barriers to a MET system. Nursing staff have a culture of recording patient vital signs and then reporting it to medical colleagues rather than acting on the findings directly. This is due in part to a long history of not being empowered to translate concern into action. In this process, nurses who find a low blood pressure, for example, will try to contact the physician responsible for that patient rather than immediately act. The exception to that rule is when the patient is found without a pulse or respiration; then the nurse may act to activate a crisis response to deal with the patient. A MET system empowers nurses to act immediately to bring a crisis response. Nurses (and physicians) may feel uncomfortable in participating in a new process that appears to change the traditional role of the nurse, and they may be reluctant to take on responsibilities that are not traditionally within their own boundaries. We have observed experienced individuals in our human simulator crisis team training course avoiding important tasks that are "not their job"—for example, no one may rescue breathe for a dyspneic patient because that is the job of anesthesia or critical care staff. Creating new processes for MET responses will challenge traditional roles and responsibilities, which is a potential barrier to the system's implementation.

Just as remaining mindful of one's profession may prove a barrier to the correct response, being mindful that one's performance may be criticized will alter behavior. Junior medical staff, who are trying to learn and impress their seniors, are likely to see calling for help as a sign of weakness. Junior doctors traditionally look after their own patients no matter how sick they are and call for help only when they have insight into their own inadequacies and the potential consequence of this for patients. The problem is that until one is knowledgeable, one can neither appreciate these possibilities and dangers nor recognize when they are "in trouble." Medical trainees often do not possess the skills, knowledge, or experience necessary to recognize and resuscitate seriously ill patients (22,23).

Physicians, nurses, and others in the hospital have operated in hierarchical and separate teams, creating an important barrier that needs to be acknowledged and understood. A nurse may recognize trouble and ask for input from other, more experienced nurses; when the situation is deemed to be beyond the capabilities of the nursing chain, they will call a physician. That physician will respond based on his or her skills and priorities. When that person finds the problem exceeds their skills, a second call is made, and a third or a fourth, until finally all the resources are assembled. This knowledge and skills ladder is hierarchical in nature and builds in delays in response. Even though there are well-recognized delays, caregivers may be reluctant to go outside the chain of command when a crisis occurs. For MET responses to work, that chain must be identified as a systematic barrier to rapid and effective care of a patient in crisis. This tacit statement that the current hierarchy is a source of error and harm could prove a barrier to accomplishing implementation of the system.

Traditional medical and nursing education is also a potential impediment to the MET system, since it teaches that learning is best when one thinks through a problem on one's own, and then learns from the successes and mistakes. Crisis response teams optimally intervene rapidly and with appropriate expertise. The response may be so fast that trainees may not have the opportunity to think it through and decide for themselves what are the most important considerations and best course of action. There may be a belief that not allowing mistakes somehow impedes learning. Since many advocate that education is an important component of medicine and nursing care, causing a situation where teachers believe learning is not possible will create concern.

The belief that an error results from an individual's actions, and not because of a failure of the "system" to prevent error, is a major barrier to MET implementation (24). Recognition that a faulty system permits error and harm to a patient is relatively advanced thinking in today's medical world. The Morbidity and Mortality (M & M) conference structure often concentrates on individual errors rather than contextualizing it into "system thinking." The failure to recognize that a system that permits errors is a faulty system is a fundamental barrier to implementing METs. It always will be easier to blame an individual than a system in such traditional M & M conferences, and so the need for a "system fix" remains unrecognized. As long as this perception persists, there will be a significant barrier to creating a new process that threatens established hierarchy and current practice patterns.

Strategies to Overcome Hurdles

The authors have noted a number of strategies to overcome a variety of hurdles. Some strategies may operate optimally during the implementation phase and others are more appropriate for systems maintenance. There is no data to support which barriers need to be overcome first, nor any to determine which strategies are most effective, easiest, or surest.

Both authors have found that hospital "stories" of failures or near misses can become the basis for a forum where an alternative system approach can be discussed. There are 2 types of stories that tend work. The first is the "cause celebre," in which some tragic event occurs, demanding analysis and action—for example, the wife of a staff physician who dies from an error involving an opioid overdose, after which careful analysis reveals that the death was due to both a life-threatening situation (the opioid dosing) but also to the hospital system's failure to respond to the event. The second is a compendium of smaller stories—for example, analysis of a series of people who had adverse events in a 6-month interval all due to opioid adverse events can be a powerful motivator to action. While it is easy to attribute a single adverse event to a single faulty practitioner, analysis of many events together will demonstrate a myriad of causes. This method makes it clear that the *system* is faulty if so many mistakes can occur, each mistake by a different individual, at a different step in the process, and at different times. This makes the need for a system response more evident. It is in this context that the person promoting a MET response must propose a system that may prevent serious adverse events no matter what their cause. Successes with 1 type of crisis tend to lead to the recognition by others that the system may work well for other types of problems. In this way the MET response becomes the system's "goal-keeper" to rescue patients when other error-detection mechanisms have failed. A major selling point for MET responses is that they can prevent deaths and serious complications from myriad causes that result in patient deterioration.

Using data is effective for motivating change: data is impersonal, and can track harm and the benefits of process change. Possibly the most important data to track is the frequency and duration of delays in care. Reviewing the 24 hours prior to a crisis or cardiac arrest event for delays in delivery of appropriate treatment is possible once standards for response times and severity of illness are created. Crisis criteria enable reviewers to determine how long after the criteria were met that it takes to deliver the definitive treatment, or even get the responsible and capable person to the bedside of the patient in crisis (19). Analysts can then graph delays by frequency, duration, location, service, day of week, time of day, etc. This data is provides a powerful tool to recognize system deficiencies and motivate process change. We believe that delays in delivering definitive treatments are the hallmarks of systems without a MET response program. Continued data collection and analysis will demonstrate effectiveness of process change in removing delays in care from an institution.

Both authors have encountered individuals who remain resistant to group efforts to solve medical crisis situations. Data from the MET system can in itself facilitate the implementation and maintenance process (25), and may be processed and targeted to every level of the organization. Specific patient details are provided for individual clinicians, while departments, divisions, and the hospital would review aggregated, de-identified data. Data includes details of MET calls, number of deaths, cardiac arrests, and unplanned ICU admissions in which MET criteria had been met but no call made; these are called potentially preventable events. A graphic depiction of duration and frequency of delays from the onset of a crisis situation (determined by satisfying crisis criteria) can help target areas that need extra educational effort.

Some clinicians or departments may not like having "unconsulted" doctors assume care of their patients, creating a political barrier to implementation of the MET system. One method to overcome this concern and facilitate the implementation of a hospital emergency system is to remind staff that calling for help in cases of complex acute medicine is no different from seeking consultations from colleagues in different specialties. Guarantees that the patient's care will remain under the control of the "primary" caregivers after the crisis is resolved (or even during it) can also foster an environment where METs may be implemented successfully.

One author discovered that the director of a residency education program did nothing to promote METs, but permitted the use of METs with the caveat that it was the responsibility of the MET response organizers to "make sure my residents get taught." After the trainees reported decreased stress when caring for sick patients, and improved understanding of the management of suddenly critically ill patients—learned during observation of and working with the MET responders—the education director relented. Residents found that with METs they could learn in a context where they had help, and they could observe the "right way"; on the other hand, they did feel that losing the opportunity to learn by doing took away from their educational program.

The MET system can help to cost effectively treat patients. For example, nursing infrastructure required to care for seriously ill patients on a general ward can detract from other routine activities. The MET response not only provides timely and expert care at all times but can decrease the burden on the rest of the staff having to care for the seriously ill in inappropriate environments. The average time for a MET response is approximately 30 minutes (1). Thus a patient who is deteriorating can be assessed, treated, and if necessary triaged in short order. This allows the nursing unit routine to remain relatively undisturbed in spite of the crisis event.

The MET system improves the safety of patients on floors with patients in crisis. We have observed what we call "domino codes," where a second patient medical crisis occurs because staff either fails to deliver treatment or adequately monitor patients while they are coping with the first patient in crisis. METs decrease "domino codes" because they swiftly bring new critical care resources to the unit, and they either rapidly resolve the crisis or triage the patient elsewhere. Identifying these unit-based resource issues and recognizing the successes that occur after MET implementation are great motivators to overcome pockets of resistance.

Adding or increasing MET responses means increased work for the response team, because each MET response brings critical care workers from other areas to treat a single patient. It may seem a daunting task to marshal the resources to take on the task of responding to all patient medical crisis events. Both authors' hospitals offer a service similar to the traditional cardiac arrest team: that is, resuscitate first, discuss after, and return the patient to the care of the primary doctor immediately after the crisis is resolved. By using the cardiac arrest team, no new resources need to be identified—the current resources are just taxed a bit more. Recognition that many emergency patients may go on to become cardiac arrest patients can help motivate responders to arrive early, before the heart stops. Early calls improve outcome and decrease the effort needed to restore homeostasis. Critical care admissions may be avoided, decreasing the down-stream work of the ICU staff. On balance, responding to crises early and effectively reduces workload for hospital staff.

In hospitals, education is a continuous and essential activity needed to maintain quality care. Find opportunities to educate staff about METs. For example, new staff orientation should include a module on crisis management and proper use of METs. New staff will accept the process based on accepted practice. In contrast, existing staff needs to be re-educated in why a systematic approach makes more sense than ad hoc processes to build crisis intervention teams for each critical event. New systems of care must be perceived by existing staff to be both easier and more effective than current practice or the new process will fail. MET rules must be made simple and objective. Any "interpretable" rules will not be consistently followed; MET response should be viewed as "one-stop shopping" for management of any medical crisis. Buist et al. have found that "caregivers 'worried' about a patient" is a common trigger for a MET response (3). Reliably rescuing staff members who have patient concerns will reinforce use of the response in the future.

For managers of the MET system, positive and negative reinforcement can foster culture change. Congratulate those who "call for help"; tell them, their bosses, and their colleagues how a life was saved. The University of Pittsburgh used e-mail for this feedback to effect culture change (19). Private notification of superiors about failure to trigger the MET response will demonstrate the impact of the failure. It is essential that MET responders reinforce the call as well; it will do no good if superiors praise calling for help while the MET responders criticize the same action. Every criticism of a MET call must trigger re-education of those individuals. All members of the institution must view a MET call as an act of heroism: it is putting patient care above ego. Other reinforcing educational strategies include placing MET criteria in all parts of the hospital and on pocket cards for responders and staff, and notifying patients and families about the MET system to protect the patients.

As noted previously, "calling for help" can be perceived as a sign of weak-ness, and this perception is promoted when the criteria for what constitutes a crisis are subjective or ambiguous. As such, the request is an indirect measure of competency: the person perceiving the patient in crisis defines crisis by his or her inability to manage the situation alone. To prevent this barrier, objective and readily recognized crisis criteria must be adopted. With objective criteria, the person who finds the crisis is merely notifying others that the crisis exists (following hospital policy), and this does not imply that the person's ability to manage the situation is inadequate. Instead, the MET call becomes a mark of excellence in patient care and clinical judgment. Hospitals that have utilized crisis criteria have shown an increase in MET response frequency and a decrease in delays to treat-ment.(Foraida, Buist)

Summary

Implementing a MET response system in a hospital will likely alter the culture of care and threaten the status quo. There are many potential psychological, emotional, sociological, and economic barriers to bringing a new system of care to a stable environment. Nevertheless, strong data indicate that such a system of care will decrease unexpected mortality in a variety of hospital settings. Therefore, the key question with which hospital leadership must grapple is how to implement the system, not whether to implement it. There is no strong data to define the particular barriers, nor how to overcome them. Instead, in this chapter we have proposed strategies that have been effective in our hospital environments and may benefit others as well.

References

1. Lee A, Bishop G, Hillman KM, Daffurn K. The medical emergency team. *Anaesth Intensive Care.* 1995;23:183–186.
2. Bristow PJ, Hillman KM, Chey T, et al. Rates of in-hospital arrests, deaths, and intensive care admissions: the effect of a medical emergency team. *Med J Aust.* 2000;173:236–240.
3. Buist MD, Moore GE, Bernard SA, Waxman BP, Anderson JN, Nguyen TV. Effects of a medical emergency team on reduction of incidence of and mortality from unexpected cardiac arrests in hospital: preliminary study. *BMJ.* 2002;324: 387–390.
4. Bellomo R, Goldsmith D. Postoperative serious adverse events in a teaching hospital: a prospective study. *Med J Aust.* 2002;176:216–218.
5. Nathens AB, Jurkovich GJ, Cummings P, Rivara FP, Maier RV. The effect of organized systems of trauma care on motor vehicle crash mortality. *JAMA.* 2000;283:1990–1994.
6. Lecky F, Woodford M, Yates DW; the UK Trauma Audit Research Network. Trends in trauma care in England and Wales 1989–97. *Lancet.* 2000;355: 1771–1775.
7. Mullins RJ, Veum-Stone J, Helfand M, Zimmer-Gembeck M, Trunkey D. Outcome of hospitalized patients after institution of a trauma system in an urban area. *JAMA.* 1994;27:1919–1924.
8. Plsek PE, Greenhalgh T. The challenge of complexity in health care. *BMJ.* 2001; 323:625–628.
9. Eccles FR, Grimshaw J. Why does primary care need more implementation research? *Fam Pract.* 2001;18:353–355.
10. Dellinger RP. Fundamental critical care support: another merit badge or more? *Crit Care Med.* 1996;24:556–557.
11. Cook RI, Render M, Woods DD. Gaps in the continuity of care and progress on patient safety. *BMJ.* 2000;320:791–794.
12. Schneider EC, Lieberman T. Publicly disclosed information about the quality of health care: response of the US public. *Qual Saf Health Care.* 2001;10:96–103.

13. Beyea SC. Implications of the 2004 National Patient Safety Goals. *AORN J.* 2003;78:834–836.
14. Griffith JR, Knutzen SR, Alexander JA. Structural versus outcomes measures in hospitals: a comparison of joint commission and medicare outcomes scores in hospitals. *Qual Manag Health Care.* 2002;10:29–38.
15. Landis NT. Government finds fault with hospital quality review by joint commission and states. *Am J Health Syst Pharm.* 1999;56:1699–1700.
16. Scanlon M. Computer physician order entry and the real world: we're only humans. *Jt Comm J Qual Saf.* 2004;30:342–346.
17. Pugliese G. In search of safety: an interview with Gina Pugliese. Interview by Alison P. Smith. *Nurs Econ.* 2002;20:6–12.
18. Cors WK. Physician executives must leap with the frog. Accountability for safety and quality ultimately lie with the doctors in charge. *Physician Exec.* 2001;27: 14–16.
19. Foraida M, DeVita M, Braithwaite RS, Stuart S, Brooks MM, Simmons RL. Improving the utilization of medical crisis teams (Condition C) at an urban tertiary care hospital. *J Crit Care.* 2003;18:87–94.
20. Hourihan F, Bishop G, Hillman KM, Daffurn K, Lee A. The medical emergency team: a new strategy to identify and intervene in high-risk patients. *Clin Intensive Care.* 1995;6:269–272.
21. Lee KH, Angus DC, Abramson NS. Cardiopulmonary resuscitation: what cost to cheat death? *Crit Care Med.* 1996;24:2046–2052.
22. McQuillan P, Pilkington S, Alan A, et al. Confidential inquiry into quality of care before admission to intensive care. *BMJ.* 1998;316:1853–1858.
23. Goldhill DR, White SA, Sumner A. Physiological values and procedures in the 24 hours before ICU admission from the ward. *Anaesthesia.* 1999;54:529–534.
24. Reason J. Combating omission errors through task analysis and good reminders. *Qual Saf Health Care.* 2002;11:40–44.
25. Hillman K, Alexandrou E, Flabouris M, et al. Clinical outcome indicators in acute hospital medicine. *Clin Intensive Care.* 2000;11:89–94.

10
Overview of Various Medical Emergency Team Models

MICHELLE CRETIKOS and RINALDO BELLOMO

Introduction

Hospitals are not as safe as they could be. Many patients experience adverse events in association with their admission or elective operation (1). Some of these adverse events result in permanent disability; others cause death (2). These events have long been accepted as part of acute medical care in complex systems such as hospitals. But the system-based deficiencies that underlie such adverse events have become more noticeable as patients undergo more complex interventions, and hospitals have been slow to develop well-planned, institution-wide approaches to protect patients and maximize their safety. Only recently, and only in select hospitals, have responses been developed in an attempt to minimize the harm to patients brought about by the deficiencies of current hospital systems worldwide.

Critical care specialists are beginning to apply the principles of acute medicine and resuscitation across the hospital to provide rapid and specialized assistance to critically ill patients wherever and whenever it is requested (3). The Medical Emergency Team (MET) is an example of such an initiative providing an immediate response to at-risk patients in an acute care hospital (3). Where implemented, the MET system has replaced the cardiac arrest team that most hospitals currently employ. The MET was modeled on the idea of the trauma team (4), which has been incorporated into most large hospitals worldwide.

The aims of the MET are similar to those of the trauma team—effective triage and management of care of potentially seriously ill patients prior to the development of progressive and irreversible deterioration. In such critically ill patients, rapid assessment and early and aggressive correction of hypovolemia and hypoxemia have been demonstrated to decrease morbidity and mortality (5–7). The MET aims to provide appropriately trained personnel who are able to perform these functions on the ward early, to prevent the development of severe adverse outcomes such as multi-organ failure or cardiac arrest.

However, MET is not the only such system that has developed with the s aim of improving patient safety exist. Other systems, such as the Outreach Team concept, are being implemented in hospitals in the United Kingdom (8,9). In the United States, the new hospitalist system deals with these same problems by having a specialist trained in resuscitation available and responsible for the welfare of all hospital patients 24 hours a day (10). It may be that the MET system provides an interim solution to the problem of suboptimal care in hospitals, until such time as the hospitalist concept has been sufficiently tested, validated, and accepted.

The MET in Practice

The Medical Emergency Team in the tertiary hospital setting usually consists of at least an intensive care unit (ICU) registrar (a critical care fellow in the United States), and an ICU nurse. In some hospitals, others may assist the MET, including the receiving medical registrar (in the United States, the admitting internal medicine fellow or chief resident). In smaller hospitals, the MET may consist of as few as two nurses trained in advanced resuscitation. The nursing and medical staff are encouraged to call the MET whenever they are seriously concerned about a patient's condition, or if a patient's signs or symptoms meet any 1 or more of the well-defined physiological calling criteria (Table 10.1).

The response team will assess the patient and institute any therapy that is immediately necessary. The patient may then be given an active medical management plan and left on the ward, with or without a do-not-resuscitate order in place, after appropriate discussion. Alternatively, if the patient is not responding to initial therapy or is judged to be too sick for

TABLE 10.1. Example of Medical Emergency Team calling criteria

Airway	Threatened
Breathing	All Respiratory Arrests
	Respiratory Rate < 5
	Respiratory Rate > 36
Circulation	All Cardiac Arrests
	Pulse Rate < 40
	Pulse Rate > 140
	Systolic Blood Pressure < 90
Neurology	Sudden fall in level of consciousness
	(Fall in GCS of <2 points)
	Repeated or prolonged seizures
Other	Any patient you are seriously worried about that does not fit the above criteria

the wards, the patient may be transferred to an area capable of higher-level care. If the patient is judged safe to remain on the wards, the ongoing care and management responsibility is transferred back to the consultant or attending physician in charge of the patient's hospital admission.

The aims of the MET are to reduce the rates of unexpected death (i.e. death without a do-not-resuscitate order), cardiac arrest, and unplanned admission to the intensive care unit. The MET has been shown to reduce the rates of cardiac arrest (11,12), unanticipated ICU admission, (13,14), and overall in-hospital mortality (12).

In summary, the key components of the MET system include:

1. Clear, simple calling criteria, including a subjective criterion
2. Activation of the MET by any staff member
3. Inclusion of both medical and nursing staff on the team
4. An immediate response by appropriately trained staff
5. Continuous monitoring and feedback of adverse events, as part of the system response

Culture Change in the Acute Care Hospital

The potential benefit of the MET system is not limited to a reduction in the rate of adverse outcomes, as discussed above; it is also capable of facilitating a change in attitude and in systematic thinking across the hospital. Implementation of the MET system results in a generally less rigid, more patient-centered approach within the hospital. By empowering all staff to call for help when required, the MET system permits staff to display initiative and be proactive when confronted by seriously ill patients. The MET also provides a sense of support and security for the junior medical and nursing staff, and an environment that is supportive and less stressful facilitates more effective learning (15).

The MET system also acts as a driving force to increase the documentation of do-not-resuscitate orders at an earlier stage. This leads to decisions concerning acute care in a more considered and controlled fashion, and this may, in turn, lead to a reduction in the rate of futile and inappropriate cardiac arrest calls. The MET system may also encourage a better quality of end-of-life care for patients and their families, by de-emphasizing acute medical management in favor of more active and holistic care of the dying (16).

In addition, the MET system incorporates a basis for clinical governance by providing information and feedback on patients suffering serious adverse events that were heralded by MET criteria but not acted on appropriately (17). This provides a framework for the continuous monitoring of hospital quality, patient safety, and medical errors. With the MET system, feedback processes may be put in place to enable corrective action where both sporadic and systematic adverse events and errors are detected (18).

The MET and the Outreach Team: Different Team-Based Approaches

Systems other than the MET have been developed in an attempt to address the problem of preventable adverse events on general hospital wards. In the United Kingdom, Outreach Team systems have become a mandatory part of every hospital structure (9). The team, usually skilled in critical care, has the responsibility of caring for patients that have been identified as at-risk. Generally these patients are identified using a "track and trigger" system such as the Early Warning Scoring System (EWSS) (19,20), the Modified Early Warning Score (MEWS) (21–27), Patient At-Risk Teams (PARTs) (8,28,29), or other local variations (30,31). Occasionally, a system of calling criteria much like that of the MET is used. All of these different approaches fall under the banner of the Outreach Team system in the UK (9,32–36).

In the United States, 3 systems for responding to patients in crisis are being implemented. The first is referred to as the ICU Outreach Team, and the second is known as the Medical Crisis or "Condition C" team (37–39) which essentially is identical to a MET (Table 10.2). There is also a third, slightly different approach known as the hospitalist system, which is not team-based. This system relies on 24-hour, on-site hospitalist consultant to cover all hospital patients (10). In these approaches, the systematic responses may differ in the method of activation of the team, in the team composition and availability, and in the specific set of activation criteria (Table 10.3). However, for all of them the basic principle is recognizing and responding quickly to patients identified as at-risk.

In the Outreach Team system, the major difference between its method of activation and the MET calling criteria is that the majority of Outreach

TABLE 10.2. Team approaches that broadly fit under the MET/Outreach classification

MET	Outreach
Medical Crisis Response team	Modified Early Warning Score (MEWS)
Code Blue	Medical Early Response Team (MERT)
Condition C	Early Warning Scoring System (EWSS)
Pre-arrest team	Patient-At-Risk Team (PART)
	Patient Emergency Response Team (PERT)
	Assessment Score for Sick Patient Identification and Step-up in Treatment (ASSIST)
	Critical Care Outreach Team (CCOT)

TABLE 10.3. Differences between MET and Outreach systems

- The MET is generally composed of at least 1 doctor (with advanced life-support skills) and 1 nurse, and is available 24 hours a day. An outreach team may be as little as 1 nurse, and may only be available for specific hours during the day.
- The criteria for calling the MET is a yes/no system for **any** of the criteria e.g is the heart rate >140 beats/minute? The criteria for an Outreach team is usually a graded system, where a patient has to be scored and reach a certain threshold before the team can be called.
- In the MET system, any member of staff can activate the team. In some Outreach systems, only a doctor of registrar grade or above can activate the team.
- A MET is sent to review the patient immediately upon receiving a call. The Outreach team may respond immediately, within a few hours, or may review patients as part of a planned ward round of the hospital.
- The MET criteria usually incorporate a subjective "seriously worried" criterion, which can be used to activate the team for nonspecific or life-threatening emergencies not covered by the other criteria. The early warning scores generally have no subjective component, and no facility for calling the team if the set threshold is not attained by the designated criteria.
- Although variations to the MET calling criteria do exist, they generally conform to heart rate, systolic blood pressure, respiratory rate, level of consciousness, and "worried" criteria. The Outreach teams use a variety of more complex calling criteria. Outreach criteria may include urine output, oxygen saturations, respiratory support, temperature, and sometimes biochemical markers, as well as specific symptoms such as chest pain.

"track and trigger" systems incorporate a graded response (9). Individual clinical observations are scored and summated, and if a threshold is reached the Outreach Team is called (Table 10.4) (25). As an example, a score of 1 point requires more frequent nursing observations and recalculation of the patient's score, a score of 2 requires the primary team to review the patient, and a score of 3 activates the Outreach Team (Table 10.5) (40). The set of activation criteria and the threshold score differ by hospital and region. In

TABLE 10.4. Modified Early Warning Score (MEWS) system

	Points						
	3	2	1	0	1	2	3
Systolic blood pressure; mmHg	<70	71–80	81–100	101–199		≥200	
Heart rate; beats/min^{-1}		<40	41–50	51–100	101–110	111–129	≥130
Respiratory rate; breath/min^{-1}		<9		9–14	15–20	21–29	≥30
Temperature; C		<35		35–38.4		≥38.5	
Neurological score				Alert	Reacting to Voice	Reacting to Pain	Unresponsive

Source: Subbe CP, Davies RG, Williams E, Rutherford P, Gemmell L. Effect of introducing the Modified Early Warning score on clinical outcomes, cardio-pulmonary arrests and intensive care utilisation in acute medical admissions. *Anaesthesia*. 2003;58:797–802.

TABLE 10.5. The graded clinical response table

Score	Action	Sensitivity (%)	Specificity (%)
1	Observe Repeat TPR, BP, SpO$_2$, GCS, calculate urine output last 2 hours (if known)	100	17
2–3	Now recalculate (if same, observe closely)	98–94	36–61
4	Bleep patient's senior house office to attend within 30 min)	89	7
5–7	Confirm with senior nurse then fast bleep senior house officer of patient's specialty	84–64	89–96
8	Inform senior nurse then call MET	52	99

Source: Hodgetts TJ, Kenward G, Vlachonikalis IG, Payne S, Castle N. The identification of risk factors for cardiac arrest and formulation of activation criteria to alert a medical emergency team. *Resuscitation*. 2002;54:125–131.

contrast, the criteria for calling the MET are objective and elicit a binary (yes/no) response for *each* of the criteria: e.g. is the heart rate >140 beats/minute? If the answer to any question is yes, the team is called (41).

In general, the "track and trigger" systems used by Outreach are more complicated than the MET calling criteria. The benefit is that the threshold for activation of the Outreach team may be set for higher specificity, thereby decreasing the number of times the team is activated. It may also provide a mechanism for nursing staff to identify and respond to an objective deterioration in a patient's clinical condition. In general, the MET calling criteria have lower specificity but a higher sensitivity to patients who are clinically deteriorating, and therefore provide a guaranteed and immediate expert review to a greater proportion of patients that have been identified, either subjectively or objectively, as at risk.

The MET criteria also usually incorporate a subjective "seriously worried" criterion, which can be used to activate the team for non-specific or life-threatening emergencies not covered by the other criteria. The "track and trigger" systems generally have no subjective component and no facility for calling the team if the set threshold is not attained by the designated criteria (9). In the MET system, any member of the staff can activate the team, but some Outreach systems may only be activated by a doctor of registrar grade (fellow or chief resident in the United States) or above, or by a senior nurse under exceptional circumstances. This is the case for the activation of the Patient-At-Risk Team, a version of the Outreach Team (Table 10.6) (8).

The MET is generally composed of at least 1 doctor (with advanced life support skills) and 1 nurse, and is available 24 hours a day (41). By contrast, the make-up of the Outreach Team can vary markedly among hospitals. It may be composed of a single critical care nurse who will review a patient upon request during normal working hours only (Monday through

TABLE 10.6. The Patient-at-Risk team calling criteria

A: The senior ward nurse should contact the responsible doctor and inform them of a patient with:

  Any 3 or more of the following:
  • Respiratory rate ≥25 breaths/min (or <10)
  • Arterial systolic pressure <90 mmHg
  • Heart rate ≥110 beats/min (or <55)
  • Not FULLY alert and oriented
  • Oxygen saturation <90%
  • Urine output <100 mL over last 4 hours
  OR a patient not FULLY alert and oriented AND
  respiratory rate ≥35 breaths/min OR heart rate ≥140 beats/min

Unless immediate management improves the patient, the doctor should consider calling the team.

Exceptionally (in emergency when responsible doctor not immediately available) the senior ward nurse may contact the team directly.

B: A doctor of registrar grade or above may call the team for any seriously ill patient causing acute concern. This will normally be carried out after discussion with the patient's consultant.

The consultant responsible for the patient must be informed as soon as practical that the team has been called.

Source: Goldhill DR, Worthington L, Mulcahy A, Tarling M, Sumner A. The patient-at-risk team: identifying and managing seriously ill ward patients. *Anaesthesia*. 1999;54:853–860.

Friday, 9 AM to 5 PM); or it may be a nurse-doctor team that performs a scheduled ward round of the hospital daily and accepts referrals; or it may be more similar to the MET in the form of a doctor-nurse team based in the ICU or emergency department that will respond to a call immediately, 24 hours a day, in the manner of a cardiac arrest team (34,42).

Upon receiving a call, the Medical Emergency Team is sent to review the patient immediately. The Outreach Team may respond immediately, or it may review patients as part of a planned ward round of the hospital, thereby constituting a delayed response (34). In one UK hospital, upon receiving a call triggered by MEWS, doctors were instructed to review a patient as soon as possible but no later than within 60 minutes (25). In some cases, the primary function of the Outreach Team is to follow up with patients who have been recently discharged from the intensive care unit (42–44).

Although variations to the MET calling criteria do exist, they generally consist of heart rate, systolic blood pressure, respiratory rate, level of consciousness, and "worried" criteria. The Outreach Team trigger systems consist of a profusion of complex calling criteria and grades of response, where criteria may include urine output, oxygen saturations, respiratory support, temperature, and sometimes biochemical markers. They may also include symptoms such as chest pain, markers of illness, and level of respiratory support (Table 10.7 and 10.8) (20,22,25,28,32,34,40).

TABLE 10.7. Modification of the MEWS

	Score						
	3	2	1	0	1	2	3
Heart rate; beats/min^{-1}		<40	41–50	51–100	101–110	111–130	>130
Systolic blood pressure; mmHg	<70	71–80	81–100	101–179	180–199	200–220	>220
Respiratory rate; breath/min^{-1}		<8	8–11	12–20	21–25	26–30	>30
Urine output in last 4h; ml	<80	80–120	120–200		>800		
Central nervous system			confused	awake and responsive	responds to verbal	responds to painful stimuli	unresponsive
Oxygen saturations; %	<85%	86–89%	90–94%	>95%			
Respiratory support/ Oxygen therapy	bi-PAP CPAP	hi-flow	oxygen therapy				

Temperature has been removed and replaced by the degree of respiratory support ranging from supplemental oxygen <15 L/min^{-1}, supplemental oxygen >15 L/min^{-1} (hi-flow) or requiring positive airway pressure support (CPAP / Bi-PAP).
Source: Pittard AJ. Out of our reach? Assessing the impact of introducing a critical care outreach service. *Anaesthesia*. 2003;58:882–885.

TABLE 10.8. Hodgetts' activation criteria for the Medical Emergency Team

Symptoms	4	3	2	1	0	1	2	3	4
Nurse concern			NEW						
Chest pain		NEW							
AAA pain		NEW							
Short of breath		NEW							
Physiology									
Pulse	<45	45–49	50–54	55–60	N	90–99	100–119	120–139	>139
Temp–core (rectal/tympanic)	<34	34.0–34.5	34.6–35.0	35.1–35.9			38.5–39.9	40.0–40.4	>40.4
RR (adult)	<8	8–9	10–11		R	21–25	26–30	31–36	>36
SpO₂ (O2)	<88	88–91	92–95		M				
SpO₂ (Air)	<85	86–89	90–93	94–96	A				
SBP (mmHg)	Falls to <90	Falls to 90–99	Falls to 100–110			Rises by 20–29	Rises by 30–40	Rises by >40	
or	Falls by >40	Falls by 31–40	Falls by 20–30		A	Pulse pressure narrows 10	Pulse pressure narrows >10		
GCS changes			13–14		N		confused or agitated		
Urine output	<10 mls/hr for 2 hrs	<20 mls/hr for 2 hrs					>250 mls/hr		
Biochemistry									
K⁺		<2.5	2.5–3.0				5.6–5.9	6.0–6.2	>6.2
Na⁺	<120	120–125	126–129			146–147	148–152	153–160	>160
pH	<7.21	7.21–7.25	7.26–7.30	7.31–7.34		7.46–7.48	7.49–7.50	7.51–7.60	>7.60
pCO₂ (acute changes)		<3.5	3.5–3.9	4.0–4.4				6.1–6.9	>6.9
SBE	<–5.9	0.9	1	–16.7					
pO₂ (acute change)	<9.0	9.0–9.4	9.5–9.9	10-Nov					
Creatinine						121–170	171–299	300–440	>440
Hb	<80	80–89	90–100						
Urea			<2	2.0–2.4		7.6–20	21–30	31–40	>40

Source: Hodgetts TJ, Kenward G, Vlachonikalis IG, Payne S, Castle N. The identification of risk factors for cardiac arrest and formulation of activation criteria to alert a medical emergency team. *Resuscitation*. 2002;54:125–131.

Some of the teams, such as the Patient-At-Risk Team described in a study by Goldhill (1999) (8) and the Medical Emergency Team as described by Hodgetts (2002) (40), are hybrids of the MET and Outreach Team approaches.

The MET as a Way Forward

The MET system reinforces who and what physiologically constitutes a critically ill patient, and therefore helps to direct attention to those at risk. Along with the ongoing overall hospital education and awareness processes that a MET system entails, this means that the staff becomes more skilled and confident in their initial response to critically ill patients. They also no longer have to deal with these extremely stressful situations—and with their potentially adverse outcomes—alone. It may be these more intangible benefits that explain the positive attitude of nursing staff toward the MET concept (45).

The problems of suboptimal care and preventable death in hospitals have been identified in many countries around the world; they are real, and they must be constructively addressed. We need to direct our attention to devising ways of providing effective and timely care to all critically ill and at-risk patients in the hospital, rather than only to those located within the designated critical care areas. The MET system is a promising step forward in this direction.

References

1. Brennan TA, Leape LL, Laird NM, Hebert L, Localio AR, Lawthers AG. Incidence of adverse events and negligence in hospitalized patients: results of the Harvard Medical Practice Study I. N Engl J Med. 1991;324:370–376.
2. Wilson RM, Runciman WB, Gibberd RW, Harrison BT, Newby L, Hamilton JD. The Quality in Australian Health Care study. Med J Aust. 1995;163:458–471.
3. Hillman K, Bishop G, Bristow P. Expanding the role of intensive care medicine. Vincent JL, ed. In: Yearbook of Intensive Care and Emergency Medicine. Berlin: Springer-Verlag; 1996:833–841.
4. Thoburn E, Norris P, Flores R, Goode S, Rodriguez E, Adams V. System care improves trauma outcome: patient care errors dominate reduced preventable death rate. J Emerg Med. 1993;11:135–139.
5. Lundberg JS, Perl TM, Wiblin T, et al. Septic shock: an analysis of outcomes for patients with onset on hospital wards versus intensive care units. Crit Care Med. 1998;26:1020–1024.
6. Blow O, Magliore L, Claridge JA, Butler K, Young JS. The golden hour and the silver day: detection and correction of occult hypoperfusion within 24 hours improves outcome from major trauma. J Trauma. 1999;47:964–969.
7. Rivers E, Nguyen B, Havstad S, et al. Early goal-directed therapy in the treatment of severe sepsis and septic shock. N Engl J Med. 2001;345:1368–1377.

8. Goldhill DR, Worthington L, Mulcahy A, Tarling M, Sumner A. The patient-at-risk team: identifying and managing seriously ill ward patients. *Anaesthesia*. 1999;54:853–860.
9. Department of Health (UK). Critical care outreach. 2003.
10. Wachter RM, Goldman L. The hospitalist movement 5 years later. *JAMA*. 2002;287:487–494.
11. Buist MD, Moore GE, Bernard SA, Waxman BP, Anderson JN, Nguyen TV. Effects of a medical emergency team on reduction of incidence of and mortality from unexpected cardiac arrests in hospital: preliminary study. *BMJ*. 2002;324:387–390.
12. Bellomo R, Goldsmith D, Uchino S, et al. A prospective before-and-after trial of a medical emergency team. *Med J Aust*. 2003;179:283–287.
13. Bristow PJ, Hillman KM, Chey T, et al. Rates of in-hospital arrests, deaths, and intensive care admissions: the effect of a medical emergency team. *Med J Aust*. 2000;173:236–240.
14. Salamonson Y, Kariyawasam A, van Heere B, O'Connor C. The evolutionary process of Medical Emergency Team (MET) implementation: reduction in unanticipated ICU transfers. *Resuscitation*. 2001;49:135–141.
15. James P. Stress and adult learners. In: Athanasou JA, ed. *Adult Educational Psychology*. Aust.: Social Science Press; 1999:321–323.
16. Lawler PG. The do-not-attempt-resuscitation ("DNAR") order: a lever to improve outcome and deliver preventative care. *Anaesthesia*. 1999;54:923–925.
17. Hillman K, Alexandrou E, Flabouris M, Brown D, Murphy J, Daffurn K. Clinical outcome indicators in acute hospital medicine. *Clin Intensive Care*. 2000;11:89–94.
18. Braithwaite RS, DeVita MA, Mahidhara R, Simmons RL, Stuart S, Foraida M. Use of medical emergency team (MET) responses to detect medical errors. *Qual Saf Health Care*. 2004;13:255–259.
19. Odell M, Forster A, Rudman K, Bass F. The critical care outreach service and the early warning system on surgical wards. *Nurs Crit Care*. 2002;7:132–135.
20. Morgan RJ, Williams F, Wright MM. An early warning scoring system for detecting developing critical illness. *Clin Intensive Care*. 1997;8:100.
21. Goldhill DR. The critically ill: following your MEWS. *QJM*. 2001;94:507–510.
22. Rechner IJ, Odell M, Forster AL, et al. The use of MEWS as an outreach tool to identify hospital patients requiring critical care. *Intensive Care Med*. 2002;28(S1):S21.
23. Carberry M. Implementing the modified early warning system: our experiences. *Nurs Crit Care*. 2002;7:220–226.
24. Manimaran N, Baishev F, Kapila A, Odell M, Farouk R. Role of modified early warning score in elective colorectal resection. *Colorectal Dis*. 2003;5(suppl2:):29.
25. Subbe CP, Davies RG, Williams E, Rutherford P, Gemmell L. Effect of introducing the Modified Early Warning score on clinical outcomes, cardiopulmonary arrests and intensive care utilisation in acute medical admissions. *Anaesthesia*. 2003;58:797–802.
26. Stenhouse C, Coates S, Tivey M, Allsop P, Parker T. Prospective evaluation of a Modified Early Warning Score to aid earlier detection of patients developing critical illness on a general surgical ward. *Br J Anaesth*. 2000;84:663.

27. Subbe CP, Kruger M, Rutherford P, Gemmel L. Validation of a modified Early Warning Score in medical admissions. *QJM*. 2001;94:521–526.
28. Wright MM, Stenhouse CW, Morgan RJ. Early detection of patients at risk (PART). *Anaesthesia*. 2000;55:391–392.
29. Cooper N. Patient at risk! *Clin Med*. 2001;1:309–311.
30. Subbe CP, Hibbs R, Williams E, Rutherford P, Gemmel L. ASSIST: a screening tool for critically ill patients on general medical wards. *Intensive Care Med*. 2002;28(S1):S21.
31. Cook J, Phillips E, Singer M, Webb A, Adam S. Using algorithms in critical care outreach: UCLH Trust Patient Emergency Response Team (PERT) algorithm for heart rate >125. *Care Crit Ill*. 2002;18:158–159.
32. Ball C. Critical care outreach services—do they make a difference? *Intensive Crit Care Nurs*. 2002;18(5):257–260.
33. McArthur-Rouse F. Critical care outreach services and early warning scoring systems: a review of the literature. *J Adv Nurs*. 2001;36: 696–704.
34. Pittard AJ. Out of our reach? Assessing the impact of introducing a critical care outreach service. *Anaesthesia*. 2003;58:882–885.
35. Goldhill DR, McNarry A. Intensive care outreach services. *Curr Anaesth Crit Care*. 2002;13:356–361.
36. Robson W. An evaluation of the evidence base related to critical care outreach teams—2 years on from comprehensive critical care. *Intensive Crit Care Nurs*. 2002;18:211–218.
37. Braithwaite RS, DeVita M, Stuart S, Foraida M, Simmons RL. Can cardiac arrests be prevented in hospitalised patients? Results of a medical crisis response team (Condition C). *J Gen Intern Med*. 2003;18(suppl1):222–223.
38. Foraida MI, DeVita MA, Braithwaite RS, Stuart S, Brooks MM, Simmons RL. Improving the utilization of medical crisis teams (condition C) at an urban tertiary care hospital. *J Crit Care*. 2003;18:87–94.
39. Scales DC, Abrahamson S, Brunet F, et al. The ICU outreach team. *J Crit Care*. 2003;18:95–106.
40. Hodgetts TJ, Kenward G, Vlachonikalis IG, Payne S, Castle N. The identification of risk factors for cardiac arrest and formulation of activation criteria to alert a medical emergency team. *Resuscitation*. 2002;54:125–131.
41. Lee A, Bishop G, Hillman K, Daffurn K. The Medical Emergency Team. *Anaesth Intensive Care*. 1995;23:183–186.
42. Ball C, Kirkby M, Williams S. Effect of the critical care outreach team on patient survival to discharge from hospital and readmission to critical care: Non-randomised population based study. *BMJ*. 2003;327:1014–1016.
43. Leary T, Ridley S. Impact of an outreach team on re-admissions to a critical care unit. *Anaesthesia*. 2003;58:328–332.
44. Fox N, Rivers J. Critical care outreach team sees fall in cardiac arrests. *Nurs Times*. 2001;97:34–35.
45. Daffurn K, Lee A, Hillman K, Bishop G, Bauman A. Do nurses know when to summon emergency assistance? Intensive Crit Care Nurs. 1994;10:115–120.

11
Early Goal-Directed Therapy

David T. Huang, Scott R. Gunn, and Emanuel P. Rivers

Introduction

The transition from sepsis to severe disease frequently develops well before admission to an intensive care unit (ICU), often in the emergency department. However, optimal care may be delayed for many reasons, including lack of recognition, emergency department overcrowding, long wait times for ICU beds, or lack of intensive care technology and expertise in the emergency department. For years we have recognized that delay in care negatively impacts outcome for trauma, myocardial infarction, and stroke (1–3). Now there is growing evidence that treatment delay can also negatively impact outcome in sepsis (4,5). This chapter will review the evidence for early intervention in sepsis, models of delivery, and potential obstacles. Medical Emergency Teams (Mets) may provide a possible mechanism for providing a rapid, coordinated response to patients presenting to the hospital with signs of sepsis.

Early Goal-Directed Therapy

Recently, Rivers et al. showed that Early Goal-Directed Therapy (EGDT) provided in the emergency department at the most proximal stages of severe sepsis and septic shock produced significant outcome benefit (Table 11.1) (5). Although all the interventions stipulated by EGDT were commonly used ICU therapies, what was novel was earlier application of these therapies in the emergency department within 1 hour of presentation. EGDT is an algorithmic approach to resuscitation designed to correct and prevent the hemodynamic and oxygen delivery instability of severe sepsis/septic shock within the first 6 hours of hospital care (Figure 11.1). It is a resuscitation strategy based on early recognition and resolution of inadequate systemic oxygen delivery and subsequent global tissue hypoxia. EGDT targets achieving normal oxygen delivery by optimizing preload using central venous pressure monitoring, afterload using mean arterial

TABLE 11.1. Entry criteria for EGDT (5)

Clinical suspicion of infection
Plus
Two of 4 systemic inflammatory response syndrome (SIRS) criteria (1) Temperature ≥38°C or <36°C (2) Heart rate >90 beatsmin $^{-1}$ (3) Respiratory rate >20 breathsmin $^{-1}$ or $PaCO_2$ < 32 mmHg (4) White blood cell count >12 000ml $^{-1}$ or <4000ml $^{-1}$ or >10% immature forms
Plus either
Hypotension (systolic blood pressure <90 mmHg after a 30 mlkg $^{-1}$ bolus) or Arterial lactate >4 mmolL $^{-1}$

pressure, and oxygen delivery guided by central venous oxygen saturation ($S_{CV}O_2$) in order to ameliorate global tissue hypoxia.

Patients presenting to the emergency department with severe sepsis and septic shock were randomized to standard therapy versus an EGDT protocol. Mean emergency department length of stay was 6.3 hours versus 8.0 hours, respectively. The standard therapy group received volume resuscitation and vasoactive therapy guided by central venous pressure and arterial pressure monitoring. The EGDT group received the same volume resuscitation and vasoactive therapy, but resuscitation in this group was guided by $S_{CV}O_2$ monitoring (Edwards Lifesciences, Irvine, CA) to assess global tissue hypoxia despite normalized central venous pressure, blood pressure, and urine output. Additional fluid resuscitation, blood transfusions, ventilatory support, and inotropic therapy were used to reach a goal $S_{CV}O_2$ of 70%. All patients received the same standard of care after admission to the ICU, with no further involvement by the emergency department or the investigators. The intensive care clinicians who assumed care were blinded to the randomization order. A significant absolute hospital mortality reduction of 16% was observed in the EGDT group. The EGDT group also required significantly less mechanical ventilation and pulmonary artery catheterization after admission to the ICU. Of the patients who survived, the EGDT group had significantly shorter hospital and ICU lengths of stay.

Implementing EGDT

Implementing EGDT requires several factors: (1) early recognition of severe sepsis, (2) mobilization of resources for the required interventions, (3) performance of the interventions, (4) a continuous quality improvement (CQI) program, and (5) a continuing education program. As with any therapy, a collaborative team approach is required, with integration of medical, nursing, and support staff from both the emergency department and ICU. Effective EGDT teams are based on reliable mobilization of

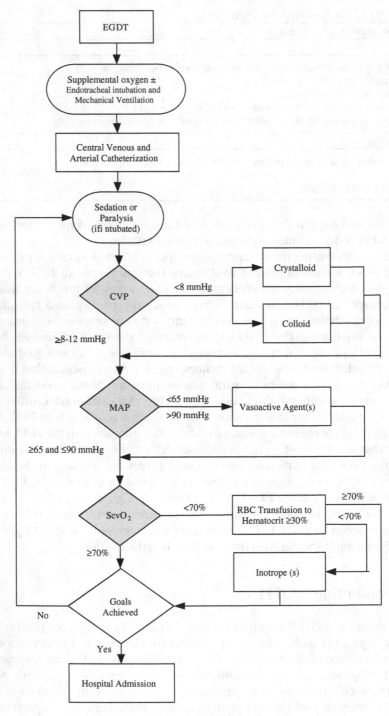

FIGURE 11.1. The EGDT protocol.

resources—both personnel and equipment—to perform the required tasks. In addition, an appropriately sized pool of health care providers (both physicians and nurses) who can effectively deliver EGDT is a key to successful implementation. Most importantly, a local "champion" is needed to be responsible for EGDT implementation and to communicate effectively with both the emergency department and ICU personnel.

Although all successful EGDT programs are collaborative between the emergency department and ICU, there are basically 3 models of implementation: (1) an emergency department-based model, (2) a mobile ICU, team-based model, and (3) a completely ICU-based model. In all models, it is the emergency department's responsibility to identify patients with sepsis that require EGDT. In the emergency department-based model, the emergency department staff would then perform all the necessary steps to deliver EGDT, before admission to the ICU. This is the model followed at Henry Ford Hospital in Detroit, MI, where the original study was carried out. However, this may not be practical or feasible for other hospitals.

For some hospitals, an ICU-based "mobile sepsis team" model may be a better fit. In this model, an ICU-based physician or a surrogate would be notified by the emergency department and would go there to begin delivery of EGDT, prior to transfer to the intensive care unit. EGDT would be continued from the emergency department to the ICU, and transfer to the ICU would occur as soon as possible. In this regard, the "sepsis team" is essentially a specialized MET, organized to provide EGDT. Hospitals that have already successfully implemented a MET may be able to expand its role to the provision of EGDT. This model requires significant cooperation between the emergency department and intensive care unit, along with 24-hour availability of health care providers capable of obtaining thoracic central venous access. It would likely work best in hospitals with a significant ICU bed wait-time in the face of the pressures for a rapid emergency department turnaround.

Lastly, an ICU-based model would entail emergency department notification and then as rapid transfer as possible to the ICU, where EGDT would be instituted only after arrival in the ICU. In effect, this model is the method that most hospitals follow for critically ill patients (i.e. emergency department recognition and initial stabilization of critically ill patients, followed by ICU admission for definitive care). The primary limitation of this model is that ICU beds may not be readily available (6), leading to delays in initiating potentially life-saving therapy.

Barriers to Implementation of EGDT

As with any new therapy, implementation of EGDT would face the familiar barriers of inertia, skepticism, and lack of resources (7). However, EGDT also faces several unique challenges. Successful delivery of EGDT requires open communication between the emergency department and intensive care unit, by both physician and nurses. Potential problems include miscommunication around such issues as billing and transfer of care between providers. Importantly, each department's autonomy must be respected to avoid resentment and non-cooperation. Both teams of health care providers (emergency department and ICU) need to develop a sense of joint "ownership" of patients presenting with sepsis, similar to how patients with ST-segment elevation myocardial infarction (STEMI) are managed today (early emergency department recognition, workup according to protocol and care in the emergency department, early cardiologist notification, with choice of revascularization technique determined by local resources) (8).

EGDT also requires the routine implementation of technologies that may be seen as "ICU-based" by many health care providers, such as measurements of central venous pressure, blood pressure (noninvasive and invasive), as well as continuous monitoring of $S_{CV}O_2$; up to 50% will be mechanically ventilated as well. The successful use of these technologies outside the ICU may require new levels of expertise among health care providers, outside of their usual domain.

Conclusion

In a single center, randomized controlled trial, EGDT has been shown to reduce mortality by 16% in patients presenting to the emergency department with sepsis or septic shock. However, widespread implementation of EGDT will require a collaborative effort between multiple disciplines (physicians, nurses, allied health personnel) as well as multiple specialties (emergency medicine and critical care medicine). This effort is best led by a local "champion" who can scientifically and diplomatically communicate with all the stakeholders. Models of EGDT delivery can be emergency department-based, team-based, or ICU-based. The team-based approach is similar to a MET and could be an extension of an already existing MET service. It may also be the most amenable to a fluid delivery of care from the emergency department to the intensive care unit. Other effective solutions may be dictated by local resources.

References

1. Nathens AB, Jurkovich GJ, Maier RV, et al. Relationship between trauma center volume and outcomes. *JAMA*. 2001;285:1164–1171.
2. Anderson HV, Willerson JT. Thrombolysis in acute myocardial infarction. *N Engl J Med*. 1993;329:703–709.
3. Marler JR, Brott T, Broderick J, Kothari R, Odonoghue M, Barsan W, et al. Tissue-plasminogen activator for acute ischemic stroke. *N Engl J Med*. 1995;333:1581–1587.

4. Han YY, Carcillo JA, Dragotta MA, et al. Early reversal of pediatric-neonatal septic shock by community physicians is associated with improved outcome. *Pediatrics*. 2003;112:793–799.
5. Rivers E, Nguyen B, Havstad S, et al. Early goal-directed therapy in the treatment of severe sepsis and septic shock. *N Engl J Med*. 2001;345:1368–1377.
6. Mccaig L, Burt C. National Hospital Ambulatory Medical Care Survey: 2001 emergency department summary. Advance data from vital and health statistics, Center for Disease Control and Prevention, National Center for Health Statistics; 2003: 335.
7. Berwick DM. Disseminating innovations in health care. *JAMA*. 2003;289: 1969–1975.
8. De Luca G, Suryapranata H, Ottervanger JP, Antman EM. Time delay to treatment and mortality in primary angioplasty for acute myocardial infarction: every minute of delay counts. *Circulation*. 2004;109:1223–1225.

12
Nurse-Led Medical Emergency Teams: A Recipe for Success in Community Hospitals

KATHY D. DUNCAN

When initiating the Medical Emergency Team (MET) concept and developing the team roles, often a critical care medicine physician is not an option. Community hospitals may not have physician coverage, either intensivists or hospitalists, in the facility around the clock. Instead, they must look within their current facility resources for rapid-response team personnel. When no physician is available, the development of the team requires not only delineation of specific team roles but also a treatment leader. This can be difficult because of the traditional professional roles in which health care workers have been constrained. In this chapter, I will describe characteristics and logistics of MET implementation in a community hospital, without an on-site physician readily available to be the team leader.

Identification of Hospital Resources

The development of team roles depends on several factors:

1. Availability: It is crucial that the staff of the hospital can call for a MET whenever needed: 24 hours per day, 365 days per year. Small community hospitals may have difficulty identifying available resources; they must look at several areas of the hospital that *could* provide resources to the Medical Emergency Team but currently do not. When the MET is called, the need is immediate, so the team members must be able to stop whatever they are doing and respond to the call. If the team members— especially the leader—have to prioritize tasks and make a snap decision, they may make incorrect choices. For example, they may choose to complete their current activity, and not make the priority the unseen patient who has begun to deteriorate, and thus the goal of intervening early in the patients' downhill spiral is doomed before the response even starts.

2. Accessibility: Calling the MET should be easy—1 number, 1 call. Staff members will not call for the "small things" if it is difficult. For example, if there are different numbers to call on the day shift or the weekend, it will

become more of a chore to call and more easy to make mistakes. Training becomes much more complex as the number of methods (phone numbers) to activate the crisis response increases. Simplicity and standardization are key. If the team is easy to reach, the staff is more likely to call at the first hint of trouble.

3. Ability/Skills: The team members must possess skills that match the tasks they are being asked to complete. It makes no sense to delegate the role of airway manager to someone who is untrained, inexperienced, and unskilled. To form a treatment plan, each team member must be able to assess the patient quickly and critically, perform their specified duties, and be confident in their decision-making skills. The team leader must not only be clinically competent in diagnosis and treatment of patients in crisis, but must also possess and be confident in the skills needed to lead a small group in crisis.

Nursing Leadership of Crisis Response Teams

With these factors in mind, an experienced nurse may best fill the leadership role in a small hospital. Critical care units, emergency departments, and post-anesthesia recovery rooms offer nurses great opportunities to develop vital skills, such as:

•The ability to accurately diagnose and collect key laboratory data;
•The ability to quickly assess a variety of complex patients;
•The opportunity to implement evidenced-based protocols and observe immediate patient outcomes;
•The ability to quickly respond and effectively perform in critical patient situations;
•Confidence in ability and motivation by the urgency of the patient populations;
•The ability to work with physicians in consultation rather than at the bedside.

Nurse-led Medical Emergency Teams have been successful in various hospital settings, from the small community hospital to the very large tertiary referral center. Jewish Hospital, a 442-bed facility in Louisville, KY, implemented a registered nurse (RN) Respiratory Therapist team in June 2003. Using 2 ICU-charge RNs and 1 respiratory therapist, the MET team responds to concerns about patient condition in the intermediate and medical surgical areas of the hospital within 10 minutes of a call. Several hospitals in Memphis, including Saint Francis Hospital and the Regional Medical Center, have also created nurse-led teams who have successfully treated numerous patients. METs are an important tool that can help to promote a culture of safety in the entire facility, and the absence of a physician on hand does not imply that METs cannot be implemented.

Support for the Nurse-Led Medical Emergency Team

A MET team that is led by a nurse must have structure and processes in place to provide resources for the patient. Three components of such structure and processes must include:

- Communication tools
- Specific protocols
- Chain of command process

With these components, resources will evolve and multiply as the MET process evolves and areas of need are identified. The facility will need to consistently review the trends noted in the calls and make adjustments to meet the needs of the patients.

Communication Tools: A common barrier is the ability of the bedside nurse to communicate a concern to the patient's physician, especially by telephone. Frequently the physician is not familiar with the patient, and the nurse will only relate the issue that is of concern. For example, the nurse may call and say "Mr. Smith's temperature is 101.4." The physician may ask for more information but without the entire picture of the patient, and this may result in an incorrect order of treatment, or in directing the nurse to "watch him and call if he gets worse." It is imperative that a nurse-led MET have a standardized, concise method of communicating with physicians by phone. This tool should be brief and include several aspects that construct a complete picture of the patient for the physician who is not in the room. For example, a tool utilizing the acronym SBAR (Situation, Background, Assessment, and Recommendation) allows the staff nurse or the leader of the MET to gather all the information and communicate all aspects to the physician (Table 12.1).

Specific Protocols: When a MET response is under the direction of an experienced nurse, protocols are essential because only certified nurse practitioners are allowed to prescribe medications in the absence of a physician. Treatment protocols and algorithms that have the force of physician orders can be used by nurses to deliver medications even when a physician is not present. These protocols are facility specific and approved by the appropriate departments and medical staff committees (Figure 12.1). At a minimum, protocols should be developed to address respiratory and cardiac events. They should be highly detailed: as specific as the approval to start an IV and move to a higher level of care. Saint Francis Hospital in Memphis has implemented several simple protocols that allow the MET registered nurse to order initial interventional and diagnostic procedures early in a call. Table 12.2 is an example of the procedure for the protocols, and Table 12.3 are actual physician orders that have been approved by the medical staff structure for use by the MET registered nurse. Dr Ed Taylor, critical care director, has been influential in guiding the medical staff of Saint Francis Hospital to anticipate the use of these protocols and the support of the team in

TABLE 12.1.

SBAR

Tool for calling physicians

Before calling the physician:
1. Assess the patient
2. Review the chart, ID correct physician
3. Read most recent progress notes
4. Heve available: chart, allergies list, MAR, lab results

S
Situation:
State your name and unit
"I am calling about: (patient name and room number)"
"The problem I am calling about is:"

B
Background:
State the admission diagnosis and date of admission.
State the pertient medical history.
Brief synopsis of treatment to date.

A
Assessment:
Most recent vital signs
BP:_____   Pulse:_____   Respirations:_____ Temp:_____
Any changes from prior assessments:
Mental status: Resp. rate/Quality   Pain
Skin color: Pulse/rhythm change Wound drainage
Neurologic changes: BP: N/V, output

R
Recommendation:
Do you think we should: (state what you would like to see done)
For example:
Transfer the patient to ICU?
Come to see the patient at this time?
Ask for a consultant to see the patient now?
Do you need any tests like CXR?ABG?EKG?CBC?

NOTIFICATION

Medical Response Team – patient care protocols

Stat Arterial Blood Gases
This may be ordered by the Medical Response Team registered nurse for the patient with
suspected pulmonary status deterioration. Patients who are anticoagulated with a continuous
heparin infusion or within 24 hours of thrombolytic or antiplatlet agent must have a
physician's order to obtain arterial blood gases by arterial puncture. Pressure will be held
unitl hemostasis occurs, at least 10 to 15 minutes or longer.

Stat Electrocardiograms
A 12 lead electrocardiogram may be ordered by the Medical Response Team registered
nurse for patients with severe prolonged chest pain and or significant monitor changes.
Chest pain emergency department physician will read the EKG if no cardiologist is
assigned to patient. The primar physician must be notified of 12-lead results.

Stat Portable Chest X-Rays
This may be ordered by the Medical Response Team registered nurse for the suspected
displacement of invasive lines, ET tube displacement, and for sever dyspnea or other signs
of respiratory distress.

Noninvasive Temporary Pacing (Transcutaneous Pacing)
Medical Response Team registered nurse may initiate noninvasive temporay pacing when
the patient condition requires.

Oxygen Therapy
Oxygen via binasal cannula at 2 L/min may be placed on any patient with chest pain or
cardiac equivalent, or for shortness of breath or increased work of breathing.

FIGURE 12.1. Saint Francis Hospital Patient care services policies and
procedures.

TABLE 12.2. Medical Response Team—patient care protocols

Stat arterial blood gases: This may be ordered by the Medical Response Team registered
nurse for the patient with suspected pulmonary status deterioration. Patients who are
anticoagulated with a continuous heparin infusion or within 24 hours of thrombolytic or
antiplatlet agent must have a physician's order to obtain arterial blood gases by arterial
puncture. Pressure will be held until hemostasis occurs, at least 10 to 15 minutes or longer.

Stat electrocardiograms: A 12-lead electrocardiogram (EKG) may be ordered by the
Medical Response Team registered nurse for patients with severe prolonged chest pain and
or significant monitor changes. Chest Pain Emergency Department physician will read the
EKG if no cardiologist assigned to patient. The primary physician must be notified of the
12-lead results.

Stat portable chest x-rays: This may be ordered by the Medical Response Team registered
nurse for the suspected displacement of invasive lines, endotracheal tube displacement, and
for sever dyspnea or other signs of respiratory distress.

Noninvasive temporary pacing (transcutaneous pacing): Medical Response Team registered
nurse may initiate noninvasive temporary pacing when the patient condition requires.

Oxygen therapy: Oxygen via binasal cannula at 2 L/min may be placed on any patient with
chest pain or cardiac equivalent or for shortness of breath or increased work of breathing.

TABLE 12.3.

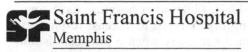 Saint Francis Hospital
Memphis

Medical Response Team protocols

Decreased level of consciousness	Respiratory distress
• Start saline lock • Pulse oximetry-oxygen to keep saturation above 92%. If history of COPD get oxygen saturation to 88-90% • If hemodynamically unstable** or orthostatic hypotensive give 250 mL bolus of normal saline • EKG • CBC, basic metabolic panel, urinalysis, arterial blood gas, accuchek, Physician Signature:_____ Date:_____ Time:_____	• Pulse oximetry-oxygen to keep saturation above 92% if history of COPD get oxygen saturation to 88-90%. • Arterial blood gas, chest Xray(for respiratory distress), complete blood count, complete metabolic panel • Begin nebulized albuterol 2.5 milligrams-one time treatment • Cardiac monitor if in moderate or serious distress • Start saline lock • Heart rate and oxygen saturation to be documented after albuterol treatment. Notify physician of HR above 140 or oxygen saturation less than 92 %. Physician Signature:_____ Date:_____ Time:_____
Chest Pain	**Seizures non-pediatric**
• Stat electrocardiogram and have read by critical care physician immediately • Place on cardiac monitor • Start saline lock • Pulse oximetry-oxygen to keep saturation above 92%. If history of COPD get oxygen Saturation to 88-90%. Physician Signature:_____ Date:_____ Time:_____	• IV saline lock • Pulse oximetry-oxygen to keep saturation above 92% if history of COPD get oxygen saturation to 88-90%. • Place on cardiac monitor • Accuchek • Anticonvulsant drug level if applicable • Pad bedrails Physician Signature:_____ Date:_____ Time:_____
Gastrointestinal bleed	**Additional Orders**
• Start IV with normal saline with large bore # 18 or larget at keep vein open • If patient is hemodynamically unstable**, start a second large bore IV and call critical care physicain to bedside • Send STAT complete blood count, complete metabolic panel, protime, PTT, and type and screen • If hemodynamically unstable**, change type and screen to tyep and crossmatch for 2 units packed red blood cells • electrocardiogram • Pulse oximetry • Place on cardiac monitor Physician Signature:_____ Date:_____ Time:_____	 Physician Signature:_____ Date:_____ Time:_____

** Hemodynamically Unstable: HR Greater than 120
or systolic blood pressure less than 90

providing urgent care for the patient. Missouri Baptist Hospital uses several Respiratory Care Protocols (Table 12.4), while other hospitals have competencies that enable a trained respiratory therapist to increase respiratory support and even intubate a patient if necessary when a physician is not available. Writing a protocol that calls for unavailable skills will be a fruitless exercise at the patient's bedside. Therefore the protocol development will guide the team development, and vice versa. While all team members should have critical care skills, they will be responding to a variety of sites such as an orthopedic floor, post-operative unit, or the radiology depart-

TABLE 12.4. Missouri Baptist Medical Center Respiratory Care Department oxygen therapy protocol

1. Purpose: To provide protocol-driven respiratory therapy to evaluate, treat, and monitor appropriate oxygen administration for all non-mechanically ventilated patients, with the intent of treating or preventing the symptoms and manifestations of hypoxia.
2. Patient type: All patients currently receiving oxygen will be evaluated with the following exclusions:
   • Patients receiving bleomycin treatments.
   • Patients with CO poisoning for first 12 hours.
   • Acute myocardial infarction patients for first 72 hours.
   • Premature infants.
   • Patients with specific orders not to change or titrate oxygen.
   • Patients using oxygen at home who have met home oxygen requirements established by doctor.
3. Clinical area: All patient care areas.
4. Equipment needed: Pulse oximeter.
5. Guidelines:
   A. The following guidelines will be used in selecting an appropriate oxygen delivery device:
      1. High-flow systems provide an adequate flow of oxygen to meet/exceed patients inspired flow rate needs.
      2. Low-flow systems will only provide flow of oxygen to supplement the patients inspired flow rate needs.
      3. Criteria for use of a high-flow system:
         a. Required $FIO_2 > 0.45$.
         b. Tidal volume <300 ml.
         c. Respiratory rate >25 breaths/minute.
   B. Types of low-flow devices:
      1. Cannula
         a. Delivers FIO_2: approximately 0.24–0.45.
         b. Most appropriate initial device for patients with chronic obstructive pulmonary disease.
      2. Simple oxygen mask: Delivers FIO_2: 0.40–0.50
      3. Non-rebreather mask: Delivers FIO_2: 0.60–0.95+
   C. Types of high-flow devices:
      1. Venturi mask: Delivers FIO_2: 0.24–0.50
      2. High-flow aerosols: Delivers 0.24–0.95+

ment, and the floor staff must remain and participate in the MET response to provide important history, assessments, and specialty knowledge that the team may not possess.

Chain of Command Process: In a community hospital most likely there will be limited physician resources in the hospital during the off hours. If staff is unable to reach the patient's physician, the nurse leader must be well versed in the facility's physician chain of command. An important task for the MET leadership and the physician leadership is to work out the chain of command and document it for ready reference by MET members. The nurse leader must be able to demonstrate the ability to use the established chain of command to get the physician direction needed. Some medical staff departments have included intensivists, medical directors, and emergency department physicians as resources for the MET, so that treatment is not delayed.

Benefits of a Nurse-Led Medical Emergency Team

Experienced nurses in the leadership role of a Medical Emergency Team bring many benefits to the team and the MET process. Nurses spend more time with patients than any other health care team member, and often have an instinctive and experiential ability to sense a patient's deterioration although they may lack the diagnostic skills to understand why. Experienced critical care nurses also demonstrate a patient-centered focus: a steadfast determination to get the failing patient the treatment needed.

In an acute care hospital environment, often staff nurses are overwhelmed with multiple and complex patients. When a MET is called to assess a patient, and the team leader is a colleague with a sense of collaboration for the good of the patient, everyone wins. The call to a MET should not trigger feelings of judgment as to what did or did not happen before the call—that someone may have missed a crucial element in the assessment, or that the nurse does not know what he or she is doing. The nurse leader—the right nurse leader—will keep the discussion and actions focused on what is best for the patient and refrain from judgment or criticisms. This attitude of mentoring is a great learning opportunity for the staff.

It is important that the MET not "take over" the care of the deteriorating patient. The role of the MET is to provide needed resources emergently to prevent death. Staff nurses who have cared for this patient for possibly the last several days will not learn from the event if they are pushed out of the way and the MET takes over completely. The team led by an experienced nurse should be able to guide that nurse to assist with or observe the assessment, intervention, and communication with the physician. This spirit of collaboration may be lost with a physician-led team (although some hospitals delegate an ICU nurse to include the floor nurse into the response team). Frequently a physician is focused on inserting a central line or getting the patient to the operating room quickly, and consequently may not nurture the needs of the nursing staff. A nurse leader with the right attitude will assist the staff nurse in becoming more confident and comfortable in managing patients in crisis, and these skills will benefit the patients the staff nurse cares for in the future.

A second benefit is that this is a proven mechanism to respond to patients in crisis when physician resources are not available. At Saint Francis Hospital, the MET has received over 700 calls in just under 10 months (Table 12.5), and in the majority of these calls the patient did not require an admission to the critical care area. The nurse-led team spends an average of 62 minutes on each call, assessing, implementing treatment plans, coaching, and observing outcomes, thus rescuing the patients from an acute event and often an ICU stay. Dave Archer, CEO at Saint Francis, states: "The Medical Emergency Team has had a tremendous impact on nursing self-image and morale by having the needed resources readily available." Institutions who do not have physician resources thus should be able to conclude from this report that METs are both possible and effective when staffed and led by non-physician health care professionals.

TABLE 12.5.

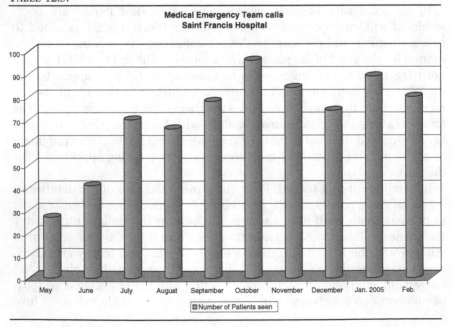

Medical Emergency Team calls
Saint Francis Hospital

Nursing Leadership and Mentoring after the MET Call

Several models of nurse-led METs provide a follow-up visit after the initial MET call is completed. The follow-up visit is made by the nurse 12 to 24 hours after the initial visit and is an intentional redundancy that provides another safety net for the patient. During this visit, the nurse assesses the patient and reviews the events that have occurred since the visit, to ensure the interventions were effective and the level of care is appropriate for the patient. This also provides an opportunity for a debriefing with the staff involved in the patient's care. The discussion and review of the patient during a less-urgent time provides a great opportunity for learning for staff members, and is a rare opportunity for collaboration of professionals to discuss the care of their patient. These discussions build relationships between nurses from different areas of the hospital and offer an opportunity to work together and learn from each other. This follow-up evaluation is noted on the call tool, which is used in data collection and given to the front-line management team of the area initiating the call for further learning.

Data Collection

Data should be gathered from each MET call; for this purpose we use a "MET call tool." This data can be analyzed later at the individual unit level as well as at the hospital level to identify a variety of system failures. The completed tool should describe the MET event in several stages:

•Reason for the call (why did the staff call)
•Assessment of the patient (Patient clinical findings)
•Background of the patient (Medical history and events leading up to the deterioration)
•Recommendations and interventions (Treatments delivered)
•Outcomes (for example, transferred to a higher level of care, cardiac or respiratory arrest, and survival)

Hospital leadership can use these completed sheets as case studies to validate the recognition of the subtle changes in the patient and the call to the MET, which may have saved the patient's life. Validation that the MET call was beneficial gives nurses the confidence to respond to their instincts and ensures this behavior will be repeated. By reinforcing the behavior of attempting to rescue the patient, it will encourage placement of calls and making calls even earlier in the patient's deterioration.

Review of the data collected from MET calls by a nurse leader may reveal system failures that can be helpful in finding subtle problems or rare but significant events that fail to reach "statistical significance." Retrospective review of multiple calls may demonstrate trends that need to be addressed through hospital channels, including:

Missouri Baptist Medical Center

Rapid Response Team Record

Date:_____ Room Number / Location:_____ Time called:_____ Arrival time:_____ Event ended:_____

Primary reason for call:	Situation: _____

Primary reason for call:

☐ Staff concerned / worried
  Specify:_____

☐ HR less than 40   ☐ HR greater than 130
☐ SBP less than 90 mmHg ☐ Acute mental status change
☐ RR less than 8   ☐ RR greater than 24
☐ SpO$_2$ less than 90% ☐ FiO$_2$ 50% or greater
☐ Acute significant bleed ☐ Seizures
☐ Failure to respond to tx

Recommendations/interventions:

Airway/breathing   Circulation

☐ Oral airway   ☐ IV fluid bolus
☐ Suctioned   ☐ Blood
☐ Nebulizer treatment   ☐ electrocardiogram
☐ Intubated   ☐ CPR
☐ NPPV   ☐ Defibrillation
☐ Bag mask   ☐ Cardioversion
☐ O2 mask/nasal   ☐ No intervention
☐ ABG
☐ CXR
☐ No intervention

Medication(s):_____

Other interventions
Specify:_____

Outcome: ☐ Stayed in room   ☐ Transferred to ICU
☐ Transferred to SDU   ☐ Other:_____

☐ Notified physician:_____ Time:_____
                    (name)

Signature:
PA_____

RN_____

RT_____

Situation: _____

Background: _____

Assessment:

Temp____ BP____ HR____ RR____ SpO$_2$____ GCS____

Follow-up report:
_____

Signature:_____Date/Time:_____

FIGURE 12.3. Data collection tool.

1. Communication failures (for example, in nurse-to-physician or nurse-to-nurse communication, communication between departments, or failure to reach the provider)
2. Recognition failures (may include failure to note a change in heart rate, blood pressure, respiratory status, behavior change, or change in level of consciousness)

3. Planning failures (level of care issues, failure to diagnose, or failure to assess or reassess the patient)

Once such trends are identified, nursing leadership can implement changes to address these system-wide failures and improve processes. For example, failure to recognize a crisis might lead to the development of mnemonic tools like pocket cards or posters, and the institution of educational opportunities to foster better knowledge and performance. The use of data gleaned from MET events and the institutional response to shortcomings can make the hospital environment safer for all patients. Missouri Baptist Medical Center in St. Louis uses a data collection tool (Figure 12.3) that incorporates these core elements as well as important elements needed for outcomes measurement.

Conclusion

Nurses can lead MET responses. Special tools may be necessary to make them most effective, including communication pathways, treatment protocols, specialized training in crisis response skills, physician chain of command documentation, and post-event debriefing of involved staff to improve patient care. The outcomes of nurse-led MET programs and physician-led MET programs are similar, and no hospital should refuse to implement METs simply because no physician is available to respond. Indeed, nursing brings a unique perspective to the leadership role in a MET process. Experience, instinct, determination, and a spirit of collaboration with the nurse at the bedside are attributes that can sustain a MET process and over time can change the environment of the facility.

13
ICU Without Walls: A New York City Model

VLADIMIR KVETAN and BRIAN CURRIE

Chance favors a prepared mind.

—Louis Pasteur

Introduction

This chapter is a case study of development of the critical care medicine (CCM) service and outreach system at a major university hospital in New York over the past 20 years. While the focus of this review will be the major milestones in development of the CCM team activity outside of the intensive care unites (ICUs), general developments and influences will be briefly discussed as well. This review makes a point of the need for and feasibility of close and effective collaboration between clinical services and institutional administration based on common language and goals. The case study is meant to be a useful teaching tool for young intensivists and administrators, to help them learn from our experiences and apply them to institutional benefit. The core references may be routine for practicing intensivists, but the goal includes having them available to non-clinician administrators. Montefiore Medical Center currently staffs 2 university hospitals with 66 adult medical and surgical ICU beds and a 24/7 in-house team of attending intensivists and fellows in an Accreditation Council for Graduate Medical Education (ACGME)-accredited training program. It provides an ICU-without-walls concept of care, with rapid bedside response to all acute requests outside of the ICU within 30 minutes. The CCM service system has been ranked in the top 100 as 1 of 2 national benchmark critical care hospitals in New York City and has demonstrated positive performance parameters including a 45% increase in emergency department volume and elimination of ambulance diversion over the past 5 years, in addition to the best regional outcomes in surgical specialties targeted for increased intensivist staffing. The ICU-without-walls model allowed for critical care medicine physicians to practice their skills to maximal institutional benefits, and the management structure responded by allocating the necessary resources based on objective performance. The hospital was the most profitable hospital in New York City in 2003.

Under the urging of the committed Leapfrog group of the Fortune 500 companies and the Institute for Healthcare Improvement, recently mainstream business publications such as the *Wall Street Journal* have begun to pay attention to the stakes of mismanaged ICU stay. Yet critical care medicine is one of the most exciting and highest impact areas of medicine that consumes some 10% of hospital beds and 30% of hospital budgets in the United States, with failure to reach expedited conclusion of stay resulting in 10% of ICU outlier patients consuming 50% of ICU fiscal resources (1). There is a large regional and international variation in allocation of resources to critical care medicine service. The potential human cost of not using therapies known to reduce mortality in ICU patients has been estimated at more than 167000 lives per year (2). As of the last analysis, up to 54000 patients in the United States die in hospitals due to medical error secondary to inadequate ICU physician staffing; this is accentuated by analysis showing a growing shortage of ICU physicians (and nurses), and the simultaneous graying of America with the potential for a doubling of the Medicare ICU population by the end of the decade. The clinical and fiscal benefits of high levels of intensivist staffing have been proven clearly for the ICU populations (3–5); the problem is to document the benefit of intensivists outside of the ICU.

Currently only 1 academic department of critical care medicine in the United States, at the University of Pittsburgh, has as one of its strategic goals the development of a primary, rather than subspecialty, training track for critical care. This service is based in a surgical intensive care unit system comprising 25% of primary university hospital beds heavily staffed by internists, with separate pulmonary and critical care service responsible for medical ICUs. The department has recently developed a functional 24/7 external response team known as Condition C (for "crisis") (6,7). While this department is an academic powerhouse and a great academic career goal for young intensivists, it also points to the need to offer other models of CCM service that unite adult ICUs under a standardized umbrella with alternate management structures. One of the goals of this discussion is to consider CCM model options ranging from a full academic department to a highly functional community hospital. This case study demonstrates how patients' needs may change over time within a hospital, and that the way hospitals meet patient needs may require different strategies and resources.

Montefiore CCM Service: Lessons Learned During Its Development

For 20 years the CCM service has been active in the provision of training to critical care medicine fellows and delivery of care to adult patients from all specialties under a unified philosophy. In many ways, the positive developments are based on the evolving needs of the fellowship program, which has graduated some 200 intensivists to date. The discussion below is designed in 5-year milestones of learning and development.

1983–1988

During the first 5 years, CCM service focused on developing a training program with 4 fellows at the primary university hospital, with 20 medical-surgical ICU beds for the sickest multi-organ failure cases, and a nearby community teaching hospital with a 20-bed medical-surgical ICU. Prior to institution of a unified team with 24/7 in-house fellow coverage, the performance parameters demonstrated length of stay more than double that of the current, over-utilization of technical and clinical services, and mortality almost 4 times higher than current (8). Aggressive collaboration of anesthesiology, medicine, surgery, and nursing produced rapid improvement, and management became comfortable with critical care problem solving and allowing new graduates to manage resources. In addition, the impact of staffing on mortality for syndromes such as septic shock was demonstrated at the teaching affiliate (9). The program was one of the first in New York State to be accredited by ACGME by the end of this period. Administrative collaboration focused on adjusting the system to implement a diagnostic-related group (DRG)-based method of hospital compensation and chronic respiratory failure services were provided throughout the hospital without geographic clustering through the institution of respiratory therapy/CCM ward rounds. During this period, CCM service team responded to cardiac arrest team calls and the bedside critical care consult response was limited to the sickest patients only, frequently those already intubated and on vasopressors, with the acceptance rate in excess of 80%. This milestone was a fairly standard development for most services in the United States.

1988–1993

At this stage, CCM service had a critical mass of staff and was able to provide rapid response to national and international emergencies and disasters requiring deployment of a fully equipped and staffed ICU team overseas in an unfamiliar environment (10–12). This required our service to organize and deploy both general and specialized teams in situations with marginal infrastructure support. An intense period of learning followed, with staff members developing the ability to function outside of the stable academic ICU environment for prolonged periods. The CCM service went through a period of national recognition and efforts were made to organize volunteer teams based in the training programs that were willing to work outside of their ICU silos. A number of academic relationships in trauma surgery and anesthesia, emergency medicine, and military medicine, led to new teaching models, such as daylong tabletop crisis management simulations provided for a number of professional societies. Internally, there was expansion of intensivist presence in providing more general and specialized consultative and procedural services, including nutritional support and transport. This milestone provided management with insight into the dynamics of a critical care team and its ability to respond to most needs. The major lessons during this milestone included building of self-confidence to function outside of the ICU silo structure, to the point of providing ICU services for prolonged periods away from the primary hospitals.

1993–1998

The CCM service identified 3 major areas requiring improvement for better performance. The first was based on the analysis of the fellowship training guidelines from the perspective of nonclinical education in administration and management (13). The CCM specialty required high-grade skills for management of large portions of hospital budgets, yet neither curriculum nor training for program directors was developed or implemented. The CCM service organized a series of national and regional postgraduate courses and symposia on business management of ICUs, with faculty including a number of intensivists working as presidents/CEOs and chairs at other institutions (14,15). This program allowed for the closely knit group of faculty and fellows to apply management standards acceptable to administration. While not the first to recognize the need for administrative training in critical care medicine, the CCM service developed a focus on physician training and faculty competence in leadership and performance. The second need identified was that while most ICU care in developed countries is practiced in community hospitals without high-intensity academic intensivist staffing, most critical illness worldwide is based in the populations of developing countries. While developed countries routinely participate in educational and consensus programs allowing them to share scientific principles and advances, they do not necessarily include intensivists from developing countries. The CCM service worked through the chair of the International Liaison Committee of the Society of Critical Care Medicine with the aim of developing functional relationships with the 54 CCM societies worldwide (16). It identified the need for inclusion of the CCM societies of developing countries and has organized consensus conferences directed toward countries with limited health care budgets and ICU resources. In addition, the faculty of the critical care medicine symposium established a journal, which is now the official journal of the Western Pacific Association of Critical Care Medicine (17). Although the CCM service had successful training fellowship rotations in all relevant specialties, it was deemed time for organizational expansion. The major learning was the ability to reach consensus and unification of language in a challenging environment. At the same time local pressure was mounting in the area of graduate medical education funding: Montefiore was responsible for one of the largest graduate medical education budgets in the United States, and restrictions on training positions as well as in the clinical time allowed for during training were having a real impact. The management team also sponsored this milestone, and this allowed the CCM service team to advance its skills in resource management and consensus development. The CCM outreach system was providing a stable rate of some 200, consultations per month, but it was clear that redesigned pressures, mandated by the institution in the 1980s as part of overall reorganization into care centers and service lines, would require increased CCM service presence in potential bottleneck areas such as the emergency department, postoperative care units, and specialty area units such as neurosciences. The third major area of focus was the recognition of the need for close collaboration between ICU physicians and nurses in delivering a coordinated response to critically ill patients outside of the ICU. During this period, a pilot study using a senior ICU nurse responding jointly with an ICU physician to calls showed optimal results for the interventions and for the satisfaction of family members and external teams.

1998–2003

The institutional management team challenged the CCM service team to completely redesign delivery of ICU services. It was recognized that the organizational models of anesthesia and critical care and of pulmonary and critical care as academic divisions did not fit. After a period of analysis, the CCM team committed itself to the ICU-without-walls concept, based on non-geographic critical care, thus reducing dependence on residencies while increasing the non-physician practitioner teams, uniting all adult ICUs into a single administrative and clinical entity, and demonstrating regional competitive performance status. Close cooperation was established between the CCM service team and the vice president for medical affairs, the vice president for emergency medicine services, the vice president and chief operations officer, and medical director. In addition, external relationships with a number of community and teaching hospitals, which were being provided with clinical teaching services, were eliminated. The focus was on collaboration in achieving drastic increases in emergency department volume and eliminating diversion-related losses, and improving safety of care in surgical and medical environments by reducing the risk of medical errors that result in multi-organ failure. The model of a service line that reports directly to the corporate leadership and provides administrative, clinical, and academic services to all departments and care centers based on need was chosen. CCM team was granted clinical department budgetary status and responsibility, with frequent governance reporting. The ability to provide critical care clinical response anywhere in the hospital was an absolute priority—5 years ago, the CCM team was providing 18 hours per day faculty coverage and 24/7 coverage by fellows in training.

The institutional management team was well apprised of the 1999 Institute of Medicine's *To Err is Human* report, as well as the 1999 Committee on Manpower for Pulmonary and Critical Care Societies report on critical care manpower and the 2000 Leapfrog Group Fortune 500 response urging computerized physician order entry and intensive care unit physician staffing; it was also familiar with the 2001 Agency for Healthcare Research and Quality and the Clinical Advisory Board recommendations on critical care (18,19). Conservative analysis of clinical literature on the impact of staffing intensity and distribution resulted in gradual and consistent allocation of increased resources, mainly payroll support. In the United States, the Leapfrog Group and Health Grades reported the minimal staffing threshold was reached in 1998, and computerized physician order entry was fully implemented by early 2002 with the institution being among the top 3.1% of the most computerized medical centers. While intensive care unit physician staffing reached 24/7 faculty staffing, simply focusing on ICU care and adjusting staffing to acuity was not thought to be effective.

The key became expansion of the ICU-without-walls team of intensivists, who are in-house 24/7 and provide 30-minute bedside response to all critically ill adults at Montefiore outside of the ICU. The benefit of a rapid response of under 5 minutes attending to the high-acuity and at-risk patient (those in cardiac and neurologic surgery, patients with ventricular assist devices or heart transplants, etc.) was obvious and validated. Our own experience with CCM consultant response was carefully compared with the potential of other systems, such as the Outreach Team in the United Kingdom, and the Australian and New Zealand Intensive Care Society MET team (20–24). The scope was rapidly expanded from highest severity response and triage to provision of a high-level progressive care and procedural services.

The major advance was collaboration with the emergency medicine department directed at eliminating ambulance diversion due to ICU bottlenecks, which resulted in a 45% increase in emergency department visits, a 20% increase in institutional discharges, but only a 5% increase in CCM discharges; similar focus was established at other major institutions (25) (Figure 13.1). The consultation service arranged ICU admissions for 50% of patients, for whom primary services were requested by the CCM team. The remaining 50% were triaged to either intermediate care after stabilization or comfort care with the palliative team. When we reviewed the impact of the triage system, the CCM-sensitive DRG analysis using the new Clinical Looking Glass information system showed no increase in length of stay or 30-day mortality. The volume of calls to the CCM consultants increased to over 4000 formal calls per year (Figures 13.2 and 13.3). At this point, the CCM resources were overwhelmed. While nursing leadership was able to provide a senior CCM nurse to function as a part of the outreach team for a number of years, with focus on managing the most unstable and reversible patients prior to transfer to the ICU, this capability was lost due to a continued critical care nursing shortage. In general, an integrated response from an intensivist physician and an intensivist nurse provide the best performance of the outreach team. The CCM team strongly supported

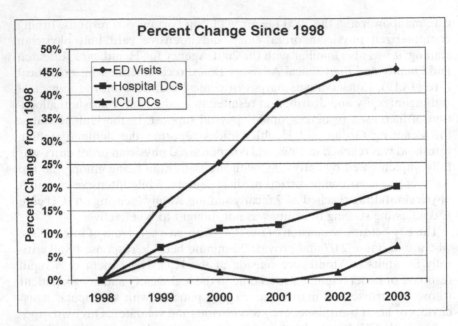

FIGURE 13.1. Impact of ICU without walls within the hospital emergency department and ward discharge structure.

the addition of a palliative care service in 2001, and surgical hospitalist service in 2002. The institution had already established a teaching hospitalist model in medicine, which was instrumental in providing the hospital with the best length-of-stay results in our region. The palliative care service was fully integrated with the CCM service. The primary university hospital set up a modular staffing pattern for all 3 adult ICUs with 34 ICU beds, and

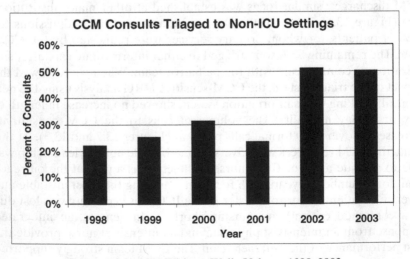

FIGURE 13.2. ICU Without Walls, Volume 1998–2003.

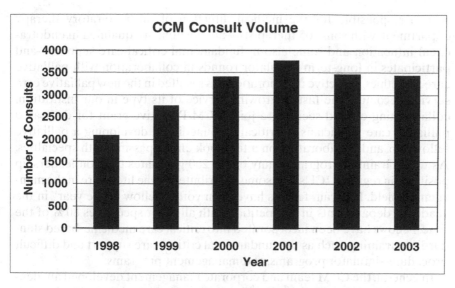

FIGURE 13.3. ICU Without Walls, Triage 1998–2003.

after establishing 24/7 staffing, it was also introduced in the secondary university hospital with 28 ICU beds. The secondary university hospital was expanding a new 911 ER, and removing the medicine house-staff from the 14-bed medical-surgical intensive care unit. The CCM team was instructed to develop staffing based on attendings, fellows, physician assistants, and a limited number of daytime anesthesia residents. A full-time team for the adjacent 18-bed cardiovascular intensive care unit was established. The CCM service for all adult ICUs was unified and standardized; rotation of faculty between all 5 ICUs and both hospitals created team recognition standard. It should be noted that while the ICU beds were being increased nationally, this medical center remained at the same ICU-bed level for more than 10 years.

During this period, the CCM team covering 5 adult ICUs and the CCM consultants received external risk adjusted recognition with the Solucient Top 100 ICU study published in 2001 comparing the 6100 US hospitals, and more specifically, the US hospitals with CCM fellowship programs (26). Montefiore was 1 of only 2 national benchmark hospitals identified in New York City. After additional investment in 24/7 coverage and supplementary training, the Alliance 2004 Report Card/New York Department of Health noted that the outcomes of coronary artery bypass surgery in our secondary university hospital were the best in New York State, at 0.8% mortality, and neurosurgery craniotomy results were the best in New York City (27).

CCM service currently functions as an institutional product/service line reporting to the vice president of medical affairs, who is responsible for coordinating the governance and collaborative practice issues among all consumers of level-1 ICU services including the emergency department, medicine, surgery, neurosurgery, and cardiothoracic surgery. The CCM team is also responsible for the medical direction of the respiratory therapy department, with some 65 therapists—all of whom are qualified in endotracheal intubation and some also in fundamental critical care support—and participates in long-term ventilator rounds in collaboration with palliative care and ethics. Effective collaboration has resulted in the new palliative care service becoming the fastest growing service of its type in our institution, collaborating on and securing a joint CCM-Palliative grant for dedicated palliative care physicians in critical care medicine, developing a palliative fellowship, and collaborating on a textbook encompassing both specialties. As to the training program, many of the 200 graduates took on leadership positions in regional ICUs, and some contributed to the literature in the management field. Program fellows have been voted "fellow of the year" in the academic departments in competition with all other specialties 80% of the time. Fellows have been incorporated into critical care medicine-based standardized training, such as the fundamental critical care support and difficult procedure-simulator programs, and management programs.

In general, the CCM team and corporate management developed an identical agenda, and implemented it to institutional benefit. Advancing the 24/7-coverage system in conjunction with mandatory ICU-without-walls response allowed for performance to improve in areas beyond simple ICU-based control. The supply crisis of physician staffing (28) was managed by maintaining an accredited fellowship program and a pool of competent graduates for recruitment, in addition to the consistent additions of external experts with backgrounds in transplant and cardiothoracic surgery, nephrology, infectious diseases, and pulmonary medicine. Economy of scale evaluations showed that while the service of 16 intensivists is an expensive undertaking, unification allowed for reduction in redundant coverage and expenses and the economic argument of intensivist staffing was accepted (5). Demand crisis was handled with a system for rapid delivery of critical care medicine expertise to the bedside anywhere (29), including stabilization, triage, and the continuous ability to provide alternate, post-stabilization routine hospitalization or humane comfort measures. And an expanding program targeting patient-family satisfaction, ranging from installing Internet stations and videoconferencing phones in the waiting rooms to a functional critical care medicine-ethics-palliative care team, has been established.

Where does the CCM service go clinically from this point, and what is the role of the ICU-without-walls outreach system? After implementing high-intensity staffing, computerized physician order entry, consensus standards, unification of medical and surgical systems, electronic morning report teleconference, and developing non-physician teams, the major opportunities are in exploring technology advances (crisis simulation, telemedicine [30]), options for regionalization of service (trauma and neonatal ICU models) urged by national experts (31), and quantitative triggers for services such as the consult team (MET standard). The business rationale for high-intensity intensivist staffing, and institutional profitability of the service/product line was developed and implemented some 5 years before the recent series of excellent publications (32), but continuing time-motion analysis and adjustments of staffing to activity are required. Our service collaborated with others on assessing the national level of administrative training and problem solving in critical care medicine fellowships; it is clear that improved management training for the leaders of tomorrow will be required (33). We hope that this case study offers a learning tool for practical development of CCM service for large teaching hospitals and an alternative approach to model development.

References

1. Annual New York metropolitan symposium on managing critical care medicine systems: chronic critical illness. Syllabus. Kvetan V, chair. Montefiore Medical Center/Albert Einstein College of Medicine; 2004.
2. Pronovost PJ, Rinke ML, Emery K. Interventions to reduce mortality among patients treated in intensive care units. *J Crit Care.* 2004;19:158–164.
3. Pronovost PJ, Jenckes MW, Dorman T, et al. Organizational characteristics of intensive care units related to outcomes of abdominal aortic surgery. *JAMA.* 1999;281:1310–1317.
4. Young MP, Birkmeyer JD. Potential reduction in mortality rates using an intensivist model to manage intensive care units. *Effective Clin Pract.* 2000;3:284–289.
5. Pronovost PJ, Needham DM, Waters H. Intensive care unit physician staffing: financial modeling of the Leapfrog standard. *Crit Care Med.* 2004;32:1247–1253.
6. Foraida MI, DeVita MA, Braithwaite RS, Stuart SA. Improving the utilization of medical crisis teams (Condition C) at an urban tertiary care hospital. *J Crit Care.* 2003;18:87–94.
7. DeVita MA, Braithwaite RS, Mahidara R, Stuart S, Foraida M, Simmons RL. Medical Emergency Response Improvement Team (MERIT). Use of medical emergency team responses to reduce hospital cardiopulmonary arrests. *Qual Saf Health Care.* 2004 Aug;13(4):251–254.
8. Jackson BS. A one-year mortality study of the most acutely ill patients in a medical-surgical ICU: toward developing a model for selection of recipients of intensive care. *Heart Lung.* 1984;13(2):132–137.
9. Li TC, Phillips MC, Shaw L. On-site physician staffing in a community hospital intensive care unit. Impact on test and procedure use and on patient outcomes. *JAMA.* 1984;252:2023–2027.
10. Pesola GR, Baystok V, Kvetan V. American critical care team at a foreign disaster site. *Crit Care Med.* 1989;17:582–585.
11. Kvetan V. Operation Desert Storm: task force on disasters and critical care. *Crit Care Med.* 1991;19:854–856.
12. Angus DC, Kvetan V. Managing critical care systems in adverse environments. *Crit Care Clin.* 1993;9(3):521–524.
13. Kvetan V. Management and administrative issues in critical care. *Curr Opin Crit Care.* 2000;5:332–338.
14. First New York metropolitan symposium of critical care management: costs, quality and outcomes. Syllabus. Kvetan V, chair. Montefiore Medical Center/ Albert Einstein College of Medicine; 1995.

15. First SCCM Leadership Program. Post-graduate course on management of critical care systems. Syllabus. Kvetan V, chair. Society of Critical Care Medicine; 1997.
16. International perspectives in critical care. In: Kvetan V, Vincent JL, Dobb G, eds. *Critical Care Clinics.* 1997;13(2): W.B. Saunders (Philadelphia).
17. Kvetan V, Mustafa I, Dobb G. First Asia Pacific consensus conference on critical care. *J Crit Care Shock.* 1999;1:57–74.
18. Clinical Advisory Board. Intensivist programs: Elevating the standard of critical care. The Advisory Board Company; 2001.
19. Pronovost PJ, Angus DC, Dorman T. Physician staffing patterns and clinical outcomes in critically ill patients: a systematic review. *JAMA.* 2002;288:2151–2162.
20. Bright D, Walker W, Bion J. Clinical review: outreach—a strategy for improving the care of the acutely ill hospitalized patient. *Crit Care.* 2004;8:33–40.
21. Bellomo R, Goldsmith D, Uchino S. Prospective controlled trial of effect of medical emergency team on postoperative morbidity and mortality rates. *Crit Care Med.* 2004;32:916–921.
22. Bellomo R, Goldsmith D, Uchino S, Buckmaster J. A prospective before-and-after trial of a medical emergency team. *Med J Aust.* 2003;179:283–287.
23. Kause J, Smith G, Prytherch D, Parr M. A comparison of antecedents to cardiac arrests, death, and emergency intensive care admissions in Australia and New Zealand, and the United Kingdom—the ACADEMIA study. *Resuscitation.* 2004;62:275–282.
24. Braithwaite RS, DeVita MA, Mahidhara R. Medical Emergency Response Improvement Team (MERIT). *Qual Saf Health Care.* 2004;13:255–259.
25. Pronovost PJ, Morlock L, Davis RO, Cunningham T, Paine L, Scheulen J. Using online and offline change models to improve ICU access and revenues. *Jt Comm J Qual Improv.* 2000;26:5–17.
26. 100 Top Hospitals™: ICU benchmarks for success—2000. Available at: http://www.100tophospitals.com/studies/icu00/winners/.
27. Adult cardiac surgery in New York State 1998–2000. New York State Department of Health; 2004. Available at: http://www.health.state.ny.us/nysdoh/heart/pdf/1998–2000_cabg.pdf
28. Angus DC, Kelly MA, Schmitz RJ. Current and projected workforce requirements for care of the critically ill and patients with pulmonary disease. *JAMA.* 2000;284:2762–2770.
29. Rivers E, Nguyen B, Havstad S. Early goal-oriented therapy in the treatment of severe sepsis and septic shock. *N Engl J Med.* 2001;345:1368–1377.
30. Breslow MJ, Rosenfeld BA, Doerfler M, et al. Effect of a multiple-site intensive care unit telemedicine program on clinical and economic outcomes: an alternative paradigm for intensivist staffing [erratum appears in: *Crit Care Med.* 2004;32:1632]. *Crit Care Med.* 2004;32:31–38.
31. Angus DC, Black N. Improving care of the critically ill: institutional and healthcare systems approaches. *Lancet.* 2004;363:1314–1320.
32. Bekes C, Dellinger RP, Brooks D. Critical care medicine as a distinct product line with a substantial financial profitability: the role of business planning. *Crit Care Med.* 2004;32:1207–1214.
33. Brilli RJ, Kvetan V. Teaching ICU administration during critical care medicine training—a national survey. *Crit Care Med.* 2003;29(suppl):A75.

14
Hospital Size and Location and the Feasibility of the Medical Emergency Team

Daryl Jones and Rinaldo Bellomo

Change is not made without inconvenience, even from worse to better.
—Samuel Johnson
We do not experience and thus we have no measure of the disasters we prevent.
—JK Galbraith

Introduction

Modern hospitals are complex institutions that treat increasingly unwell patients with multiple co-morbidities. The aim of such institutions is obviously to improve the outcome of the patients they treat. Unfortunately, up to 1 in 5 patients in hospital systems in the United States (1,2) and Australia (3,4) will suffer a serious adverse event or an unexpected death during their admission. Although little data is available on such events outside of these countries, there is no reason to believe that this problem does not exist in other health care systems throughout the world.

The frequency and nature of serious adverse events and unexpected deaths is likely to be affected by factors such as the number of patients treated by the institution, the patients' general health status, and the nature of the services provided (e.g. trauma and cardiac surgery versus elective day surgery). Thus, it is probable that university-affiliated teaching hospitals will experience a greater burden of serious adverse events or unexpected deaths than smaller regional hospitals.

On the other hand, reports from the United States suggest that the risk of operative death is related to the total number of procedures that the hospital performs each year (5). Smaller or medium-sized regional hospitals may have a higher rate of postoperative complications for any given procedure, even if the total number of events is lower. Hence, serious adverse events and unexpected deaths are likely to be a ubiquitous phenomenon that all hospitals must somehow aim to prevent. At our Austin Health in Melbourne, we have implemented a Medical Emergency Team

145

(MET) to identify and treat acutely ill ward patients. This chapter outlines the various approaches for the early warning systems that have been employed to prevent serious adverse events and unexpected deaths, and how METs can be implemented in different locations and in hospitals of different size.

Antecedents, Cardiac Arrests, and Criteria for Medical Emergency Team Activation

The logic behind the concept of an early warning system that identifies acutely unwell hospital patients has been outlined in detail in other chapters in this book. A number of studies have demonstrated that serious adverse events and unexpected deaths are preceded by a period of physiological instability (6–8) manifesting in derangements of commonly measured observations and vital signs. These physiological derangements are often present for some time before deterioration occurs, thus allowing time for appropriate intervention. Accordingly, criteria for the activation of early warning systems are typically based on acute changes in heart rate, respiratory rate, blood pressure, conscious state, urine output, and oxygen saturation derived from pulse oximetry.

At Austin Health, 82% of the MET reviews are initiated by a nurse (9). It is perhaps not surprising that analysis of the timing of 2568 MET reviews that have occurred at Austin Health in the 3.5 years since the introduction of the MET service revealed that MET activation is more likely to occur during periods of routine nursing observation and nursing shift handovers (Figure 14.1). These findings emphasize the need for simple criteria in activating review of an unwell ward patient, regardless of the personnel that comprise the team that performs the review.

Models, Location, and Size

The structure and personnel comprising the team that review acutely unwell ward patients must by necessity vary among hospitals according to local resources, patient acuity, and the frequency of serious adverse events and cardiac arrests.

In well resourced, university-affiliated teaching hospitals, the high degree of patient acuity and complexity demands an intensive care–based team. In hospitals or district general hospitals with fewer resources that service patients of lower acuity, alternative models may be adopted (Table 14.1). In addition to variations in the team personnel, the team's goals and objectives may differ among the models.

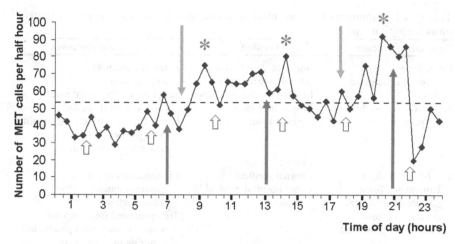

FIGURE 14.1. Number of MET calls made per half hour over a 24-hour period in relation to aspects of daily nursing and medical routine for 2568 episodes of MET review. Arrows demonstrate periods of nursing handover (↑), beginning and end of daily medical shift (↓), and periods of routine nursing observations (⇧). The dotted line represents the average number of MET calls made per half hourly interval. Statistically significant ($p < 0.05$) levels of increased activity are also indicated (*).

Teaching Hospitals

MET systems in teaching hospitals are typically composed of intensive care-based staff. At Austin Health the MET includes an intensive care fellow and nurse, as well as the admitting medical care fellow of the day. In the last 12 months, our MET service was called to review 809 patients. At the peak of activity, in April 2004, the MET was summoned to review almost 1 in 12 of all surgical admissions. In the 3.5 years since the MET's introduction, 2568 reviews have occurred (an average of 734 calls per year). The distribution of these calls was relatively even throughout the week, indicating that the MET is an important mechanism for managing unwell ward patients in the periods not staffed by the parent unit doctors. This information also makes it clear that a model created for a teaching hospital must deliver the service with uniformity 24 hours a day, 7 days a week.

DeVita et al. (10) recently have reported a retrospective analysis of 3269 MET ("Condition C" team) responses in a 622-bed university medical center occurring over 6.8 years (an average of 480 calls per year), further highlighting the specific high-resource requirements associated with a MET service at a large institution.

TABLE 14.1. Summary of various models of emergency teams for reviewing acutely unwell hospital patients

Description of team	Personnel	Roles and objectives
Intensive are-based Medical Emergency Team e.g. university teaching hospital (9–12)	Intensive care fellow Intensive care nurse Internal medicine fellow Respiratory care practitioner	Advanced medical resuscitation Safe transfer to critical care environment if needed Formulate and coordinate ongoing management plan for patients remaining on the ward
	Level 1	
Dual-level Medical Emergency Team e.g. Secondary referral center with limited criticalcare personnel	Internal medical fellow and hospital medical officer	Identification of patients requiring intensive care fellow review Treatment and follow-up for acutely unwell ward patient not requiring intensive care review or admission
	Level 2	
	Intensive care fellow and nurse	Activated at the discretion of ward staff or following review medical fellow
Emergency department-based MET e.g. district general hospital (14)	Emergency department Hospital medical officer (Consultant and/or registrar attend if available)	Resuscitation conducted by emergency department doctor Ongoing management by ward doctors or visiting medical practitioner
Intensive care liaison nurse e.g. District general hospital, in conjunction with MET (13)	Intensive care nurse	Review complex patients prior to MET criteria developing Follow-up of patients discharged from the ICUI Consultation service

Although larger institutions have a greater need for a MET service, resulting in a greater demand on resources, they typically also have more resources at their disposal to meet such demands.

The role of the MET in a university teaching hospital is to provide advanced resuscitation for the patient, and to decide the location of a patient's continued care. If the patient is to remain on the ward, a management plan is communicated to the medical fellow and the parent unit caring for the patient. Each institution needs to develop protocols for intensive care medical handover of ward patients requiring MET review, as well as protocols for the management of care for patients receiving multiple MET reviews during a single admission episode.

In a university-affiliated teaching hospital, the MET system may *reduce* the incidence of unplanned intensive care admissions (9–11). At other institutions with fewer critical care personnel and resources, the MET may *facilitate* the process of intensive care referral and admission.

Secondary Referral Centers

Several different models of review have been adopted for patients fulfilling early warning system criteria in secondary referral centers. The MET may supersede the existing cardiac arrest team (e.g. Lee et al. [12]) so that it reviews all medical emergencies in the hospital. In this model, the criteria for calling the MET are expanded to include criteria similar to those described previously (9). This is an effective way to meet the resource challenge by simply redeploying those resources to intervene at an earlier time in the evolution of critical illness. As most hospitals have a cardiac arrest team, this is an easy initial way of allocating the necessary resources for a MET service.

In centers with limited critical care personnel, the MET can be divided into 2 levels or tiers (Table 14.1). The first tier ("MET review—medical") involves review by the medical fellow for patients who fulfill MET calling criteria but are not critically unwell. The second tier ("MET review—intensive care") is activated at the discretion of the nurse initiating the call, or following review by the medical fellow.

The implementation of a MET initially could be restricted to a limited number of wards. In this model, wards with the highest incidence of cardiac arrests and serious adverse events could be targeted to obtain maximum impact, with minimal outlay of resources.

Alternatively, an intensive care nurse who is specifically trained can perform the initial review of the unwell ward patient (13).

In all of these models, one of the aims of the MET review is to improve the process of identification and referral for patients who require intensive care management.

If a cardiac arrest team is deployed to provide a MET service, it is likely that its workload will increase as it attends more patients. This may require subsequent minor adjustments in resources. In addition, because the demands of acute patient care under more complex circumstances require a wider array of interventions and knowledge, specific nursing and medical expertise and training may be required. These will have to be assessed in each institution on the basis of patient characteristics and acuity.

District General Hospitals

For institutions with very limited or no critical care facilities, the MET can be comprised of emergency department staff who review the ward patient and then communicate with the patient's visiting medical practitioner (14). This system is appropriate for hospitals in which there are no dedicated ward medical staff, and in which the overall number of MET calls is not excessive. Daly et al. (14) reported on the implementation of such a model at the Swan District Hospital in Western Australia. Over a 12-month period, there were 68 reviews for 63 patients. The system reduced the time delay for recognition of a life-threatening incident and improved the process of communication with the visiting medical practitioner. This model required the emergency department staff to be trained in advanced resuscitation. This experience provides proof that an effective MET service can be provided in a small hospital. It also emphasizes the need to employ resources that are already available by re-engineering their use and underlines the need to provide adequate training.

Small City Hospitals with an Intensive Care Unit

The authors have recently implemented a MET service for a small private city hospital in Melbourne containing a 7-bed intensive care unit (ICU) with 24-hour coverage by an in-house ICU fellow. The hospital has approximately 120 beds and is adjacent to a university teaching hospital with an established MET service. The hospital services a mixed population of surgical patients (including open heart surgery) and medical patients (mostly cardiology and oncology). It does not have an emergency department, and patient care outside of the ICU is provided by visiting specialists. In response to the occurrence of cardiac arrests (approximately 1 per month) and other serious adverse events, the medical advisory committee in conjunction with the ICU staff introduced a MET using the available resources. The ICU fellow and an ICU nurse became the Medical Emergency Team and hospital nursing staff was educated to the benefits of the MET; additionally, the calling criteria were made known and available throughout the hospital. The system was taken up rapidly, and over a 6-month period the number of MET calls became stable at approximately 10 per month.

The service has proved sustainable and a preliminary review of data shows that over a 6-month period there were only 2 cardiac arrests and the lives of an estimated 6 patients probably were saved by the availability of the MET. As the number of events is small, it is not possible to demonstrate a statistically significant reduction in cardiac arrests. However, the benefits of the MET service are already visible to nursing and visiting medical staff, and the system is already fully supported by both groups of stakeholders. Although the system is not perfect and may require additional resources, as well as better auditing, it delivers a much better level of care than was previously available to acutely ill patients on the hospitals wards.

Summary

Despite the best efforts of hospital medical and nursing staff, serious adverse events and unexpected deaths are an unfortunate facet of medicine in the modern-day hospital. Although the overall burden of such events may be higher for teaching hospitals, all medical institutions can develop a system for the identification of and care management for seriously unwell ward patients, and are likely to benefit from its introduction. This system should be tailored to meet the burden of events and to incorporate the most appropriately trained personnel available within the hospital. A somewhat imperfect system may initially be deployed, but this should not be a justification for inaction. Even an imperfect early intervention system is likely to be better than what is normally available in most institutions. The need for ongoing auditing and modification of the system cannot be overemphasized.

References

1. McGlynn EA, Asch SM, Adams J, et al. The quality of health care delivery to adults in the United States. *N Engl J Med.* 2003;348:2635–2645.
2. Brennan TA, Leape LL, Laird N, et al. Incidence of adverse events and negligence in hospitalised patients: results of the Harvard Medical Practice Study I. *N Engl J Med.* 1991;324:370–376.
3. Wilson RM, Runciman WB, Gibberd RW, et al. The quality in Australian health care study. *Med J Aust.* 1995;163:458–471.
4. Bellomo R, Goldsmith D, Russell S, Uchino S. Postoperative serious adverse events in a teaching hospital: a prospective study. *Med J Aust.* 2002;176:216–218
5. Birkmyer JD, Siewers AE, Finlayson EV, et al. Hospital volume and surgical mortality in the United States. *N Engl J Med.* 2002;346:1128–1137.
6. Buist MD, Jarmolowski E, Burton PR, et al. Recognising clinical instability in hospital patients before cardiac arrest or unplanned admission to intensive care. A pilot study in a tertiary-care hospital. *Med J Aust.* 1999;171:22–25.
7. Franklin C, Mathew J. Developing strategies to prevent in-hospital cardiac arrest: analyzing responses of physicians and nurses in the hours before the event. *Crit Care Med.* 1994;22:244–247.
8. Schein RMH, Hazday N, Pena M, et al. Clinical antecedents to in-hospital cardiopulmonary arrest. *Chest.* 1990;98:1388–1392.
9. Bellomo R, Goldsmith D, Uchino S, et al. A prospective before-and-after trial of a medical emergency team. *Med J Aust.* 2003;179:283–287.
10. DeVita, Braithwaite S, Mahidhara R, et al. Use of medical emergency team responses to reduce hospital cardiopulmonary arrests. *Qual Saf Health Care.* 2004;13:251–425.
11. Bellomo R, Goldsmith D, Uchino S, et al. Prospective controlled trial of effect of medical emergency team postoperative morbidity and mortality rates. *Crit Care Med.* 2004;32:916–921.
12. Lee A, Bishop G, Hillman KM, Daffurn K. The Medical Emergency Team. *Anaesth Intensive Care.* 1995;23:183–186.
13. Green A. ICU liaison nurse clinical marker project. anj. 2004; Available at: http://www.anf.org.au/pdf_anj/0402_clin_update.pdf. Accessed February 5, 2005.
14. Daly FF, Sidney KL, Fatovich DM. The Medical Emergency Team (MET): a model for the district general hospital. *Aust NZ J Med.* 1998;28:795–798.

15
Medical Emergency Teams in Teaching Hospitals

HELEN INGRID OPDAM

Introduction

Like other large organizations, hospitals are complex places. Providing medical care for patients requires the coordination of a large number of people, services, and interventions. The human involvement is immense, as is the potential for error.

Teaching hospitals have additional dimensions of intricacy due to their large size, a case mix high in subspecialty patients receiving sophisticated treatments, and the employment of a rotating, and often inexperienced, junior workforce.

Such an environment is ripe for critical illness and adverse events. A high frequency of adverse events in acute care hospitals has been reported, many of which are preventable. Earlier recognition of critical illness and timely intervention may prevent adverse events, and when they do occur, limit their impact on patient outcome. For a process of earlier detection to endure, a systematic change is necessary, such as the introduction of a Medical Emergency Team (MET). The introduction of the MET in teaching hospitals has particular challenges but can result in reduced adverse events and improved outcome for patients.

The Nature of Teaching Hospitals

Teaching hospitals share the complexities of other health care facilities and large organizations, with the added dimension of a large number of incompletely trained caregivers and perhaps a higher likelihood for error. Errors in teaching hospitals may be augmented because of their typically larger scale and more complex case mix.

Teaching hospitals are the training ground for junior health care workers and as such, there is a high turnover of medical, nursing and allied staff. Junior staff may rotate to a new position every few months (in essence, removing them from an area of practice as soon as they have become competent, which ensures a progression of incompetence within teaching hospital systems.) This changes the nature of the patients they care for and requires them to provide unfamiliar treatments and follow new protocols; in addition, trainees must regularly adjust to working with a different team of people in an unfamiliar setting. This need to adapt to a new environment is an even greater problem for foreign trainees, who comprise a significant portion of the workforce in some teaching hospitals.

Junior staff are not only "knowledge deficient," they are also "skills deficient:" they perform procedures that are new to them. This initial learning curve is associated with a greater risk of complications, which may be reduced with adequate supervision but, unless training procedures are dramatically altered, will probably never be as safe as when performed by experts. In addition, junior trainees may be reluctant to request support from senior staff members with whom they have not had an opportunity to develop rapport.

The constant shuffle of junior and inexperienced staff creates a permanent situation akin to a sports team playing together for the first time. Because of the lack of interpersonal knowledge that often occurs in teaching hospitals, supervisors and trainees may not be aware of each other's skill levels and weaknesses, and consequently there is a reduced ability to compensate for less competent staff members. A third problem with trainees is they are "judgment deficient"—that is, they lack high-level judgment skills that enable them to recognize and react to situations in a safe and consistent manner. In particular, they may fail to recognize when they—or, more to the point, their patient—require additional services.

The acuity of hospital patients is also increasing, along with the sophistication and technological demands of available treatments. Hospitalized patient populations are now older and sicker, and face financial pressures requiring them to have shorter hospital stays. Such patients will be more prone to critical illness and adverse events. Junior and senior medical staffs need to stay abreast of the growing range of complex therapies, and the consequences of such medical advances include heightened expectation from the community and better-informed, more demanding consumers.

The hospital's physical structure and layout may contribute to adverse events, since older hospitals were not designed for modern equipment and workflows. For example, transporting a ventilated patient with an intra-aortic balloon pump or extracorporeal membrane oxygenation to a computed tomographic scanner becomes a logistic feat in older hospitals that have small elevators and narrow corridors. Similarly, the historical evolution of clinical groups, training programs, and patient ward rounds may not be best suited to modern workflows. The typical surgical unit, in which the junior doctors are expected to spend long hours assisting after an early-morning ward round, is a typical example. This clinical workday may have been suitable decades ago, when the care of postoperative patients was perhaps relatively straightforward. Today, surgical inpatients often require much more frequent medical review because of medical co-morbidities or the complexity of the surgery performed.

Teaching hospitals do have the advantage of better staffing in the form of around-the-clock medical coverage. However, it is the most junior staff member who is first called to review a sick patient. The typical notification from the least trained to the person with the most knowledge and skills causes inevitable delays that hinder timely intervention. In a system of this structure, it seems surprising that so many crises are averted.

The reluctance to overhaul this faulty system resides in the desire to expose junior trainees to situations that they need to master in order to become expert physicians. To date, no better system has been conceived or developed for training. Perhaps there is also a reluctance to move away from what is known and familiar. A teaching hospital has all of the politics and powerbases common to large organizations, and individuals will resist change if they believe the proposed alteration to the system will impact them negatively.

Lastly, any major change to the system will have associated costs. In a resource-poor system, which is typical of many teaching hospitals, there will be financial restrictions due to fixed budgets. The potential for a system change to improve patient outcome and save lives may, in itself, not be sufficient argument for its implementation. Any proposal for change will need to be supported in terms of cost efficiency. Frequently, in systems where additional funds are not available, savings in terms of hospital bed days and other cost markers must be demonstrated to obtain executive approval for implementation.

A Milieu Ripe for Adverse Events

In the complex environment of a teaching hospital, it is inevitable that errors will occur and result in adverse outcomes for patients. It is known that adverse events in hospitals commonly occur and result in patient death on a scale approximating 10 times the national road death toll in Australia. Adverse events may be defined as an injury caused by medical management—rather than the underlying disease—that results in disability, death or prolonged hospital stay (1,2).

The Harvard Medical Practice Study reviewed 30 121 patient hospital records in New York State in 1984 (1). They reported that adverse events occurred in 3.7% of hospitalizations, and that 27.6% of these were due to negligence and 13.6% led to death. In 1992, a similar study in Australia, the Quality in Australian Health Care Study reviewed the medical records of over 14 000 admissions to 28 hospitals (2). Adverse events occurred in 16.6% of admissions, of which 51% were considered highly preventable. Of the adverse events, 13.7% resulted in permanent disability and 4.9% in death (Figure 15.1).

This data raises 2 important questions: are adverse events predictable, and is there an opportunity to intervene and prevent their occurrence? There is evidence in cardiac arrest literature to suggest that warning signs precede the cardiac arrest in a large proportion of cases. A study of consecutive hospital cardiac arrests in a Miami hospital showed that 84% had documented observations of clinical deterioration within the 8 hours preceding the cardiac arrest (3); in addition, most of the patients who suffered the cardiac arrest had underlying disease processes that were not in themselves fatal. The most commonly observed forms of clinical deterioration among the patients included worsening respiratory and mental functions, and metabolic derangement. A study of 150 cardiac arrests in Chicago had similar findings (4): in 66% of the cases, a nurse or physician documented deterioration within 6 hours of the cardiac arrest. Premonitory signs and symptoms included neurologic and respiratory deterioration. An Australian study showed that critical events (cardiac arrest/unplanned intensive care admission) were preceded by warning clinical signs for an average of 6.5 hours (5). Warning signs included abnormal physical observations and laboratory test results (Figure 15.2).

Other studies have suggested that the response to critical illness in general hospital wards may be suboptimal (6). This may be due to both failure to recognize critical illness and a lack of knowledge about how to appropriately respond to critical illness. It has been suggested that more than 50% of intensive care unit (ICU) patients with emergency admissions receive inadequate pre-ICU care (7).

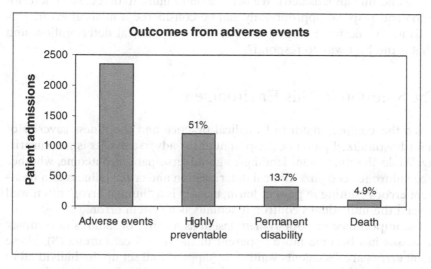

FIGURE 15.1. Diagram of the outcomes of adverse events in Australian hospitals. From data in Wilson et al. (2)

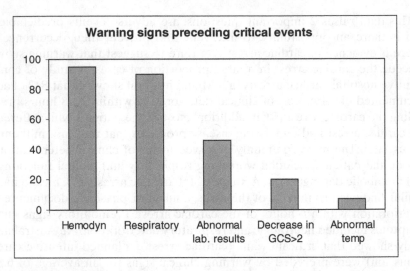

FIGURE 15.2. Hemodynamic changes included systolic blood pressure <90 or >200 mmHg, pulse <50 or >130 beats/min; respiratory included rate >30/min, oxygen saturation <85%; abnormal laboratory results included pH <7.2, Na⁺ <125 or >150 mmol/L, K⁺ >6 mmol/L; abnormal temperature <95°F or >104°F. GCS = Glasgow Coma Score. From data in Buist et al.(5)

So it appears that some adverse events, such as cardiac arrests, may be anticipated by the presence of preceding clinical deterioration (and the cardiac arrest itself is a final result of a clinical deterioration that was undetected and uncompensated). We believe that failure to detect such deterioration and respond appropriately can be considered a medical error. This leads us to ask: what is the best way to detect clinical deterioration, and what is the best way to respond?

The Solution in This Environment

Given the complex nature of medical practice and the illness severity of many hospitalized patients, the potential for adverse events is not surprising. While the final event leading to an adverse patient outcome, whether it be failure to recognize clinical deterioration and critical illness or a treatment error resulting in patient harm, usually is a "human error" often well beyond the individual's control, it actually is a system error.

The importance of poor *system* design as a cause of failures in complex processes has become more apparent in the health care arena (8). These latent errors are "accidents waiting to happen" and set up the individual to fail. Such conditions include junior staff being expected to operate beyond their level of expertise, inadequate supervision, unrealistic workloads, and inadequate training. Common to this system is the lack of a uniform approach, often involving a multitude of ways of providing the same treatment, frequently without written guidelines. Other conditions typical of the hospital environment include a dependence on people for vigilance (for example, to follow up on investigation results) and lack of use of available technology, such as electronic prescribing with built-in protections against incorrect drug dosing, drug interactions, etc. (9).

The importance of recognizing and responding to antecedents to adverse outcomes has been understood in the aviation and nuclear power industries and has led to the introduction of system changes that take the emphasis off the individual and hence limit the potential for human error. This has also contributed to the safety of both industries, creating a degree of safety that is several magnitudes greater than that which exists in the health care industry.

Clinical medicine's slowness to recognize this and respond appropriately may be related to a lack of awareness of the severity of the problem. To date, unlike plane crashes or nuclear disasters, hospital-acquired injuries and adverse events are not reported in the newspapers. And unlike nuclear and aviation events, hospital errors are difficult to discover, and result usually in a single death at a given time. Individual staff members may only see occasional isolated and unusual events. It may be difficult to distinguish between a poor patient outcome that is inevitable due to the underlying disease and that which results from an error of omission or commission.

In addition, doctors and nurses may perceive a pressure to handle all situations; and in a sense, failure (or a request for help) can be seen as a sign of intellectual or psychological weakness. Denial when things are going wrong and erroneous hopeful thinking that everything will be all right may prevail. There may be pressure on both junior doctors and nurses not to seek help outside of the clinical unit. Even if requested, senior help may not be readily available.

When things clearly have not gone well and the clinical deterioration of a patient's condition has not been recognized and responded to appropriately, there is a tendency to blame the individual closest to the event. The cause of the error may be attributed to a lack of experience, knowledge, or judgment; a typical response may be that the individual, "having learned from this experience," will prevent similar occurrences in the future. This focus on the individual is a poor solution, especially when a new, similarly inexperienced junior staff member will be in the same decision-making position with the next staff rotation.

Successful intervention is not based on training or changing the behavior of individuals. What is required is a system and cultural change. One such change that has the potential to meaningfully improve outcomes is the introduction of a Medical Emergency Team. This single strategy bypasses a number of barriers that prevent the provision of expert timely care. One such stumbling block is the reliance upon junior staff to recognize and appropriately act upon critical illness. Another is the barrier to nursing and junior staff that prevents them from obtaining sufficient senior and skilled medical review of a critically ill patient in a timely manner; calling for help must be viewed as an act of heroism, not weakness. This cultural change is no small matter to accomplish.

Introducing a Medical Emergency Team System in a Teaching Hospital

Implementing a MET successfully into a teaching hospital has more to do with producing a cultural change than setting up the logistics. The logistics are relatively straightforward, and their exact nature depends on the particular institution.

Acceptance of the MET Within the Hospital

With any introduction of change to a system, there will be resistance from those individuals who may perceive it as having the potential to negatively impact upon them. For the change to be accepted and implemented successfully, such concerns must be addressed and alleviated. The MET should be introduced only after consultation with all the stakeholders. Presentation of the proposal to all major hospital groups, followed by an open discussion that encourages concerns (voiced and unvoiced) to be addressed, is a prudent approach. Possible concerns include that patient care will be "taken over" by the MET, or that ward staff will become deskilled in managing acute illness. An underlying fear is that the doctors feel that they will look deficient and will "lose control" of their patient. To overcome this hurdle, senior staff of clinical units must be reassured that they will be consulted if a MET call results in an altered care management plan for their patient. Junior staff of the admitting unit must be involved in the MET review, and MET team members must behave in a professional, collegial, and inclusive manner.

Setting Up the Team

The key members of the team should be sufficiently skilled in recognizing and appropriately responding to critical illness. Both medical and nursing expertise is required. Medical staff should be able to diagnose the cause of the clinical deterioration and implement appropriate therapies. Required capabilities may include intubation, obtaining (central) intravenous access, and the administration of fluids and emergency medications quickly. Nursing assistance may be required for instituting vital-sign monitoring, drawing up medications, and applying other treatments like oxygen or assisted ventilation. Medical staff of the admitting clinical unit should also be notified at, or soon after, the time of the call. This promotes an inclusive environment and facilitates patient assessment by having staff present that know the patient.

In Austin Health, the team includes an intensive care nurse and registrar, the medical registrar and, if required, ICU consultant backup. The junior doctor for the clinical unit under which the patient has been admitted is also expected to attend. Finally, most teams in the United States have a respiratory therapist to assist oxygenation, ventilation, and intubation, and to set up respiratory treatments like beta-agonist nebulizers.

Activating the Team

The ward staff needs to be educated as to when and how the MET should be called. A poster with the MET criteria and how to call the MET should be prominently displayed in every ward. Prior to the MET's introduction, nursing and junior medical staff should become familiar with the MET process through preparatory education sessions.

Our Experience with the MET

A number of reports have described the benefits of the MET (10–13). Data was collected at Austin Hospital before and after introduction of the MET to assess its impact on cardiac arrests, serious adverse events, and hospital mortality. Studied over 2 comparative 4-month periods, for surgical patients the introduction of an ICU-based MET was associated with a 65% reduction in hospital cardiac arrests and 26% reduction in hospital mortality (14) (Figure 15.3). A number of serious adverse events were studied in a cohort of patients undergoing major surgery during these same periods. The MET was associated with a statistically significant reduction in the frequency of severe sepsis, respiratory failure requiring ventilation, stroke, emergency ICU admission, and acute renal failure requiring renal replacement therapy, and also in the number of postoperative deaths (15) (Figure 15.4). Substantial cost savings, far exceeding the cost of implementing the MET, were estimated based on reduced length of hospital stay for patients undergoing major surgery and reduced bed occupancy related to cardiac arrest.

Equally important to a hospital with a teaching mission, senior and junior medical and nursing staff in Austin Hospital have embraced the MET. Positive feedback is regularly received regarding the MET, thereby providing great support to ward staff and serving to educate junior members that learn from the attending MET staff. Trainees report an equivalent or improved teaching environment because of improved supervision, especially in critical situations, and because of improved psychological atmos-

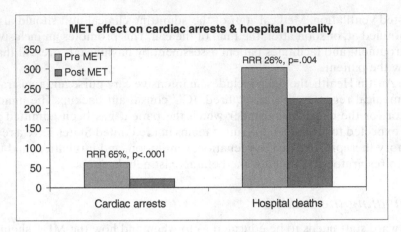

FIGURE 15.3. Illustration of the effect of the MET on cardiac arrests and hospital mortality. From data in Bellomo et al. (14)

phere: they do not perceive themselves to be abandoned as they are trying to simultaneously care for patients and learn.

The introduction of the MET has not been without some drawbacks. It has increased the workload of the regular intensive care staff members who comprise the MET, at times calling them away from responsibilities and patient care within the ICU. There are currently 794 MET calls per year (roughly 2 per day), necessitating the employment of an additional ICU registrar/fellow.

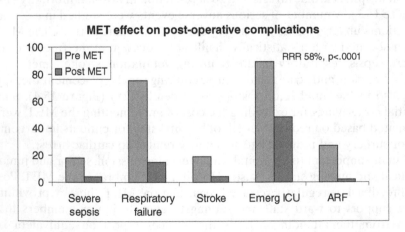

FIGURE 15.4. Representation of the effect of the MET on major adverse events. (Emerg ICU = Emergency intensive care unit admission; ARF = Acute renal failure requiring renal replacement therapy). From Bellomo et al. (15)

Although most MET calls are justified, there are also occasions when MET calls are made inappropriately. However, to promote getting help early, every MET call must be approached as if it were correct. This fosters trust (that the MET caller will not be reprimanded) and safety (that the patient's needs are always met, even if too many resources occasionally are brought to bear).

In Austin Hospital, the MET has been a victim of its own success, with nursing staff knowing they can obtain prompt medical attention instead of persisting with trying to page the covering junior doctor, who may be slow to respond. Of course, this safety mechanism creates pressure for the trainee programs to develop more efficient methods of responding to nursing requests. Additionally, calls in response to patient deterioration at night can lead to early discovery of patients for whom cardiopulmonary and other invasive critical care interventions should not be employed. The intensive care staff then conducts an end-of-life discussion with families that should ideally have been managed in-hours by the attending team.

Similarly, there are many occasions when the MET has not been called despite the patient having MET call criteria. This has lead to a delay in providing appropriate treatment and may have resulted in a worse patient outcome.

These points highlight the need for some level of ongoing education of the MET users, which includes formal or informal feedback about their use of, or failure to use, the MET.

In our teaching institution, the MET has been very successful, but this has been dependent upon the approach taken: a careful and thorough introduction and much ongoing support from medical and nursing staff. It is possible, and even likely, that a less enthusiastic implementation and lower level of service would not have produced the same beneficial outcomes.

Conclusion

The MET system has great potential to reduce adverse patient outcome through improving the early recognition and appropriate response to critical illness in teaching hospitals. Fundamental to its effectiveness is that it is a system change that allows any attending health care provider to trigger the rapid mobilization of appropriately skilled personnel. Its success depends upon appropriate implementation, which must involve consultation with all the stakeholders, widespread education of hospital staff, and enthusiastic MET providers. The MET is not incompatible with a teaching environment, and in our experience, it seems to augment the educational value of providing in-hospital care.

References

1. Brennan TA, Leape LL, Laird NM, et al. Incidence of adverse events and negligence in hospitalized patients: results of the Harvard Medical Practice Study I. 1991. *Qual Saf Health Care*. 2004;13:145–151; discussion 151–142.
2. Wilson RM, Runciman WB, Gibberd RW, et al. The Quality in Australian Health Care Study. *Med J Aust*. 1995;163:458–471.
3. Schein RM, Hazday N, Pena M, et al. Clinical antecedents to in-hospital cardiopulmonary arrest. *Chest*. 1990;98:1388–1392.
4. Franklin C, Mathew J. Developing strategies to prevent in-hospital cardiac arrest: analyzing responses of physicians and nurses in the hours before the event. *Crit Care Med*. 1994;22:244–247.
5. Buist MD, Jarmolowski E, Burton PR, et al. Recognising clinical instability in hospital patients before cardiac arrest or unplanned admission to intensive care. A pilot study in a tertiary-care hospital. *Med J Aust*. 1999;171:22–25.
6. Hillman KM, Bristow PJ, Chey T, et al. Antecedents to hospital deaths. *Intern Med J*. 2001;31:343–348.
7. McQuillan P, Pilkington S, Allan A, et al. Confidential inquiry into quality of care before admission to intensive care. *BMJ*. 1998;316:1853–1858.
8. Leape LL. Error in medicine. *JAMA*. 1994;272:1851–1857.
9. Bates DW, Leape LL, Cullen DJ, et al. Effect of computerized physician order entry and a team intervention on prevention of serious medication errors. *JAMA*. 1998;280:1311–1316.
10. Bristow PJ, Hillman KM, Chey T, et al. Rates of in-hospital arrests, deaths and intensive care admissions: the effect of a medical emergency team. *Med J Aust*. 2000;173:236–240.
11. Lee A, Bishop G, Hillman KM, et al. The Medical Emergency Team. *Anaesth Intensive Care*. 1995;23:183–186.
12. Buist MD, Moore GE, Bernard SA, et al. Effects of a medical emergency team on reduction of incidence of and mortality from unexpected cardiac arrests in hospital: preliminary study. *BMJ*. 2002;324:387–390.
13. Cretikos M, Hillman K. The medical emergency team: does it really make a difference? *Intern Med J*. 2003;33:511–514.
14. Bellomo R, Goldsmith D, Uchino S, et al. A prospective before-and-after trial of a medical emergency team. *Med J Aust*. 2003;179:283–287.
15. Bellomo R, Goldsmith D, Uchino S, et al. Prospective controlled trial of effect of medical emergency team on postoperative morbidity and mortality rates. *Crit Care Med*. 2004;32:916–921.

16
The Nurse's Perspective

Nicolette C. Mininni and Carol C. Scholle

Introduction

For emergency event response teams to be effective, an organized plan for implementation must be established. This chapter outlines the essential steps to prepare nursing staff for their roles during emergency events. The first challenge is the need to change practice. The second is the methodology to create a culture change. Finally, we will discuss the impact of the Medical Emergency Team (MET) system and how the use of METs relates to nursing empowerment, satisfaction, and retention.

Medical Emergency Teams and Continuity of Care

Although emergency events may occur anywhere in a hospital, they are most common in patient care units. The human resources needed to manage an emergency event adds to the workload to a nursing unit staff, and so to maintain the efficiency and safety of the unit, additional resources must be rapidly assembled. This sudden flux in care needs supports the need for a well-organized emergency response team. Nurse-to-patient ratios vary from unit to unit, based on the acuity of the patients' illnesses, and are calculated daily based on patient-care hours. Staffing ratios are designed to meet the patients' average or expected nursing needs and the formula does not consider adequately the potential need to staff sudden, unexpected crises. As a result, when an emergency event occurs with a single patient, the nursing care delivered to all patients on the unit is affected.

In institutions that do not have an emergency response team, usually the nurse will first assess a change in patient status and attempt to contact the physician or resident. All too often, the response is delayed. When one is obtained, it usually involves new physician orders that need to be implemented: activation of multiple resources like respiratory therapy, the electrocardiography department, consultations with other physicians, laboratory work, radiology, and perhaps a transfer to an intensive care unit

(ICU). These simultaneous needs can leave the nurse frustrated due to system flow issues while she or he is trying to rescue the patient. Implementation of these multiple steps may remove the nurse from the bedside of the patient in crisis, as well as the bedsides of all the other assigned patients, leading to a sense that the nurse is abandoning patients. Other staff nurses on the floor are also drawn away from their assignments to support the nurse and patient in crisis. This can lead to delays in delivery of treatments, patient satisfaction issues, or even delayed detection of deterioration in the condition of 1 or more other patients on the unit, resulting in what we colloquially term "domino codes."

In institutions with a MET system in place, the flow is different. The bedside nurse notes the change in the patient's condition and, cognizant of the autonomy and authority to trigger a MET response, can easily expedite the essential care that the patient needs without ever leaving the patient's room. On average the first responders at the UPMC Presbyterian Shadyside arrive within 90 seconds, and all essential personnel are assembled within 3 minutes. In some institutions the overhead speaker system calls the emergency event, enabling first responders to arrive within 30 seconds. This rapid response certainly reassures the nurse that help for the patient (as well as assistance for the nurse) is on the way. In contrast to the preceding scenario, where it may take up to 30 minutes to actually begin therapy, the MET response is usually able to stabilize or transport the patient to a better site of care within 30 minutes. The MET response process enables resources on the floor during the time of crisis to support other patients or even family members who may need assistance. This streamlined and coordinated process is efficient: it enables minimal interruption to workflow for unit staff and continuity of care delivery for all other patients on the floor.

Nursing staff are motivated and driven to care for patients to the best of their abilities: that is the essence of being a nurse. When a patient is experiencing a medical crisis, the bedside nurse wants to be able to deliver the required as quickly as possible, and employing a MET response is one way to do so. Data from our Nursing Emergency Event Response Team Survey support the use of emergency event response teams. A summary of the survey questions and responses related to nurse satisfaction are listed in Table 16.1. When asked whether they thought the implementation of an emergency event response team improves patient care, an overwhelming 89% of the 250 nurses surveyed responded "yes", and 74% of the same nurses believe that having a response team makes it a better place for nurses to work.

Changing Culture

Among hospitals within the University of Pittsburgh Medical Center health system (a university-based, integrated delivery system including 16 hospitals, thousands of practitioners, subacute care facilities, and an insurance

TABLE 16.1. Nursing Emergency Event Response Team Survey summary of nursing satisfaction

Survey question	Response of those surveyed
Have you participated in response to Condition "C" or "A"? (emergency medical response)	90% responded "yes"
Do you think the implementation of Condition C criteria improved patient care?	89% responded "yes"
Do you feel that the implementation of the Condition C criteria made this a better place to work for nurses?	74% responded "yes"
How much do you value your ability to call a Condition C?	90% responded "important," "very important," or "essential"
Would you change the Condition C criteria or the response process?	85% responded "no"
If you had the opportunity to work at an institution that did not have an emergency event response team for Condition C criteria, would you?	55% responded "less likely to take the job," or "weigh this into the decision"

product) that have adopted a MET system, nursing attitudes toward calling for an emergency event team are positive. In the emergency event response team survey, responses to the question "How much do you value your ability to call a condition C?" were equally distributed among "important," "very important," or "essential" (Table 16.1). A fourth option on the survey "not important" was not selected. Institutions that have implemented METs have been successful in changing the old behavior from a nurse individually attempting to handle a situation 1 phone call at a time, to providing 1 phone call for help. Our nurses immediately recognized the value of getting rapid assistance for a patient in crisis. A second benefit that they have identified when a MET is called is the minimal negative impact on patient care on the entire unit where the emergency event is occurring; in particular, newer nurses report great satisfaction from immediate expert support available during a crisis.

Prior to the existence of the emergency response team, it was not uncommon for staff to stay beyond the end of their shift to complete work that was deferred due to an emergency. Because of the additional resources that respond to an emergency event when called, unit staff are not stretched or thinned to the point where additional hours must be spent to catch up on work missed while the emergency was being managed.

All of these factors have led to a culture change among nursing staff: they no longer expect or are tolerant of delays in care to patients in crisis, and they are empowered to assume a fundamental nursing role effectively—being their patients' advocates.

Steps to Changing Culture

"Nursing intuition" is not a myth—it is synonymous with critical thinking. Critical thinking is defined as the blending of knowledge, skills, and attitude. It is the ability to translate subtle changes in a patient's condition into information that assists in anticipating patient needs, and is the result of years of clinical practice, expertise, and experience. Being in tune with subtle changes is what nursing intuition/critical thinking is about. The reasons that most emergency events are recognized by the bedside nurse are: (1) the nurse's sensitivity to subtle clinical changes, (2) his/her physical proximity to the patients, and (3) his/her frequent reassessment. The development and ongoing revision of the emergency response criteria come from the accumulated past experience of nurses' intuition and critical thinking skills.

In the past 2 decades, nursing culture has changed include more independent functioning recognizing the critical-thinking skills of the nurse. Nursing care is frequently guided not only by physician orders written for individual patients, but also by established protocols or treatment algorithms, standards of care, and patient care guidelines. Given criteria, algorithms, standing orders, or protocols, nurses use their assessment and critical-thinking skills to deliver the appropriate standard of care. Additionally, nurses are practicing in an arena where regulatory and documentation requirements and the hospital demographic workload (like decreased staffing ratios and increased patient acuity) have resulted in more work for staff nurses over the last 2 decades. A study of nurse staffing and adverse events in hospitals suggests that the patient load for a licensed nurse began increasing in the 1990s (1). This increased workload has occurred at a time when a relative shortage of licensed professionals has stretched personnel resources to a critical point. Carrying heavy patient loads while lacking sufficient autonomy to implement procedures and make decisions is frustrating for nurses (2). Nurses are eager to adopt programs that make their workload more manageable, especially when such programs provide safer and higher quality care to patients in their charge. For these reasons, ready adoption by nursing personnel of the emergency response team has been shown to grow steadily since its initial introduction.

However, the startup can be difficult. The MET may be perceived as interfering in the care provided by the unit physician and nursing staff. Usual reporting mechanisms and work patterns are threatened. Doctors have been known to quash calls for help, and nurses who activate a MET response anyway may fear reprisal. There are several methods to change perceptions, practice, and ultimately culture. The first step is to establish objective criteria for activation of the emergency response team (development of crisis criteria is discussed in detail in Chapter 5), for which nursing input is essential. Criteria may vary based on patient populations; e.g. pediatric versus adult patients. Having nurses participate in the criteria's development will increase their investment in the process and foster knowledge of the criteria and their purpose. Establishing objective criteria also is important: this helps to decrease the nurse's fears of appearing weak for not being able to handle patient deterioration. Instead, nurses are identifying a crisis (and requesting help) rather than being perceived as being scared, weak, or lacking knowledge. In addition, the objective nature of the criteria empowers nurses by allowing them to call for outside assistance without fear of physician reprisal. An audit of the event and the presence of the criteria are sufficient to demonstrate that the MET call was "the right thing to do for the patient," and thus the nurse becomes a hero, not a weakling.

The second phase of culture change is to redefine and enforce the bedside nurse's role and tasks after the MET is called. Prior to the team's arrival, the nurse has several basic responsibilities: assess the patient's airway, breathing, and circulation, and call for or bring emergency equipment and the patient record at the bedside. In addition to basic life-support training, UPMC has developed education regarding the bedside nurse's role and responsibilities in an emergency event (Table 16.2). Assembling key data for the arriving team can speed and increase the accuracy of the handoff of care to the MET responders, while using the acronym AMPLE (Table 16.3) simplifies the verbal report to the team.

Of the many steps that need to be taken to fine-tune the MET response, the most important step is to empower the bedside caregiver to activate the team without fear of reprisal. Consistent and obvious support of the bedside nurse by physician, nursing, and administrative leadership are important to success. Objective criteria take human emotion and ego out of the decision-making process, focusing attention on the patient in crisis. One of the most reinforcing aspects of the MET response is that all of the tools and resources needed to deal with a crisis are no further away than a single phone call.

Continuing Quality Improvement

About one-third of crisis events are preceded by errors, and another third could be prevented by some process change even though no error occurred (3). This finding was discovered in retrospective review of the 48 hours leading up to the MET response. We involve nurses in the retrospective review of emergency events because they are essential to discovering process flaws and repairing them. The goal is a redesign that might prevent future events. Once a process flaw is discovered, a multidisciplinary taskforce of content experts is created. The taskforce then focuses on

TABLE 16.2. Unit Staff Responsibilities prior to arrival of Emergency Response Team

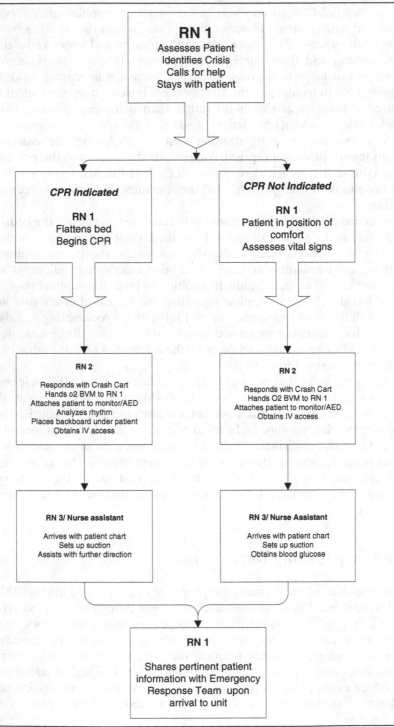

TABLE 16.3. AMPLE system for verbal report to MET on patient in crisis

	AMPLE Acronym
A	Allergies
M	Medications
P	Past medical history
L	Last meal
E	Events prior to emergency situation

deconstructing and analyzing similar events, designing a new or improved process, and leading implementation of the process. Future events are forwarded to them for further refinements.

Are METs a Recruitment and Retention Tool?

Nursing Emergency Event Response Team Surveys indicate that having the autonomy and ability to call for an emergency event team is important. Blegen and McNeese-Smith identified through their research that METs increase job satifaction and retention rates, and have an indirect effect on recruitment (4,5). Prospective nurses interviewing for employment should inquire about average length of employment of nurses, nursing involvement with decision making, ongoing educational opportunities, Magnet hospital status, and should meet nursing staff and have an opportunity to discuss job satisfaction and job stressors. The majority of nurses surveyed report that they would, if looking for a new position, inquire about the availability of an emergency response team and would weigh this information in their decision to accept or reject a new position.

At UPMC nursing recruiters and unit directors report that potential candidates are interested in attending Advanced Cardiac Life Support certification programs. Candidates are told that in addition to these programs, they will be offered the opportunity for additional MET training. The availability of continuing education has been identified not only as a retention tool but also as a recruitment tool (4–6). Currently UPMC is talking about the MET team and its value to nursing at recruitment events for the organization (Table 16.4).

Nursing Education

Education of nursing staff is dependant on specialty care area requirements (for example, nurses in a coronary step-down unit will have different needs than those in a postsurgery unit), acuity (ICU versus a general medical or

TABLE 16.4.

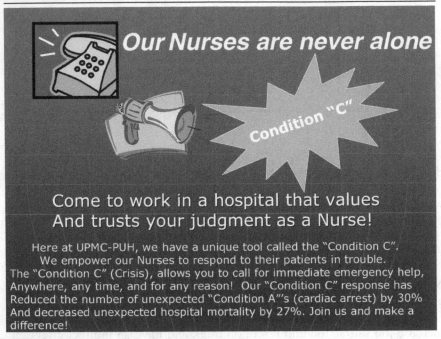

Our Nurses are never alone

Condition "C"

Come to work in a hospital that values
And trusts your judgment as a Nurse!

Here at UPMC-PUH, we have a unique tool called the "Condition C".
We empower our Nurses to respond to their patients in trouble.
The "Condition C" (Crisis), allows you to call for immediate emergency help,
Anywhere, any time, and for any reason! Our "Condition C" response has
Reduced the number of unexpected "Condition A"'s (cardiac arrest) by 30%
And decreased unexpected hospital mortality by 27%. Join us and make a
difference!

surgical unit), and experience of nursing staff. All staff should have repeated exposure to the emergency event response process. For the new nurse, part of the initial orientation process is to review: (1) the institutional culture for calling for help in a crisis (MET), (2) the criteria for recognizing a crisis event, and (3) the process for calling an emergency event. The orientation program plan should also include a review of the crash cart location and contents, as well as the proper documentation for the events leading up to and following the MET response.

The UPMC orientation program includes periodic, unit-based, educational "mock code" simulations. We use a Laerdal SimMan human simulator in a patient room. On the days prior to the mock code, we review with staff the MET criteria and unit responsibilities. We record the event on video, as well as the MET team response via the SimMan software. After the simulation, the facilitator reviews the assigned roles that every crisis response team must fill, emergency medications, use of emergency equipment (defibrillators, pacemakers, suction apparatus), and the quality of interpersonal communication and behavior during emergency events. The frequency of these reviews is based on staff needs, but occurs at least annually to ensure competency in emergency event response performance and to update any procedural changes. For example, when a new nursing unit opens, a mock code simulation is staged to assess and improve crisis response. Nursing staff that works on high-risk telemetry units or intensive care units also attend American Heart Association Advanced Cardiac Life Support (ACLS) classes offered through the institution. We have built into these skill station-based programs the required American Heart Association guidelines for interventions for specific emergency events, and also our institution's MET criteria, procedure for calling emergency events, and the MET team roles we have specified (see Chapter 21, Figure 21.2). These roles are discussed further in the chapter on simulator education for METs by Fiedor et al. (see Chapter 21). The ACLS course is multidisciplinary and is attended by attending physicians, residents, ICU nursing staff, telemetry nursing staff, respiratory therapists, and anesthesia personnel. An additional and important educational program is our simulation-based crisis team training course. Experienced ICU nurses, respiratory therapists, attending physicians, and fellow and resident physician trainees comprise the training team (along with, of course, the hospital's crisis response team). The crisis team course has been found to be the most valuable part of their training, because it adds structure and confidence to their role in an emergency event.

Summary

Nursing experiences at our organization related to the implementation and ongoing development of a MET team have been positive. A survey of nurses in the organization has shown that they value their ability to call for an emergency response team (Table 16.5).

TABLE 16.5. Nurse response to survey regarding value of their ability to call for an emergency response team

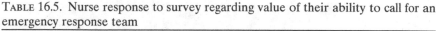
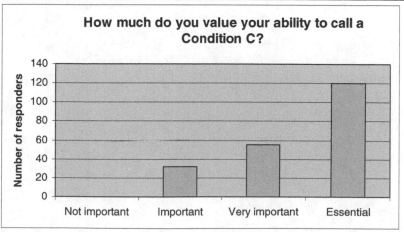

The ability to call the MET team has allowed nurses to do what they do best: give outstanding patient care by using their critical-thinking abilities, and know that they have a system that is supported by the administration.

References

1. Unruh L, Licensed nursing staffing and adverse events in hospitals. *Med Care.* 2003;41:142–152.
2. Strachota E, Normandin, P, O'Brien N, Clary M, Krukow B. Reasons registered nurses leave or change employment status. *J Nurs Adm.* 2003;33:111–117.
3. Braithwaite RS, DeVita MA, Mahidhara R, Simmons RL, Stuart S, Foraida M. Use of medical emergency team (MET) responses to detect medical errors. *Qual Saf Health Care.* Aug 2004;13(4):255–259.
4. Blegen MA. Nurses' job satisfaction: a meta-analysis of related variables. *Nurs Res.* 1993;42:36–41.
5. McNeese-Smith DK. A content analysis of staff nurse descriptions of job satisfaction and dissatisfaction. *J Adv Nurs.* 1999;29:1332–1341.
6. Mills AC, Blaesing SL. A lesson from the last nursing shortage: the influence of work values on career satisfaction with nursing. *J Nurs Adm.* 2000;30:309–315.

17
The Hospital Administrator's Perspective

CRAIG WHITE and RINALDO BELLOMO

Introduction

Hospitals are places that people usually come to for healing, for the relief of pain and, sometimes, to die. However, common health care processes sometimes encounter problems, and as a result, preventable adverse events occur, and serious morbidity and mortality are well documented (1–5). Yet efforts to improve this situation are slow to emerge and can be hard to implement (6,7). The reasons for such apathy toward change are many and are complex in nature: they involve logistical, cultural, financial, political, social, professional, and knowledge-based processes. Hospitals are places where many people also come to work and, sometimes, to learn or do research. Their work is usually complex in addition to being technically and emotionally demanding. These are intensively human endeavors. The difficulties faced by hospital administrators who are dedicated to the development of a culture of safety within their institution can be daunting. This chapter provides a backdrop for a management perspective toward the successful—but not perfect—implementation of a Medical Emergency Team (MET) system.

The Concept of a Medical Emergency Team System

The authors deliberately refer to the "MET system" rather than just the MET itself, because the successful implementation of a system change requires much more than just having a Medical Emergency Team available (8–10). As this chapter will illustrate, it is a system change that should be aimed for, not just the creation of a specific team of physicians and nurses. Moreover, irrespective of the requirements, the MET should be viewed as part of *an overarching strategic plan to make the hospital safer*. The administrator should see the introduction of a MET system as just 1 tactical component of this strategic process. Other important and simultaneously developed components of a safety strategy should, at the very least, include several other steps (Table 17.1).

In providing patient safety in hospitals, it is useful to remember the quip "every system is perfectly designed to produce the results it produces." Accordingly, to make a hospital safer for patients by earlier detection and response to physiological deterioration (11–14), we have to change the approach used to monitor the condition of as well as the response to the early signs of such deterioration. A MET system is a major and important component of such a change.

The setting for the MET system that we have developed and applied is a large academic hospital in Australia. This hospital comes with all the usual logistic, political, and administrative challenges. Acute patients are treated in 2 campuses, separated by about half a mile. One main campus has full intensive care unit (ICU) services, while the other is dedicated to more chronic services including psychiatry, geriatric medicine, and postoperative rehabilitation. This latter campus contains only 1 acute care ward, because acute services were consolidated to the first campus for financial and logistic reasons. This immediately creates additional challenges to solutions for the emergency care needs of patients admitted to the institution.

From the point of view of the administrator faced with facilitating the introduction of a MET-based safety system for patients who require rapid deployment of emergency care within such an institution, the challenges are ensuring the availability of resources, planning, and financial support for the multiple components of the process. While some components of a MET system are obvious, others may be less so. In the opinion of the authors, there are at least 5 essential components to the successful administrative implementation of such a system.

1. The team
2. Obvious clinical and management leadership commitment
3. A receptive culture
4. Performance monitoring, evaluation, and feedback
5. An ability to create and sustain change (i.e. being able to change how people do their work beyond simply adding new services or roles)

Each of these components is equally important. Without one of them, the system can easily fail.

TABLE 17.1. Fundamental components of a hospital patient safety strategy

- Continuing staff education
- Continuing optimization of information technology use
- Fully developed clinical governance processes
- Formal auditing of medical and surgical unit activities and performance
- Regular comparison of such activities to intra-hospital, regional, national, and international benchmarks
- Implementation of professional clinical outcome review committees

TABLE 17.2. Fundamental elements necessary to ensure the success of a MET system

- Appropriate level of skills within team to provide ICU level of care within minutes
- Necessary medications and devices to be delivered anywhere in the hospital
- Clinical credibility
- Availability 24 hours a day, 7 days a week
- Auditing of all emergency calls
- Excellent communication skills

The Administrative View of the Team

The MET needs to contain some fundamental elements to ensure success (Table 17.2).

First, to deliver the appropriate level of care at the highest degree available in the hospital (ICU care), the logical approach is to have a team that delivers ICU expertise. Recreating what a patient would have at the bedside if he or she were in the ICU can accomplish this. In our hospital, this means an advanced trainee in ICU medicine—a fellow in the United States, a registrar in Australia and the United Kingdom—and a trained ICU nurse. These 2 people must also be able to contact and obtain the assistance of an ICU specialist 24 hours a day, as would be the case if the patient was in ICU. Emergency equipment and medications must be immediately available. In our institution, these specialized ICU staff members take a small trolley with them that has all the necessary medications for initial emergency care (second element) and monitoring. As recently reported, this system can deliver such care to a patient within an average of 4 minutes.

The team must have clinical credibility (third element). This concept is difficult to measure but essential. It refers to the perception of the medical and nursing community within a given hospital that, when the MET arrives, it consistently delivers rapid, high-quality, clearly professional, competent, and compassionate care. This care must be perceived by other staff members to clearly and immediately help make their patient safer. If this element of competence is missing, the MET system will fail. The administrative manager must work with senior ICU practitioners to ensure that the care delivered by the MET contains each of the 5 "C's" of good medical practice—competence, care, compassion, communication, and collegiality—at all times.

This system must be available around the clock (fourth element). Patient safety must be viewed as a priority, and not a secondary concern that only operates from 9 to 5. The role of the hospital administrator and the ICU-based Medical Emergency Team is to ensure that a 24/7 patient safety approach is the only one acceptable.

Auditing (fifth element) is a vital component of this process, as is prompt and collegial communication with the primary unit that triggered the call (sixth element). It is the manager's challenge to ensure the availability of such services 24 hours a day. This can be challenging, especially because in a large institution, once the MET system matures, there can be up to 6 to 7 calls during a busy day. All MET calls must be documented. In Austin Health, this means that the MET fills out specifically designed data-collection tools with demographic, intervention, and outcome data that is later entered into an electronic database. All calls are recorded by the hospital switchboard, which acts as a source of verification for each call. Auditing must also include overall collection of information on major adverse events (cardiac arrests and deaths) in the hospital. These are collected separately via the coronary care unit, the clinical governance unit, and, of course, the hospital's electronic database of admissions discharges and deaths.

Financial Support

In a large hospital within a system like the Australian state-funded hospital system, where allocation of resources is capped, obtaining financial support often requires a multi-pronged approach. This includes better deployment of staff, optimization of rosters to provide more staff at times of greatest need, re-allocation of resources within the hospitals from areas of decreasing priority to areas of greater priority (this is difficult and politically complex), and presentation of the case for more funding from the central department of health (Department of Human Services in Australia).

In the private sector, a more direct case can be made for funding, as evidence is growing that implementation of the MET system might represent an important increase in efficiency (10). In smaller hospitals, where resources are fewer, an initial step might be rethinking the use of the cardiac arrest team. All hospitals have these teams as a matter of accreditation, and such a team should be able to deliver advanced life-support skills promptly. It would make sense to simply change the trigger for such calls from cardiac arrest to physiological instability (MET calling criteria). These are practical solutions from an administrative point of view; however, the astute manager will realize this cannot happen without clinical and managerial leadership, which is needed to overcome political barriers (patient ownership, control of process of care in each unit) as well as sociological barriers (old framework of reference, hierarchical models of care).

Additional costs beyond those related to personnel include the costs of extra equipment and medication use associated with MET calls. However, this typically requires some reallocation of funds, as the hospital itself would require such mediations and equipment for patient care anyway in the absence of a MET system. Finally, there is the cost of auditing, or the cost of infrastructure: the operators, pagers, computer use, or personnel who enter or review data. However, operators already exist and simply have to make different calls, computers are already widely available, and pagers can be readjusted; the major additional cost relates to the need for an office dedicated to MET education, auditing, data entry, and research. Typically, a nurse coordinator can complete these roles successfully.

Clinical and Management Leadership Commitment

Leadership is a difficult concept to define and measure. It is often most evident from the consequences of its absence. Unless opinion leaders and management within the hospital fully commit to the MET system, the approach will fail. Depending on the institution, leadership has to be applied at different levels. There must be board leadership and support in favor of a culture of patient safety. Physician leadership is also essential in ensuring that, across the hospital, the work of the MET is perceived as important and that there is support for its continued implementation. Administrative leadership is vital to convey to all staff that the hospital administration sees this activity as essential to the institution; this type of leadership has repercussions throughout the hospital at board levels as well as medical and nursing levels. Nursing leadership is also fundamental, as nurses are the initiators of more than 80% of MET calls. Without support and encouragement from hospital and nursing management, the system cannot develop and be sustained. There are different leadership techniques for change, and no one is necessarily right or wrong. From a management point of view, one needs to understand the organization and the stakeholders, and present the case for change gradually and in a way that emphasizes the gains to the organization's members. Education and the demonstration, through anecdotes and data, that a problem exists are important. Emphasis that the change will be gradual is important. Explanation and persuasion with an opportunity for people to express their concerns and ideas are also vital. Once the system has been changed, successes must be reported, emphasized, and celebrated. Anecdotes and data are powerful to both describe problems with the old system and successes with the new one.

Receptive Culture

Even if there is leadership and commitment, the MET system will fail in the absence of a receptive culture. If the hospital has an internal culture of "unit versus unit" antagonism, if it operates in "specialty silos" with little communication among groups of practitioners, if caregivers and their needs, agendas, or goals are allowed to take precedence over the patient's needs, then the MET will fail. It is the role of management to enforce, support, and promote a culture that is receptive to change, innovation, and greater cooperation. A favorable cultural environment is one that focuses on the system and not the individual. It is one that sees near misses as opportunities, not as defeats. It is a system where the team is celebrated, not the individual. It is one where auditing of performance is embedded in patient care, where formal structures of clinical governance exist, and in which staff are encouraged to identify areas where safety can be improved and are acknowledged for their contribution.

Performance Monitoring: Evaluation and Feedback

An ability to create and sustain change (i.e. being able to change how people do their work beyond simply adding new services or roles) is fundamental to the success of the MET. The system must have a means of monitoring outcomes, regularly reporting such outcomes to the users/callers and offering people the opportunity to provide feedback. Without the application of this constant quality cycle, it will not succeed. The reason for this is that every change requires time to become embedded in the system and become the "way we do things around here." Systems are known to naturally regress back to old practices. To overcome this natural tendency, the administrator must ensure that clear and realistic outcomes are set and that appropriate measuring tools are available to detect changes in such outcomes. In Austin Health, MET calls that highlight specific system problems are regularly presented at the surgical and medical grand rounds. A regular update on outcomes is presented to the clinical governance unit and to the hospital grand round.

The Structure of Hospitals

Many hospital structures across the Western world and their ways of organizing medical care have changed relatively little since the 19th century, despite monumental evolutions in our understanding of disease and the development of many new and effective therapies.

The traditional care provision model is one largely dependent on the knowledge and memory of the caregiver. It is an intensively human and social process, with all the potential this model creates for adverse events. Understanding this concept is an initial but fundamental step in being able to modify the system and the culture. The basis of the personal and human dimension of the doctor-patient and the nurse-patient relationships needs to be appreciated. These relationships have evolved over more than 2 millennia of medical care in the West and are based on the construct of a deep trust and professional commitment that operate at an individual level. This is a powerful, emotionally charged model but one with which patients are deeply comfortable. This model immediately identifies the "person responsible," removes the risks of impersonal care (I do not know the patient; he/she is not "my" patient; I do not know the family; I have never spoken to him; I do not know what he wants; the patient is old; etc.), and has great potential to ensure respect for the patient's wishes.

For this potential (and often realized) benefit, patients are willing to sacrifice much, and even suspend rational thought (e.g. by pretending that their doctor/nurse would *always* know the right thing to do). This model has many pluses and seems to perform reasonably well in the chronic care situation, where time allows for adjustments, consultations, change of mind, reassessment, second opinions, follow-up of initial therapeutic efforts, etc. In the acute care setting, it performs less well. Therefore, it is not surprising that hospitals are perhaps not as safe as they could be (1–5). They must, however, become safer, and this should be the administrator's viewpoint. This value judgment might mean that the traditional model of care has to be challenged. There are different tactical responses to this strategy of and need for greater safety: for example, outside the traditional model of care, the use of information technology is increasingly being explored as 1 tactical approach to providing new ways to enhance safety through better access to current knowledge, as well as more sophisticated monitoring and communications. In electronic prescribing, the evidence is supportive that information technology can deliver such increased safety. This section will not deal with information technology, but rather will focus on patient and staff needs at different levels. Managers might wish to think of a MET system, as one designed to meet people's needs, an approach that provides yet another way of thinking about safety. Simultaneously focusing on the needs of patients, clinical staff, and management provides a useful way to illustrate how such a system can work, and how the hospital can try to simultaneously meet these seemingly diverse needs. The requirements of these 3 groups might be summarized as such:

1. Patients want to be confident that they will be safe and receive excellent care.
2. Clinical staff wants to provide safe and effective care and find satisfaction in their work.
3. Management wants a safe hospital offering properly funded services, which are efficiently provided to the patients who need them.

One possible approach to simultaneously meeting these major needs within the institution is to increase safety through education. Education alone, however, is inadequate for this task because—as is the case for most things requiring personal change, like fitness, weight control, smoking, drug use, and the application of current evidence in clinical settings—the data show only very limited penetration and ability to sustain change.

A MET system, on the other hand, can be an effective and affordable means of significantly reducing preventable in-hospital death and limiting complications, thereby meeting the needs of patients, staff, and administration (4,10). While an important part of an improved "safety net" to offer tertiary prevention, it should only be part of a hospital-wide comprehensive patient safety program. This program should address all aspects of clinical safety and quality improvement (15–19).

Financial Issues

In the end, the financial aspect is a major component of the implementation of a MET system and of the institution's ability to sustain it. Health care settings have radically different funding models, each with their own incentives (some of which may even be perverse) and constraints. In Victoria (the second-largest state of Australia in terms of population, with 4 million inhabitants in the capital city of Melbourne) public hospitals are allocated funds by the state government on an output-funded, case-mix model where the total value of work being funded each year is capped. Standard prices are paid according to the procedures done and diagnoses made during the hospital stay, up to the value of the cap.

Given that the aim of a MET is to prevent more serious complications, its effectiveness will translate into shorter lengths of stay and/or fewer/less severe complications for patients admitted to the hospital. Generally, these can lead to reduced costs. However, such savings are offset by any additional costs arising from the MET itself, which includes a relatively modest investment to be able to convene a suitable team on a 24/7 basis and also any additional ICU days or investigations.

The impact on hospital revenue is likely to vary according to the local funding model. There are no direct financial incentives for the MET in Victoria's system. Indeed, there may be, on a case-by-case analysis, potential disincentives arising where there is a less favorable cost/revenue equation. Nonetheless, no matter how potentially "perverse" the funding model might be, failing to prevent adverse events or deaths would be hard to justify on financial grounds, aside from any moral or ethical considerations.

Another function of the academic hospital is the teaching and training of new professionals at undergraduate and postgraduate levels. Part of the management mandate is to ensure that these future professionals, whether they are training to be nurses, doctors, or allied health practitioners, achieve proficiency in handling clinical emergencies. Training of young professionals is becoming more difficult as reduced working hours and changed models of care also limit their exposure to emergency situations. The transition from novice to expert is thus hindered.

The astute administrator can create a synergy of needs to obtain funding for a MET system: the need for government to be seen as promoting safety, the need to deliver more cost-effective care, the need to provide an educational framework where young doctors can learn to make decisions without jeopardizing the safety of patients, and the need to promote the hospital within the community as a center of excellence that provides new and effective services. Additionally, the administration should have a risk-management strategy for the hospital, the ethical need to be seen to strive toward better patient care and the research need to be conducting continuing investigations into better ways of providing acute hospital care. All of these areas are potential sources of funding and can be used for the purpose of supporting a MET system.

The Road Ahead

Greater efforts and investment are essential to improve hospital safety. Organizations focusing only on the latest technical innovations will be exposed as inadequately addressing the need for a fundamental change in how systems of care are organized and managed. If we are to make the system and culture changes required, some attention and funding will have to be directed toward developing the capacity to achieve rapid clinical practice change and more effective leadership.

Further study of clinical and other indicators predictive of deterioration might allow even earlier detection of deviation from expected recovery, and even earlier intervention and prevention. Information technology may be able to assist this process by facilitating measurement and communication of vital signs, as well as linking with laboratory result systems. Electronic collection of patient observations within the whole hospital may represent another step toward the activation of even earlier intervention by specific teams (sepsis team, tracheostomy team, trauma team, etc.)

We know that the MET system works in Austin Health because there are so many fewer in-hospital cardiac arrests. Other hospitals will soon make similar observations. We will know that the next innovation works when we have a similar reduction in MET calls.

Clearly, the MET system is an important part of a comprehensive patient safety program and is a paradigm shift for the clinical practice system. The incremental costs of funding a MET system are modest compared with the benefits, and thus represent an excellent investment yield. Funding the MET system likely requires an imaginative solution and is dependent on the funding model and the setting. The system's success demands a receptive and change-capable organization.

Patient safety culture requires and deserves at least as much attention and management as the hospital budget. The changes necessary for the MET system to be effective require active clinical and non-clinical leadership across the entire hospital. Patients will benefit if implementation of the

MET system is thoughtful and organized. Staff will benefit from the MET system in terms of education, understanding, and job satisfaction if their patients do better and are seen to be safer. Management will benefit if it is seen to take a leadership role in patient safety initiatives, rather than always taking the role of financial gatekeeper.

References

1. Brennan TA, Leape LL, Laird N, et al. Incidence of adverse events and negligence in hospitalised patients: results of the Harvard Medical Practice Study I. *N Engl J Med*. 1991;324:370–376.
2. Leape LL, Brennan TA, Laird N, et al. Nature of adverse events in hospitalised patients: results of the Harvard Medical Practice Study II. *N Engl J Med*. 1991;324:377–384.
3. Hillman KM, Bristow PJ, Chey T, et al. Antecedents to hospital deaths. *Intern Med J*. 2001;31:343–348.
4. Bellomo R, Goldsmith D, Uchino S, et al. Prospective controlled trial of effect of medical emergency team on postoperative morbidity and mortality rates. *Crit Care Med*. 2004;32:916–921.
5. Schein RMH, Hazday N, Pena M, et al. Clinical antecedents to in-hospital cardiopulmonary arrest. *Chest*. 1990;98:1388–1392.
6. Nathens AB, Jurkovich GJ, Cummings P, Rivara FP, Maier RV. The effect of organized systems of trauma care on motor vehicle crash mortality. *JAMA*. 2000;283:1990–1994.
7. Mullins RJ, Veum-Stone J, Helfand M, Zimmer-Gembeck M, Trunkey D. Outcome of hospitalised patients after institution of a trauma system in an urban area. JAMA. 1994;27:1919–1924.
8. Lee A, Bishop G, Hillman KM, Daffurn K. The Medical Emergency Team. *Anaesth Intensive Care*. 1995;23:183–186.
9. Buist MD, Moore GE, Bernard SA, Waxman BP, Anderson JN, Nguyen TV. Effects of a medical emergency team on reduction of incidence of and mortality from unexpected cardiac arrests in hospital: preliminary study. *BMJ*. 2002; 324:387–390.
10. Bellomo R, Goldsmith D, Uchino S, et al. A prospective before-and-after trial of a medical emergency team. *Med J Aust*. 2003;179:283–289.
11. McQuillan P, Pilkington S, Alan A, et al. Confidential inquiry into quality of care before admission to intensive care. *BMJ*. 1998;316:1853–1858.
12. Goldhill DR, White SA, Sumner A. Physiological values and procedures in the 24 h before ICU admission from the ward. *Anaesthesia*. 1999;54:529–534.
13. Rapoport J, Teres D, Lemeshow S, Harris D. Timing of intensive care unit admission in relation to ICU outcome. *Crit Care Med*. 1990;18:1231–1235.
14. Bishop GF, Simmons G. Duration of life-threatening antecedents prior to intensive care admission. *Intensive Care Med*. 2002;28:1629–1634.
15. Hodgetts TJ, Kenward G, Vlackonikolis I, et al. Incidence, location and reasons for avoidable in-hospital cardiac arrest in a district general hospital. *Resuscitation*. 2002;54:115–123.
16. Goldhill DR, McNarry AF. Physiological abnormalities in early warning scores are related to mortality in adult patients. *Br J Anaesth*. 2004;92:882–884.

17. Hillman K, Parr M, Flabouris A, Bishop G, Stewart A. Redefining in-hospital resuscitation: the concept of the medical emergency team. *Resuscitation.* 2001;48:105–110.
18. Garrad C, Young D. Suboptimal care of patients before admission to intensive care. *BMJ.* 1998;316:1841–1842.
19. Goldhill OR, Worthing L, Miteaby A, Tarlng M, Summer A. The patient at-risk team; identifying and managing seriously ill ward patients. *Anaesthesia.* 1999;54:853–860.

18
Personnel Resources for Crisis Response

Andrew W. Murray, Michael A. DeVita, and
John J. Schaefer III

Introduction

Care for patients who are in a medical crisis has historically entailed management by their physician and nursing staff in a way that was somewhat haphazard and reactive. The system's success was based largely on whether the established hierarchy was followed in an appropriate and timely manner, allowing the patient to receive the required attention rapidly enough to prevent further deterioration. Staff learned how to respond to crises on the job: they were handed pagers and told to respond, but never received specific instruction regarding who else should respond, who had responsibility for what, and what was expected of them during a crisis event. It is no wonder that crisis team responses are often described as chaotic.

There is a problem with identifying the need for a crisis team response, which is deeply imbedded in medical care. A strict hierarchy has made the patient's individual attending physician the "captain of the ship." This is a great strategy for coordinating care in routine situations, but can become an obstruction to rapidly responding to changes in a patient's status. In some clinical settings, such as the operating room or intensive care unit (ICU), this hierarchical system further adds to the potential confusion when multiple "captains" are responsible for different aspects of a single patient's care. The problems with this hierarchical style of management stem partly from the commonly held belief that the hierarchy must be "ascended" instead of being "transcended." For example in, a medical education model, a nurse assistant would first call the nurse, who would then call the intern, who would call the resident, who would then call the attending physician of record, with each call occurring when the individual perceived that he or she was incapable of managing the situation. A similar problem occurs in a non-educational health care setting: the nurse assistant notifies the nurse who calls the primary physician, who then calls the consultant. For a patient with sudden onset of respiratory distress, one can imagine that it could take 30 minutes or more just to contact the person best able to manage the problem. By then, the patient's condition could have significantly deteriorated, to the point where the patient could be in extremis. These hierarchical considerations are not limited to the administrative chain of command, but are found in many settings and cultures and reflect a social hierarchy that in a crisis setting can interfere with optimal patient care. For example, a nurse responsible for a patient experiencing a crisis may feel reluctant to offer suggestions and even important information to a perceived higher authority, because they feel that it is not their "place" in the social or professional order.

The Medical Emergency Team (MET) system is a vastly improved method of providing care for these patients, because it brings the necessary individuals to the bedside within minutes and establishes a "flat" hierarchy that prioritizes the patient's immediate interests above any social or professional considerations. Unfortunately, devising strategies is less than half the battle, and change needs to occur in the minds of the caregivers to implement plans to best benefit patient. While this paradigm shift starts with individuals, to be effective it must reach the institutional level. Implementation is difficult primarily because it requires a true institutional commitment of leadership and resources, as is discussed in other chapters in this book.

Shortcomings of the Current System

It has been assumed that once physicians and nurses have completed their training, they are adequately equipped to deal with any crisis that may arise. The method of training has been based on the time-honored method of apprenticeship, which relies on individuals learning by observing more experienced individuals, assuming that the longer you are in the situation, the more expert you become. Some people do this very well and naturally, but others not at all. Inherently, this is a very time-inefficient process. The question is whether staff can be trained to a point where there is a greater pool of people able to deal effectively with crises (1). This is analogous to the concept of herd immunity—in this case, enough people are adequately trained in a system such that for any individual patient crisis, enough responders with adequate training show up so that the crisis team effectively and efficiently provides care. Most crisis responders have basic life support and/or Advanced Cardiac Life-Support training, and while this is important, crisis care is rarely delivered well by any one individual: an optimally functioning, well-coordinated team delivers optimal care. Knowledge of the causes of respiratory distress and what treatments are indicated may facilitate care management of patients. Advanced education and training in a profession, specialty, or subspecialty are also beneficial. However, an additional form of training is necessary: teamwork training. The current paradigm of delivering crisis care to a patient at risk of morbidity or mortality is analogous to asking a group of mechanics who do not know each other to show up when paged to a NASCAR pit stop, spontaneously organize into a team, get the work done as fast as a trained team, and neither hurt themselves or the driver through their action or lack thereof. No matter how capable each of the individuals, they cannot be expected to be as effective as a trained team. This type of methodology would be risky for both the patient and members of the crisis team.

Untrained crisis response individuals may make myriad mistakes that are representative of latent errors in the system and which are only discovered when the individual is being stressed. The authors have observed that when first exposed to the crisis inexperienced anesthesiology residents respond in the following ways:

1. Compulsion to do something
2. Loss of routine
3. Fixation on a task
4. Loss of effective communication

In a crisis, caregivers may feel compelled to do something to help the patient, even if they are not certain as to the best course of action. While this "need to act" is noble, it may not be done with forethought as to whether it is the most important task or what the ultimate outcome might be for the patient. The loss of the routine has the effect of putting blinders on the provider, as they no longer look at data streams and thus are unable to respond to them. When caregivers place themselves in a situation where they are engrossed in 1 action, they can often become fixated on that task and stop paying attention to the situation as a whole. Communication breaks down to the point that no direction is given to any other responders to the crisis about what has happened to the patient, what has been done to rectify the situation, or what still needs to be addressed. Planning and practice are needed to overcome both intrapersonal and interpersonal barriers to effective crisis management.

How Organization Can Help in Crisis Response

Organizing the response to a crisis is an attempt to ensure that a team of different people can respond to an unexpected event and, once there, co-operate to perform a series of mindful responses that benefit the patient. Group training creates a coordinated response that allows people to act intelligently within the bounds of the team and adapt to the differences in each situation. This concept of adaptability, or flexibility, is a highly useful team attribute considering the potential myriad and complexity of medical crises. From an educational design perspective, this concept allows one to focus on role-oriented goals and objectives for the individual as they apply to the collective team goals and objectives. To maintain integration among roles and introduce enhanced collective responsibility for the patient, the goal is not to simply perform designated tasks, but also to constantly monitor the situation and note how an individual response has to change to coordinate with that of others and to benefit the patient. From a learner perspective, this collective approach allows them to focus on their own specified set of treatment, monitoring, and communication goals. Through a focused understanding of how their actions both influence and are influenced by other team members' goals, the learner can become more efficient and flexible in both achieving individual goals and contributing to other team members' performance, all to the benefit of the patient. The institutional or system advantage of training individuals in functioning as a team is that while the individual composition of a crisis team can be expected to change, both the individual and the team training objectives are uniformly developed. As long as the responders know what their interactions should be within the group and also understand that they are to retain their own monitoring of the situation, then any combination of trained individuals can gather to solve the problem (2). This collective pool of capabilities transcends skills to include social or professional behaviors and expectations centered on the primary goal of the patient's welfare, as a counterpoint to the typical, hierarchal professional and social barriers that can decrease a team's flexibility.

The process of training responders also provides an opportunity to uncover and correct latent errors. The individuals that arrive at the scene of a crisis are usually either overwhelmed into not doing anything, or they try to correct everything that they see as a problem. Both of these responses are undesirable, the former because the patient receives no care, and the latter because the care is haphazard, at great risk for things getting missed, inadequately managed, or an additional risk (i.e. a therapy that includes risk of a complication). Individuals who feel they have to do everything run the risk of providing inadequate, if not poor, care, although this is not their intent. If they are not made aware of the pitfalls of the situation, they cannot avoid them. In the training environment, this individual performance trait can be identified, corrected, and re-evaluated.

One author's observations of anesthesiology trainees in the training environment has been that they tend to become fixated on 1 task or piece of information while the situation requires that many tasks be completed in a prioritized manner. This can be referred to as a fixation error (1) where the operator becomes so engrossed with the task at hand that all other input is actively or passively ignored or rejected. Organizing crisis responders empowers them to focus more effectively on the tasks assigned. With fewer tasks to accomplish (due to better division of labor that occurs with better design and rehearsal) they become positioned to either help with another team member's tasks or to perform their next required task. This directly improves the efficiency of both the individuals' and the team's performances, with the added potential benefit of improving the outcome for the patient.

When the position of leader is predetermined or accepted by all members of the team, it allows that person to observe the situation and make clear-minded, informed decisions regarding care. This role should be regarded more as a coordinating position than a hierarchical one. In our hospital crisis team training, each person already knows what his or her responsibility is and therefore self-assigns. Because team leaders do not have to organize personnel resources or perform a specific therapy, they can efficiently focus on the coordination of the collection of data, data interpretation, treatment prioritization and intervention, reassessment, etc. If the leader is instead focused on organizing the team, less time and thought is spent on the leader's primary responsibility: orchestrating the treatment.

Rethinking the Thinking

The thought processes involved in the management of a crisis need to be quick, reliable, and able to adapt easily to an ever-changing situation. Effective performance requires that the person be able to process simple routine tasks while simultaneously performing and using all sensory-motor input to adjust the way that they are performing. Cognitively, this implies the efficient combination of pattern recognition and reflexive response. Until now, we have expected this development to occur through experience in an apprenticeship training process. However, the author's experience with anesthesiology residency training is that often simple routines have not been established through experience and they become all-consuming (1).

The greatest challenge lies in the position of the leader. This individual needs to be able to step back from the situation and not physically do anything unless absolutely necessary. This will allow for that person to be able to survey the situation and ensure that tasks assigned are being done, that appropriate interventions are occurring, data is being collected and relayed appropriately, treatment decisions are being made, and therapy is delivered as ordered. They are functioning on 2 different levels. The first level is that of: what is happening, what are we doing about it, are our actions effective, are we causing more problems, and are we on the right track. The second level is that of oversight. They need to develop supervisory control of the amount of attention that they are devoting to any given task. This will allow the leader to decide what inputs are worth paying close attention to and create a priority list for the next point of care that needs to be addressed (1). Resource management is also included in this level of cognition., in which the leader uses all resources, human and otherwise, most effectively. This may occasionally entail changing the roles of the team members to ensure that the efficiency is maintained. An example would be calling additional help or requesting the departure of a member.

Structure

One of the keys to caring for these patients better is being able to treat the patient early in the progression of the crisis. This entails equipping the nursing staff and junior physicians with the tools and training that they need to feel comfortable asking for help at the best possible time—earlier rather than later. However, once the communication has been improved, it has to be met with a structure that creates a meaningful response.

Structure is necessary from various aspects. The obvious initial goal is deciding on the structure of the human resources to be applied to the medical emergency situation. A second aspect is the structure of team activation, from the initial call to their arrival. This needs to be reliable, constant, and unambiguous. The next aspect is the structure that needs to exist so that the patient is cared for in the most efficient manner, ensuring the best outcome from the emergent situation. This is probably the structure point that is best managed by training, so that the responders can function as a team. The final structure point should be that of the physical resources, such as intravenous fluid and supplies, medications, defibrillators, and monitoring and laboratory testing.

Human Resources

Whereas it would be very comforting to have a dedicated team that has no responsibility other than responding to crises, this does not seem feasible in a system that is already laden with costly care. Cross training is a must, and to this end the Medical Emergency Teams that have been created have consisted of people with the necessary expertise being called together at a moment's notice from different ends of the hospital to focus their collective care and attention on a single individual. The team needs to be large enough to be able to provide all the technical and knowledge resources that are required but not so big that it becomes cumbersome. The 2 required constants are a team leader and a record-keeper (1).

The treatment leader must remove him/herself from the fray to understand the larger picture of the unfolding crisis. This person's performance can be crucial in the crisis being handled appropriately and efficiently. The person needs to be able to develop situational awareness to not only monitor what is happening or evaluate what has occurred, but, most importantly, also to extrapolate the result of their current direction. The leader must be able to avoid the trap of getting fixated on the minutiae of the problem, but at the same time be able to ensure that the little things do get done as requested.

The remaining team members must assume identified roles and complete the essential tasks for each. The roles need to be designed to ensure application of monitors, airway management, intravenous access, and patient examination. The details of these roles and responsibilities are described below in terms of skills required to assume the task, and a separate chapter in this book focuses on team training in detail (see Chapter 25).

The team should consist of people who are familiar with the crisis situations and have the required knowledge. These would invariably, but not exclusively, be people who frequently are involved in the care of acutely ill patients. The authors' institution, the University of Pittsburgh Medical Center (UPMC), employs the use of intensivist physicians (fellow and attending), an intensive care nurse, and the medicine residents on call for that day. Specialists in airway management and surgical management are also available, although they do not respond to every MET activation. An additional member is an administrator to facilitate the rapid transit of the patient to an ICU location to continue care of the patient.

Activation of the MET

A system is of no use if it is not activated. The next step is to get the MET activated when a crisis develops. Herein lies a great challenge, in that the standard approach is one of individual management of the patient's care by the most junior member of the staff. This mindset needs to change so that the MET is activated instead of "business as usual." A study performed in United Kingdom examined the results of the establishment of a dedicated code team. This study showed a more rapid response to the crisis, and the survival to discharge was 10%, which falls in the range of other studies that have investigated cardiac arrests (3). The amount of time that the MET takes to respond also affects the outcome, as illustrated in a study in Italy that showed that in cases where the crisis response took longer than 6 minutes, none of the patients survived (4). Where the absolute response time has not been established in such a way that a benchmark exists, certainly the concept of "more time is worse" must be accepted.

The Ad Hoc Team

The individuals will respond to a call and instantly be inserted into an ad hoc team (Table 18.1). The members who respond to a call bring with them experience and skill sets that can be very necessary and specialized. The varying skill sets and the nature of an ad hoc team can be both a strength and a potentially a significant weakness. The strength is that enough people respond to be able to divide the workload and function as a collective mind—think in terms of the adages, "Many hands make light work" and "Two heads are better than one." The responders need to enter the situation in such a way that they understand that their primary goal is to ensure that the patient's care is the best possible, regardless of who is seen to be right or wrong in the management of the situation. The individuals need to perceive themselves as useful to the structure that has been created. They

TABLE 18.1. Roles and goals for crisis team in the operating room

Responder roles	Skills/expertise
Team leader	Experience in managing acutely ill patients, preferably current attending anesthesiologist/surgeon
	Advanced Cardiac Life Support training
Technician	Blood sampling (arterial blood gas, coagulants, thromboelastography)
	Troubleshooting equipment
	Supply equipment needs
Scribe	Keep accurate record of interventions and results
Airway management	If needed in airway emergency
Medication delivery	Knowledge of allergies
	Knowledge of ongoing medicinal therapy
	Knowledge of pharmacology
	Advanced Cardiac Life Support training
Circulatory support	Provide cardiopulmonary resuscitation support if needed
Surgeon	Surgical intervention to correct or prevent problems

need to feel that their opinion will be regarded thoughtfully and applied if appropriate.

The ad hoc structure also presents the greatest challenge. Ideally, the people who arrive upon activation of the MET previously would have practiced working together. More often than not, however, they may have only occasionally worked together and in some instances may have not even met. There needs to be a way of training and structuring so that the responders, who may have vast amounts of technical skills but very limited skills of working with the particular individuals in that situation, will be able to form a cohesive team in an extremely short period of time.

Each institution must create its own structure in response to the perceived needs that they experience on a day-to-day basis.

Changing the Existing Culture

Much of the difficulty in altering the way things are done exists in changing the minds of the people involved. The longer things are done a certain way, the stronger the culture becomes. As stated previously, the historical culture is that a knowledgeable, skilled physician should be able to deal with any crisis, and this is to be achieved with the knowledge that has been obtained during the short years of training in medical school. All too often these years have been jammed full of other competing, yet important, concepts. The management of crises has only been addressed by providing the didactic knowledge.

Accordingly, there needs to be a modification at the training level if one expects the system change to last. Medical trainees should be introduced to the concept of a team approach and team training at a very junior level.

This will allow for the development of respect for one's limitations, as well as for the contributions of other responders.

The training should stress that the concept of being "all-capable" is false: the well-trained team should perform better than the sum of its individuals. In a training setting, the student can be nurtured in an environment that is non-threatening to both the learner and the "patient," rather than having to learn from poor performance in the real world. This also opens the possibility of constructive, retrospective review of the management of crises in a way that is nurturing to all team members.

Unfortunately, human nature is often concerned with being the one with the correct answer in a given situation. While this is a noble goal, it can often be destructive in a team setting. MET system training puts much focus on the non-medical, non-technical aspects of team management of a medical crisis (5). The emphasis is on the concept of being a member of a team, a cog in the machine that is taking care of the patient.

Communication is a key concept that needs to be taught. Communication needs to be clear and organized. Speaking should be limited to what is absolutely necessary in order to minimize confusion and missed orders. Such communication should function as a closed loop, so that the individual who asks the question or gives the order is absolutely sure that they were heard, understood, and that the request is being carried out or is already completed.

Resource management is also a concept that needs practice and training. The person functioning as the leader needs to be trained so that all their resources, human and otherwise, are managed effectively and brought to bear against the problem. Some of the pitfalls that face the leader are the risk of getting too involved in the micromanagement of the patient care, forgoing the oversight function that they are responsible for, and becoming fixated on a certain aspect of the patient's problem while the patient's overall situation deteriorates. The focus must be on data acquisition, analysis, and treatment delivery.

An important component of resource management is recognizing the crisis and reliably alerting the team. The UPMC had a system in place for responding to crises for a decade, but it saw limited use while physicians were still being paged urgently and sequentially to the bedside to care for their patients. The institution then started reviewing the incidences of sequential stat pages and reminding the nursing units to use the team response, and the individuals responsible for the delay in team activation were given feedback on their actions. However, the most effective two policies that were implemented were: (1) the establishment of calling criteria, and (2) the dissemination of these criteria to the nursing units and other caregiver groups. The result was a significant positive change in MET use, with a corresponding drop in the number of sequential stat pages (6).

Because hospital resources differ, one would expect that their MET compositions would be different (Table 18.2); yet all will have to fill the needs

TABLE 18.2. Roles and goals of MET responders, Pittsburgh methodology

Responder roles	Skills/expertise
Treatment leader	Management of acutely ill patients in ER, OR, or ICU
Airway manager	Mask ventilation
	Endotracheal intubation
	Neurological assessment
	Administer medications (sedative, neuromuscular blocking agents)
Airway assistance	Mask ventilation
Bedside assessment	Attain reliable intravenous access
	Delivery of medications
	Knowledge of allergies
	Obtain vital signs
Equipment manager	Deploy medications and equipment
(crash cart)	Run defibrillator
Circulatory support	Rapid assessment of the patient's physical examination
	Mechanical circulatory support
	Place defibrillator pads
Data manager	Keep accurate recording of the events of the crisis
	Obtain key data from chart, caregivers
	Deliver data to treatment leader
Procedure physician	Check pulse, adequacy of chest compressions
	Perform procedures

of the patients in crisis. In our courses for training teams, we have identified a number of different roles that must be filled: airway manager, airway assistant, circulatory support person, someone to deliver medications, someone to deploy medications and equipment from the crash cart, a person who makes therapeutic decisions after analyzing the data, and finally, someone to collect data and record the events.

The skills and knowledge needed for each position is different. For example, the airway manager will be responsible for assessing the airway, positioning the head, choosing whether ventilation needs to be assisted, and if so, determine the methodology for that. The airway manager must know how to mask ventilate the patient, suction the airway, and intubate the trachea if necessary. In addition, because of the location relative to the patient, the airway manager should be able to assess the patient's level of consciousness, check pupils, and feel carotid pulses. Finally, the airway manager must have the capability to deliver medications for sedation, anesthesia, or neuromuscular blockade to facilitate intubation when necessary. Because of the complexity of these skills for set of duties, the airway manager role can be filled by only a few types of professionals. Usually anesthesia, critical care, and emergency medicine physicians, as well as nurse anesthetists have this capability, and so they are usually responsible for this role. Respiratory care personnel have the training and experience to non-invasively manage the airway, and at some hospitals, they also have the skills to perform endotracheal intubation using standardized physician order sets for sedation. Every team must have a person from one of these professions to manage the airway, oxygenation, and ventilation during a crisis response.

The airway manager cannot function alone, because it is difficult to both manage an airway and simultaneously set up the necessary equipment for this. An airway assistant therefore is assigned to deploy and assemble a bag-mask unit for use, connect the oxygen source to the airway devices, set up suction, assist intubation, prepare the endotracheal tube and laryngoscope prior to insertion, testing carbon dioxide in exhaled air, and connect the patient to a ventilator if necessary. In addition, because so many METs are due to respiratory causes, they must have the knowledge and skills to deliver respiratory treatments and adjust oxygen levels. Usually a respiratory therapist, respiratory technician, or nurse can tend to these duties.

Most hospitals have a crash cart that contains the medications and equipment needed for a crisis response. The medications must be located swiftly and mixed expertly, and then delivered via the appropriate route. The crash cart manager will be better able to manage the defibrillators if all of the institution's defibrillators are the same. The crash cart manager should be trained and should practice frequently. Several types of professionals have the skills to run the crash cart, including nurses, pharmacists, respiratory therapists, and perhaps physicians. Regardless of the profession, the crash cart manager must be able to operate the defibrillator efficiently and effectively, and be knowledgeable about and trained on the crash cart equipment and medications. Creating appropriate admixtures are usually in the professional skills and experience of ICU nursing staff and pharmacy staff, so they may be preferred to take on this responsibility.

Most teams have a person responsible for recording what happens during the crisis, usually focusing on the vital signs and treatments delivered. We had trained (and depended on) the crash cart manager to also keep the records. However, when the same person both manages the crash cart and the record keeping, there tend to be errors. We therefore have delegated two people to manage these responsibilities separately. We have also attempted to make the recorder a more active position, since one of the more common mistakes in a crisis response team is a failure to collect data and deliver it to the person (role) who needs that information to make decisions. In our training, we have changed the recorder into a data manager who is active, collects a database that includes recent laboratory results, electrocardiogram and chest x-ray results, and physical findings by the team.

A person is needed at the patient's bedside to deliver the medications and to obtain vital signs. Most responders should be able to take vital signs and, if this person delivers medications under the supervision of another nurse (for example, when an ICU nurse is the equipment/medication manager), then medication delivery is within the scope of this person's capabilities. We prefer the patient's bedside nurse to assume this role because she or he usually is aware of the prior state of the patient and can tell the team if findings change. The bedside nurse also is usually aware of allergies and recent medication administrations, and this knowledge if relayed to the treatment leader can prevent error or lead to a diagnosis of the etiology of the crisis.

At the UPMC, we have sufficient personnel to have 1 person assume each role. Other institutions may not have as many responders, and so 1 person may need to assume more than 1 role. In designing a crisis team response, the directors should attend to these roles, and make sure that responders with adequate skills and knowledge are assigned to them.

Redundancy needs to be built-in when establishing the teams; people should be cross-trained adequately to be able to fill in for other members until they arrive.

Operating Room Crisis Teams

Crisis teams may be needed for other purposes than a crisis on a hospital ward or lobby area. Much has been written about anesthesia (or operating room [OR] crisis teams) (1). Personnel considerations for METs need to reflect organizational and hierarchal realities from these environments to create effective training programs. OR crisis teams respond to anesthetic emergencies, such as a difficult airway with failure to ventilate, malignant hyperthermia, OR fires, massive hemorrhage, and obstetrical emergencies. In contrast to the floor crisis response teams described previously, OR personnel that could be used in a MET are often largely already present on-site or immediately available (with other duties) when the crisis emerges. A surgical team is constructed, organized, and focused on a collective task such as a surgical procedure. A typical one includes an anesthesiologist and/or anesthetist, a surgeon, a scrub nurse, and a scout nurse. The hierarchal structure is quite variable, with ranges of perceptions including a surgeon, anesthesiologist, or a nurse anesthetist who may each believe themselves to be "captain of the ship," or some combination thereof. This often changes with the introduction of a crisis, where the assumed team leader during a regular surgical procedure—usually the surgeon—switches to the case anesthesiologist for management of the crisis. Additional resources are dictated by the type or severity of a crisis and may include equipment like a defibrillator, a bronchoscope or perhaps a "difficult airway cart," central line placement kits, blood products, blood administration devices including rapid infusers, and emergency medications that require preparation, like dantrolene. The number and composition of additional personnel required, as well as specialized equipment, depends on the type and severity of the specific crisis.

For purposes of discussion, an OR crisis can be viewed as any adverse event that requires additional personnel or equipment beyond that normally anticipated for the specific surgical procedure. OR crises can either present as a sudden, obvious event that requires significant immediate resources, or can arise as a slowly escalating continuum that requires a matching escalation of resources to manage appropriately. Similarly, an OR crisis usually occurs in the setting of an ongoing surgical procedure that requires its own resources at the same time. Crisis management and personnel decisions need to take this into account, as they draw resources from the same pool—whether from personnel involved in the case during which a crisis occurs or from resources earmarked for other cases, either ongoing at the time or about to be started (Figure 18.1).

Administrative control and communication channels of these resources are site-specific and often varied. Compared to a generic MET response system and training program, design and training for OR crisis management must include significant leadership training for the anesthesia team to be able to rapidly recruit and organize resources. Institutionally, for the operating room environment the burden of this can either be left to the individuals involved in a crisis, such as the anesthesiologist (currently the most predominant method), or addressed at the system level such as with the full MET concept level. For example a hospital's OR system could systematically address: the composition of a MET for the OR; the method to activate this team and address effective cross-coverage for the responding

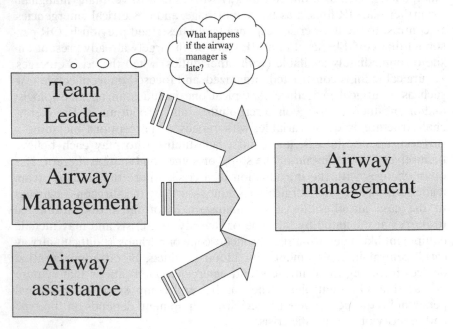

FIGURE 18.1. Resource management is the key to successful treatment of a patient with an airway crisis

members' responsibilities, so that they can focus on the crisis; and an administrative process for capturing the information about the root causes of the OR crisis, to benefit from the lessons learned. If systematically addressed, then the emphasis for training is less centered around how to de novo recruit and deploy a MET, but rather is focused on getting the optimal performance out of a MET designed for the OR.

At our facility, we train around the existing operational, administrative, and hierarchical operating room environment, where there is no highly organized MET response for a crisis. Therefore the crisis training program focuses on training the anesthesia care team, including: (1) generic patient safety principles and concepts, (2) how to rapidly tap into existing resources to organize a scalable crisis team in the setting of an ongoing surgical procedure, and (3) expanding capabilities of effectively treating uncommon and common types of crisis through simulated experiential and reflective learning methods. This is an interdisciplinary approach including all members of the anesthesia care team. Over the last 10 years we have trained approximately 1000 anesthesiology residents, student nurse anesthetists, and anesthesia technicians. The objective validity and reliability of the training methods and outcomes have still to be proven, yet the subjective survey and incidental case reports suggest a valuable outcome (7).

Conclusion

Crisis teams are an effective response system to emergency situations. For crisis teams to be effective and efficient, they must be well designed. The best design requires bringing together the personnel who will participate in the response and determine what is needed for that institution's crisis team. We have delineated the roles needed for a ward crisis and an OR crisis team. How each institution fills these roles depends on many local factors. The planning team needs to ensure that sufficient people with knowledge and skills to accomplish the task respond, and that appropriate equipment and resources are made available. Furthermore, there must be a strategy for bringing those resources to bear; simply making sure they are available is not sufficient. In addition, a plan must exist for both assembling the equipment and personnel and deploying them in a crisis. Finally, crises by their nature require more than 1 person to respond effectively; cooperation and coordination are necessary. Like any group effort, knowledge of what to do is insufficient, so group practice is needed to maximize potential. We believe that full-scale simulation is the best tool at this time to enable the responders to perform the skills needed to save lives. The difference between the knowledge of what to do and the skill of actually doing it in a group setting is huge. Developing this group skill can be life-saving.

References

1. Gaba DM, Fish KJ, Howard SK. Crisis Management in Anesthesiology. New York: Churchill Livingston; 1994.
2. Weick KE, Roberts K. Collective mind in organizations: heedful interrelating on flight decks. *Adm Sci Q*. 1993;38:325–350.
3. Lee KH. Survival after cardiopulmonary resuscitation in the general wards—the result of a dedicated "Code" team. *Ann Aca Med*. 1998;2:323–325.
4. Sandroni C, Ferro G, Santangelo S, Tortora F, Mistura L, Cavallaro F, Caricato A, Antonelli M. In-hospital cardiac arrest: survival depends mainly on the effectiveness of the emergency response. *Resuscitation*. Sep 2004;62(3):291–297.
5. Lightall GK, Barr J, Howard SK, et al. Use of a fully simulated intensive care unit environment for critical event management training for internal medicine residents. *Crit Care Med*. 2003;31:2437–2443.
6. Foraida MI, DeVita MA, Braithwaite RS, Stuart SA, Brooks MM, Simmons RL. Improving the utilization of medical crisis teams (Condition C) at an urban tertiary care hospital. *J Crit Care*. 2003;18:87–94.
7. Byrne AJ, Greaves JD. Assessment instruments used during anesthetic simulation: review of published studies. *Br J Anaesth*. 2001;86:445–450.

19
Equipment, Medications, and Supplies for a Medical Emergency Team Response

Edgar Delgado, Wendeline J. Grbach, Joanne Kowiatek, and Michael A. DeVita

Introduction

Once a patient has a crisis event, it is essential to deliver safe, accurate, and timely emergency care. Patient survival depends on the efficiency of the response (1). This response must include not only the appropriate personnel, but also the supplies, equipment, and medications that are needed. We have noted that most people who have been involved in a cardiac arrest (or Medical Emergency Team) situation characterize the crisis response using words like "disaster," or "chaos;" at best, it may be termed "ineffective." This does not have to be the case, as an organized response can be planned and achieved. This chapter will describe a methodology for providing an organized equipment and medication supply response.

Institutional Oversight of Equipment

To obtain a quality emergency response team, education of the personnel deemed responders is critical. All staff members in contact with direct patient care are required to have basic life support education, and critical care staff is also educated in advanced life support. However, depending upon the acuity of the patient's condition and observations, one may not have experience in a crisis until it actually happens, and some medical staff may not feel adequately prepared to participate in a crisis event. To help staff understand the importance of correct procedures, everyone should be educated during hospital and/or unit-based orientations regarding their specific role in a crisis. Annual competency evaluations are another method of training for crisis event management; to reinforce and test the knowledge base, we use "mock code" scenarios. The mock code can also determine system and personnel deficiencies, and promote processes to decrease or eliminate them. By using programmable, computer-based, full-scale human simulation, events can be repeated and data obtained regarding specific personnel tasks. For example, one may determine the range of how long it takes for a crash cart to get to the scene of a crisis, or how long it takes personnel to defibrillate a patient in ventricular fibrillation. This data can determine equipment needs and personnel education. By retesting, frontline staff can gain the comfort level and knowledge necessary to improve patient outcomes in any crisis situation, and hospital leaders gain confidence in the adequacy of their crisis response program.

The Medical Emergency Response Improvement Team (MERIT) committee at our hospital ensures that personnel and equipment are prepared for crisis events. The committee noted that all nursing units and clinic settings had various types of equipment stock for crisis response, including intubation equipment, individually designed and stocked crash carts, and a variety of personnel designated by individual units to respond to crisis calls. This resulted in problems related to equipment mismatch and malfunction.

First, we noted variation of the crash carts throughout the hospital, with each designed according to specific unit needs. Nursing staffs were responsible for restocking the carts after the event. At times, because of normal patient care activities, this task was delayed, perhaps posing a safety risk in that if a subsequent emergency occurred, the cart was not prepared. The organization's pharmacy and central supply were enlisted to improve medication delivery and restocking. Fully stocked crash carts were kept ready in the central supply area and exchanged for used carts, dramatically shortening the time it took a unit to have a restocked cart. When all the carts are prepared in a central area, it is possible to employ a systematic method for stocking: we use a sectional medical tray system that can quickly be changed out, thus limiting the time it takes to restock the cart.

To improve patient safety, the intubation equipment was removed from all non-intensive care units and placed in a portable orange airway bag. This bag was stocked in central supply to ensure reliable, functioning equipment. After every intubation, the old bag is exchanged for a new one. The bag was kept only by the on-call anesthesia and critical care personnel. This forced novice physicians to intubate patients under the supervision of physicians with airway management experience and training.

Personnel Response

Efficiency in personnel response during a crisis event is also desirable. There is evidence (citation: GABA, DeVita, Raemer) that teamwork during crisis events is deficient, and consequently errors may be made. Personnel response and teamwork therefore should be improved. Two models for teamwork improvement have been advanced: the first depends on the training for the crisis team leaders, and the second emphasizes a flat hierarchy wherein each team member has a specified role and responsibilities. The personnel designated to respond, the rationale for choosing those responders, and team training are discussed in Chapters 18 and 21 (Murray et al. and Fiedor et al.).

Nursing Responder Equipment

At the University of Pittsburgh Medical Center, we provide equipment from several sources. Intensive care nurse responders are designated to respond to geographic zones, resulting in a very rapid response time. Because the equipment cart may arrive after the ICU nurse if the crisis is located outside a patient care area, the nurses have created an equipment bag that contains items necessary for immediate intervention, such as a blood pressure cuff, stethoscope, gloves, and equipment for intravenous catheter insertion and intravenous fluid resuscitation. However, the packs do not contain medications. The nurses are responsible for restocking the bag afterward.

Airway Equipment

Success during a crisis response requires a secured airway and adequate ventilation and oxygenation. Therefore, personnel, equipment, and medications must all be brought to the scene within about a minute of the onset of the event.

Over the years, hen attempting to establish an airway, clinicians have been frustrated by unfamiliarity with the equipment, lack of available equipment, or lack of process standardization. This presents a significant challenge in an institution where medical students, residents, or fellows are required to learn and perform airway management. To facilitate and improve this skill set, a system was set up which uses a portable emergency airway bag (identified house-wide as the "orange bag" mentioned previously), which contains the necessary equipment to allow a clinician to quickly ensure adequate oxygenation and ventilation.

The bag's contents are standardized, so that any member of the response team will know where to find any needed item. The airway bag is divided into 2 compartments; a "quick intubation kit" and "other accessories." The division improves organization and facilitates rapid intubation, since the equipment for most intubations is placed in one location. The bag contents are in Table 19.1. They include: an intubation kit with laryngoscopes and blades, and a variety of endotracheal tube sizes, a mask with a bacterial filter for mouth-to-mask ventilation, gloves, nasal and oral airways, a CO_2 detector, syringes, tape, an endotracheal tube fixation device, Magill forceps, suction equipment, and a hand-jet insufflator in case of an emergency cricothyrotomy. A locked side compartment contains medications to facilitate intubation, including: etomidate, succinylcholine, benzocaine topical spray, and lidocaine jelly are included. The critical care medicine fellow must

TABLE 19.1. Emergency airway bag contents

Intubation kit	Other accessories
1. Surgi-lube	1. CO_2 detector
2. 6≤ Tongue blade	2. Mask with filter set-up
3. Gum bougie	3. Mask (child)
4. #3 Mac blade	4. Mask (small adult)
5. #4 Mac blade	5. Mask (large)
6. Laryngoscope handle with batteries	6. Exam gloves
	7. Suction catheter kit
7. #3 Miller blade	8. Salem sump 16 fr.
8. Adult Magill forceps	9. 1≤ tape
9. Green oral airway 80 mm	10. Nasal airway 28 Fr.
10. Yellow oral airway 90 mm	11. Nasal airway 30 Fr.
11. Red oral airway 100 mm	12. Nasal airway 32 Fr.
12. Intubation stylet	13. Syringe 30 cc Luer lock
13. Yankauer suction	14. Syringe 10 cc Luer lock
14. #9 Endotracheal tube	15. Biohazard specimen bag
15. #8 Endotracheal tube	16. Splash mask with shield
16. #7 Endotracheal tube	17. Endotracheal tube holder
17. #7 Endotracheal tube	18. 20 gauge 1.5≤ needles
	19. Jet ventilation kit

ensure the integrity of the bag at each exchange between fellows. Once the crisis event is over, the orange bag is returned to the central supply department and exchanged for a new, fully stocked one. The used bag is then sent to the pharmacy for medication restocking and medication integrity assurance by means of a numbered, red lock seal, and then returned to central supply for equipment restocking. Then the bag's contents are locked with a white plastic seal to assure the integrity of the contents.

Emergency Cart Standardization

To organize crash carts, it is essential to thoroughly review all emergency carts in hospital departments and patient units, including the operating rooms and post-anesthesia care units. Emergency carts may differ in both organization and contents (disposable supplies, durable equipment, medications, and documentation). Following a review of the differences among the hospital's emergency carts—and of individual units' special needs—a central committee (often the hospital's medical emergency response committee) can negotiate and develop a standardized emergency cart. Standardization includes medications, supplies, equipment, and layout for all general patient units, intensive care units, hospital departments, emergency department, post-anesthesia care units, operating room, and hospital-based outpatient clinics. On the outside of the cart, crisis algorithms and dosing charts can be securely attached for use by the emergency response team.

This strategy facilitates the actions of the emergency team and reduces the potential for error. For example, if one unit stocks dopamine at 8 mg per 250cc, and another stocks it at 16mg per 250cc, it is probable that a dosing mistake will occur. Another mistake is a misreading error. If magnesium is stocked on one cart, but morphine is placed in the same spot on another cart, it is more likely there will be a morphine-for-magnesium switch. In addition, the committee must decide whether certain medications that are needed in only a few sites are worth putting on the standardized cart. The cost goes up as additional medications are included, and the probability of a medication being used goes down as medications are excluded. Stocking crash cart contents are thus a collaborative and ongoing process. We continuously review and revise, and implement changes once a year. This facilitates and organizes the process for change and education.

Selecting an Emergency Cart

The emergency cart we chose as a model was an anesthesia cart, with a workstation on the top (Figure 19.1). We chose it because it was able to accommodate an oxygen tank, needle box, and backboard that our com-

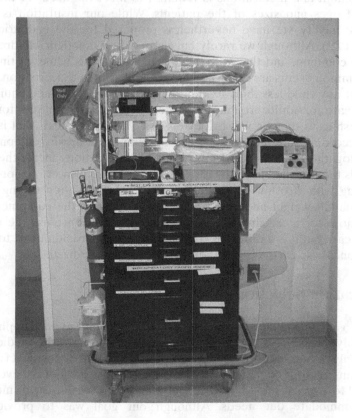

FIGURE 19.1. Adult Crash Cart.

mittee required. The emergency cart had 5 drawers, 2 for medications and 3 for supplies and equipment.

The crash cart needs to be durable, mobile, and secure; it should have sufficient capacity for the equipment and medications, and accommodate a workspace. A number of suppliers make carts that meet these specifications.

The 2 medication drawers hold trays (medication cassettes) that can be prestocked and sealed in clear plastic by the pharmacy for easy replacement. The medications contained within the cassettes are arranged alphabetically, and so can be found and viewed easily through the plastic (Table 19.2).

Because the cart has a locking mechanism that can be secured with numbered, plastic, break-way locks, reviewers can determine whether the cart is "ready for use." This facilitates central supply restocking and storage, as well as the unit auditors (every shift checks crash carts).

Need for Specialty Carts

Pediatric crash carts present difficult logistic problems because a wide array of equipment and medications is required to meet the needs of the large range of ages and sizes of the patients. While our institution is not a pediatric facility, we have nevertheless prepared for the pediatric crisis (Figure 19.2). Although we rarely have a pediatric inpatient, children visitors are common, and they may have a medical crisis while visiting. The most common events are seizures, syncope, and asthma exacerbation. Obviously, for any child less than 40 kilograms, the medications and equipment used to care for adults are inappropriate. There are 2 techniques for pediatric crash carts that we will briefly discuss. The first is a cart that is organized according to equipment type: for example, all airway equipment is stored together in a single drawer, and all medications in another. The second is the so-called Broslow cart. In this cart, each drawer is color-coded according with Broslow tape, which delineates medication dosing based on the child's weight and size. Each drawer contains the equipment and medications for a certain size child. At our institution we use the former style of cart, but it is a different color than the standard adult cart to avoid confusion. These carts, like the adult carts, are standardized.

Medication Selection

Every hospital must decide which emergency medications and supplies will be readily available in patient care areas. We referenced the medications and supply requirements from the Advanced Cardiac Life Support (ACLS) algorithms and our own clinical experience. Because 90% of the events we respond to are crises and not cardiopulmonary arrests, our cart is modified to accommodate our needs. Although our goal was to provide the

TABLE 19.2.

DATE: _____
CART NUMBER: _____

U.P.M.C. HEALTH SYSTEM
P.U.H.
STANDARD CRASH "CODE" CART
SUPPLY CONTENTS

NURSING UNIT: _____
COST CENTER: _____
ISSUE # _____

ITEM	DESCRIPTION	QTY.	ISSUE UNIT	FILLED	EXPIR. DATE
	TOP OF CART				
8740	Electrodes	2	each/box	NO CHG	
8838	Gloves, non sterile exam	1	box	NO CHG	
9289	Wipes, Alcohol	10	each/box	NO CHG	
8254	Swabs, Betadine	5	each/box	NO CHG	
8030	Tape, Adhesive 1-inch	1	roll/box	NO CHG	
8040	Tape, Adhesive 3-inch	1	roll/box	NO CHG	
8041	Tape, Transpore 2-inch	1	roll/box	NO CHG	
E051100	Tape, Mircopore 1-inch	1	roll	NO CHG	
8046	Tape, Micropore 2-inch	1	roll/box	NO CHG	
100078	Needle Box w/ Lid	1	each		
	Please secure lid onto top of needle box				
8801	Resuscitator Bag "AMBU"	1	each		
8075	Airway 90mm yellow	1	each		
8076	Airway 100mm red	1	each		

ITEM	DESCRIPTION	QTY.	ISSUE UNIT	FILLED	EXPIR. DATE
	DRAWER 3				
8962	Interlink Luer Lok	5	each		
E056600	Vac Holder(no charge)	1	each	NO CGE	
100235	Vac Needle(no charge)	3	each	NO CGE	
109730	Blood Gas Kit	5	each		
8911	Lever Lock	5	each		
8913	Threaded Lock	3	each		
6222	NACL 0.9% 30 ml	3	each		
103557	Chloraprep swabs	3	each	NO CGE	
8251	Benzoin Solution	1	each		
8806	Tourniquet	2	each		
6000	I.V., D5 w/H$_2$O 100ml	2	each		
122877	Needle, Spinal 18ga × 3-1/2	1	each	NO CGE	
122851	Needle, filter 19ga × 1-1/2	4	each	NO CGE	
8740	Electrodes	2	each/box	NO CGE	
9923	Ultrasonic gel	1	each		
109772	Vacutainer, green top	2	each	NO CGE	

Continued

TABLE 19.2. *Continued*

**** RESUSCITATOR BAG MUST BE ASSEMBLED AND PLACED IN THE DRAW STRING BAG PROVIDED				
THE RED AND YELLOW AIRWAYS MUST BE PLACED INTO THE BAG ALSO.				
THE BAG MUST THEN BE HUNG IN PLAIN SIGHT ON THE OUTSIDE OF THE CART.				
70075	Vacu, purple top no charge	2	each	NO CGE
109763	Vacutainer, red top	2	each	NO CGE
109751	Vacutainer, red top serum	2	each	NO CGE
109760	Vacutainer, grey top	2	each	NO CGE
122854	Syringe, 10cc slip-tip	5	each	NO CGE
9780	Syringe, 30cc luer-lock	1	each	
122847	Syringe, 10cc luer-lock	5	each	NO CGE
DRAWERS 1 AND 2 ARE FOR PHARMACY USE. PLEASE DO NOT PLACE				
8505	Cath. IV 14ga protective	2	each	
ANY ITEMS IN THESE TWO DRAWERS.				
8506	Cath. IV 16ga protective	2	each	
8507	Cath. IV 18ga protective	2	each	
9038	Gauze, pad 4 × 4 (2/pack)	6	pack/box	
122823	Blunt Cannula	4	each	NO CGE
122865	Needle Safety 21 GA × 1 1/2	4	each	NO CGE
122875	Needle Safety 25 GA × 5/8	4	each	NO CGE
122841	3 cc Syringe (lok)	4	each	NO CGE
DRAWER 3				
B37370	5 CC Blunt Cannula	5	each	NO CGE
B37375	3 CC Blunt Cannula	5	each	NO CGE
B37385	10 CC Blunt Cannula	5	each	NO CGE
116539	10 CC Syr Flushers	8	each	NO CGE

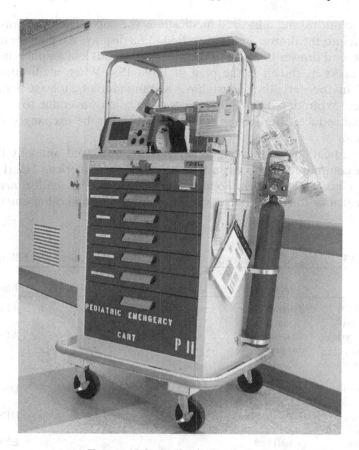

FIGURE 19.2. Pediatric Crash Cart.

necessary medications and equipment, another goal was to limit medication choices to one drug from each class where possible. The 3 reasons for
this are: fewer medications reduces opportunity for error, practice standardization also reduces error, and fewer medications means lower costs.
When medications are commercially available in a premixed dosage form
(i.e. magnesium sulfate, esmolol, dopamine), we chose that formulation to
reduce the chance for errors in admixing. A final goal was to create an emergency cart that requires minimum maintenance (except for the required
daily checks by nursing staff to ensure that the cart is intact, up-to-date, and
ready to go).

The cart is organized to improve efficiency and limit errors. Medications
on the emergency cart are arranged in alphabetical order by the generic
(not trade) drug name. The individual drug vials are placed in the vial
trays and are clearly labeled with the generic name, the drug concentra-
tion, and the stock quantity. The top medication drawer holds boxes of
needle-less emergency medication syringes, pre-mixed medication intra-

venous solutions, and odd-sized medications (i.e. topical gels or sprays that do not fit into the drawer 2 cassette). Table 19.3 displays the plan for drawer 1. The second drawer holds all of the medication vials and ampules in a vial display racks as shown in the plan in Table 19.4. When medications are stocked in the cart, they must have a minimum of at least 6 months until their expiration date. This reduces medication waste due to outdated items and reduces the frequency that carts need to be exchanged due to expiration.

The medications in the emergency cart are reviewed annually by the MERIT committee members and are based on the American Heart Association *Guidelines for Cardiopulmonary Resuscitation and Emergency Cardiovascular Care* (2). Changes to the medications and other emergency

TABLE 19.3. UPMC syringe drawer contents list, expiration dates, and billing

Medication	How supplied	Quantity stocked	Expiration date	# to bill	Mnemonic
Albuterol inhalation	5 mg/ml 20 ml vial	1			ALBT20L
Atropine syringe	1 mg/10 ml	3			ATRP1S
Topex spray (Benzocaine 20%)	54 gms	1			
Dextrose 50% syringe	50 ml	2			D5050S
Dopamine premix	800 mg/250 ml	1			DPMN800I
Epinephrine syringe	1 mg/10 ml (1:10,000)	8			EPNP10S
Lidocaine jelly	2% 5 ml	1			
Lidocaine premix	2 g/250 ml	1			LDCN8I
Lidocaine syringe	100 mg/5 ml	4			LDCN25S
Esmolol premixed bag	2.5 gm/ 250 ml or 10 mg/ml 2 50 ml	1			
Magnesium sulfate premixed bag	80 mg/ml 50 ml or 4 gm/50 ml	1			MGS80
Racemic Epinephrine inhalation	2.25% 0.5 ml	1			RCPN225
Sodium bicarbonate syringe	50 mEq/50 ml	6			SDBC50S
Hextend (place in Drawer #5 on cart)	500 ml	2			HXTD500I

TABLE 19.4. UPMC vial tray contents, crash cart medication list, expiration dates, and billing

Medication	How supplied	Quantity stocked	Expiration date	# to bill	Mnemonic
Adenosine	3 mg/1 ml 2 ml	5			ADNS6I
Amiodarone	150 mg/vial 3 ml	3			AMDR3
Aspirin, chewable	81 mg	2			
Calcium chloride	1 g/10 ml	2			CACH10I
Diphenhydramine	50 mg/1 ml 1 ml	2			DPHNI
Dobutamine	12.5 mg/ml 20 ml	2			DBT250
Epinephrine	1 mg/1 ml 30 ml (1:1000)	2			EPNPI
Syringe labels		10	N/A	N/A	N/A
Flumazenil	0.1 mg/ml 10 ml	1			FLMZ1I
Furosemide	10 mg/1 ml 10 ml	2			FRSM10S
Heparin	1,000 units/ml 10 ml	2			HPRN10I
Lidocaine	2% 20 ml	1			LD20I
Methylprednisolone	125 mg	2			MTHL125I
Metoprolol	1 mg/ml 5 ml	4			MTPR1I
Midazolam	1 mg/ml 2 ml	5			MDZL2I
Naloxone with 10 cc sodium chloride	0.4 mg/ml 1 ml	4			NLXN4I
Nitroglycerin	0.4 mg tablets SL #25	1			NTRG4
Norepinephrine	1 mg/ml 4 ml	4			NRPNI
Phenobarbital	130 mg/ml 1 ml	4			PHNB130I
Phenylephrine	10 mg/ml 1 ml	4			PHNY10I
Phenytoin	50 mg/1 ml 5 ml	4			PHNY250
Procainamide	100 mg/ml 10 ml	3			PRCN10I
Vasopressin	20´units/ml 1 ml	3			
Vecuronium	10 mg	2			VCRN10I
Verapamil	2.5 mg/ml 2 ml	4			VRPM2I
Bacteriostatic water	30 ml	1			WTR30I
0.9% sodium chloride	10 ml	5			SDCL10

cart stock are permitted only once per year, due to the workload involved in updating each of the emergency carts in the hospital.

The MERIT members, in particular a pharmacist and a critical care medicine physician, review requests to add or remove medications on the emergency cart. Medication requests that have been particularly troublesome include controlled substances (such as morphine), lorazepam (because of it activity against seizures), and insulin. Controlled substances are difficult to add to the emergency cart because the federal requirements for double locking, daily audits, and concern for diversion create too much work. Medications that require refrigeration, such as lorazepam and insulin, and have a reduced stability when not refrigerated (i.e. 30 days) should not be stocked in the crash cart. Again, the additional workload of maintaining and tracking short expiration medications on emergency carts is prohibitive. In addition, some medications (insulin) have a high propensity for error, and yet may not be required in virtually any crisis situation. While insulin may often be helpful (as in hyperkalemia), there may be other medicines that can be used with fewer risks and logistic difficulties.

Some medications in the cart require additional warning labels or information to ensure safety in preparation and administration. Examples are warning labels on phenytoin to note that the drug must be mixed in 0.9% sodium chloride solution, and specific dilution and administration instructions for use of naloxone injection to reverse opioid overdose.

Pharmacy Emergency Cart Exchange Process

Regulatory agencies like the Joint Commission on Accreditation of Healthcare Organizations (3) have outlined requirements for the emergency cart. These include: restocking, maintaining appropriate inventory, securing medications in emergency carts, and verifying that the carts themselves are secure in their location within the hospital. After opening and using medications and equipment from the emergency cart, the supplies must be replaced as soon as possible in order to be prepared for the next event. We have an exchange process to meet performance standards that was developed with all of the involved disciplines—nursing, respiratory therapy, central supply, pharmacy, and critical care medicine physicians.

Restocking Medications in the Emergency Cart

As discussed previously, medications placed on the cart must have at minimum a 6-month expiration. The outside of the cart contains the name and expiration dating of the first medication to expire in the cart. During the monthly pharmacy inspections of the patient units and hospital departments, the pharmacy checks for outdated carts and to ensure that nursing staff is performing the daily required emergency cart checks and documentation. Inside the emergency cart there are billing forms with the medication trays, so that patients can be charged for medications used, and preprinted labels denote specific emergency response team assignments during the code. Table 19.5 shows our cart replacement process. We offer it as an example; many different processes are possible, and the one chosen at a specific hospital depends on that institution's resources.

The pharmacy keeps a sufficient supply of backup emergency carts on hand for immediate exchange with units that have used their carts. In addition, the pharmacy maintains complete and sealed medication cassettes, so that the exchange process within the stocking area can be performed quickly on all shifts.

TABLE 19.5. Cart Replacement Process

Medication cart exchange process:

Emergency cart is opened by nurse caring for patient:

- At completion of crisis care, nurse calls pharmacy department to exchange the cart.
- Pharmacy technician brings new cart and a black plastic lock marked "do not use" (this denotes the cart as "used" and prevents unintentional redeployment) to central supply.
- Central supply department technician brings new cart and black seal to unit. New cart is left on unit and black seal is placed on used cart.
- Used cart is taken to pharmacy and 2 medication drawers are removed.
- Used cart is taken to central supply for cleaning and to replenish supplies and equipment. A form is placed on top of the cart stating the first expiration date of the supplies.
- Newly stocked cart is taken to pharmacy.
- Pharmacy replaces the 2 medication drawers.
- An inventory-tracking sticker is applied. The stick notes the date the cart was filled and checked, the supervising pharmacist's signature, and date and name of the first medication to expire.
- The cart is secured with red plastic lock (denotes new cart that is ready to go).

Additional Methods for Supplying Emergency Medications

In addition to the crash cart process, other methods have been developed to provide emergency medication before or during a MET response. We have created transport emergency boxes and orange airway management bags (Figure 19.3). Both contain a small assortment of medications, and the orange bag also contains intubation equipment and supplies. Transport boxes are for units that care for patients on monitors and must be transported for a test or similar transport. The box contains the 3 most highly used medications for emergencies: atropine injection, epinephrine injection, and lidocaine injection. The emergency airway bag contains a sedating agent for intubation (etomidate), local anesthetic (benzocaine aerosol and lidocaine jelly), and a neuromuscular blocking agent (succinylcholine). Other orange bag contents are described elsewhere in this chapter.

Barriers to Implementation

The potential barriers to implementation of the emergency medications, equipment, and supply exchange systems include cost, ability to standardize contents (resolving the variation), dynamic administrative backing and leadership, education and training needs, knowledge deficits, time involved, and the staff needed to maintain the processes. To break through these barriers, the focus must be on a common goal—patient safety. Our approach to standardizing the emergency carts was to define a core group who shared the need to simplify the cart restocking procedure, and improve the relia-

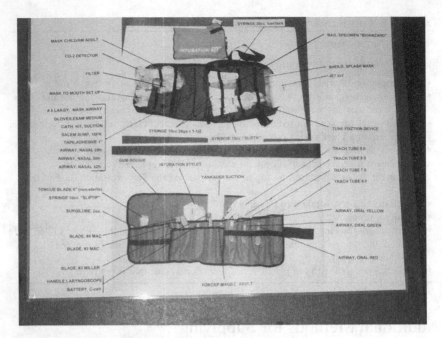

FIGURE 19.3. Emergency Bag Layout.

bility of the equipment. With administrative help, other groups that were also relatively easy to convince were included. Consensus regarding content was achieved, and the hospital administration provided the funds to purchase the carts and their content. After staff education, the carts were deployed only on those units. After observing the improved reliability and decreased effort by unit nursing staff, other units requested inclusion in the system. The few "stragglers" were then easily brought on board as their own system now fell outside the hospital standard.

There is a cost associated with crash cart standardization. In many hospitals, cart purchases are part of a nursing unit's budget, and the individual unit must prioritize purchasing a new crash cart above other expense items. Most units see use of the emergency carts as exceptions to the rule, and many may therefore consider it a low priority. The administration was essential in creating funds for the purchases and creating the imperative for units to make the appropriate purchase. While there were costs, there were also savings. First, standardizing the carts reduced the number of medications on carts, and provided a mechanism for systematically reviewing and choosing medications and supplies with global costs in mind. Second, it reduced nursing work for restocking and checking the medications. Third, less waste of outdated medications occurred. Fourth, because all the carts are the same, staff became very familiar with their contents so there were fewer episodes of 2 crash carts being opened to deal with a single crisis event.

Crisis events are low-frequency, high-stress occurrences. Therefore training is important, and performance is unreliable unless practiced frequently. Training nurses, respiratory therapists, and physicians to perform well during crisis situations is an essential component to crisis response preparedness. Standardizing the medication and equipment response dramatically facilitates training. However, if the hospital's educators are not involved in the process, there are 2 potential problems. First, they may not train people according to the hospital's process design. Second, the design team may make decisions that seem sensible from one perspective, but may create huge training issues. Overcoming this barrier is relatively simple if the education staff is included.

Supply Standardization in the Emergency Carts

The normal supply stock for the cart needs to be uniform for the same reasons as outlined above. To achieve this goal, central supply staff was enlisted to develop consistency in all crash carts. The methodology was similar: review of the current carts' contents, determine relevance and necessity, and consider which items could reasonably be provided from floor stock. The emergency cart drawers 3, 4, and 5 are standardized, which helps prevent restocking errors, limits the time crisis response staff needs to find items, and decreases the probability of error (either through misuse, or a mistaken impression that the equipment is not present). Table 19.6A and 19.6B show the equipment drawer configuration and contents.

Emergency cart standardization in all areas of the institution is an important patient safety methodology. In our opinion, the most important piece

TABLE 19.6A. Syringe Drawer Layout

Drawer 1 Layout: 1 Dopamine 800 mg/250 ml premixed bag will be placed on the top of the Bicarb

Atropine 1 mg/10 ml Syringe 3	Dextrose 50% 50 ml Syringe 2		Sodium Bicarbonate 50 meq/50 ml Syringe 6
Epinephrine 1 : 10,000 1 mg/10 ml Syringe 8	Lidocaine 2 g/250 ml premix bag 1		Magnesium Sulfate Premix 80 mg/ml 50 ml 1
	Lidocaine Jelly 2% 5 ml 1		Esmolol Premix 1 2.5 gm/ 250 ml
Lidocaine 100 mg/5 ml syringe 4	Albuterol Inhalation 5 mg/ml 20 ml vial 1	Topex SPRAY 57 gm 1	Racemic Epinephrine Inhalation 2.25% 0.5 ml 1

TABLE 19.6B. Vial Drawer Layout

Drawer 2 Vial Layout						
Procainamide 100 mg/ml 10 ml	Procainamide 100 mg/ml 10 ml	Vasopressin 20 units/ml 1 ml	Vecuronium 1 mg/ml 10 ml	Vecuronium 1 mg/ml 10 ml	Verapamil 2.5 mg/ml 2 ml	Verapamil 2.5 mg/ml 2 ml
1	1	3	1	1	2	2
Naloxone 0.4 mg/1 ml with 10 cc NSS	Naloxone 0.4 mg/1 ml with 10 cc NSS	Naloxone 0.4 mg/1 ml with 10 cc NSS	Nitroglycerin 0.4 mg SL #25 Tab bottle	Norepinephrine 1 mg/ml 4 ml	Norepinephrine 1 mg/ml 4 ml	Norepinephrine 1 mg/ml 4 ml
1	1	1	1	1	1	1
Flumazenil 0.1 mg/ml 10 ml	Furosemide 10 mg/ml 10 ml	Furosemide 10 mg/ml 10 ml	Heparin 1,000 units/ml 10 ml	Heparin 1,000 units/ml 10 ml	Lidocaine 20 mg/ml 2% 20 ml	Methylpred 125 mg
1	1	1	1	1	1	1
Adenosine 3 mg/ml 2 ml	Adenosine 3 mg/ml 2 ml	Amiodarone 150 mg 3 ml	Amiodarone 150 mg 3 ml	Aspirin 81 mg Chewable	Calcium chloride 1 g/10 ml	Calcium chloride 1 g/10 ml
3	2	2	1	2	1	1

of equipment to standardize was at first overlooked by our MERIT members. All crash carts in the institution are mandated to hold a defibrillator (with monitoring, pacing, defibrillation and synchronous cardioversion capabilities); however, they were not initially standardized. If cables, pads, paddles, and defibrillators are not standardized, mismatches result and the equipment cannot be used. Further, if the responding staff is not familiar with a particular model, an inability to use the equipment could result. Both problems might appear to be "equipment failure" although the equipment might be in perfect working order. At one point, a survey of all defibrillators in this institution yielded up to 8 different varieties. Figure 19.4 shows several models, including the required assortment of pads, paddles, and cables that they use, and it is possible to imagine the confusion that might result from an assortment of equipment in an emergency. While stopgap measures like writing "No Pacing" or colored stickers to prompt recognition of compatible equipment might be enticing, they are unlikely to prevent error. Instead, standardized defibrillators provide an important patient safety measure.

Standardization facilitates education. Unfamiliarity may contribute to hesitation on the part of less experienced staff to perform defibrillation without an expert clinician. To address this, we chose to purchase "hands-free" and "auto-analyze" defibrillators. Because pads and not paddles are used, the staff is more willing to perform a "quick look" maneuver with the

Drawer 2 Vial Layout

Bacterio-static Water 30 ml	0.9% Sodium Chloride 10 ml	0.9% Sodium Chloride 10 ml	0.9% Sodium Chloride 10 ml	0.9% Sodium Chloride 10 ml	0.9% Sodium Chloride 10 ml
1	1	1	1	1	1
Norepinephrine 1 mg/ml 4 ml	Phenobarbital 130 mg/ml 1 ml	Phenylephrine 10 mg/lml 1 ml	Phenytoin 50 mg/ml 5 ml	Phenytoin 50 mg/ml 5 ml	Procainamide 100 mg/ml 10 ml
1	4	4	2	2	1
Methylpred 125 mg	Metoprolol 1 mg/ml 5 ml	Metoprolol 1 mg/ml 5 ml	Midazolam 1 mg/ml 2 ml	Midazolam 1 mg/ml 2 ml	Naloxone 0.4 mg/1 ml with 10 cc NSS
1	2	2	3	2	1
Diphenhydramine 50 mg/ml 1 ml	Dobutamine 12.5 mg/ml 20 ml	Dobutamine 12.5 mg/ml 20 ml	Epinephrine 1 : 1000 (1 mg/ml) 30 ml INJECTION	Epinephrine 1 : 1000 (1 mg/ml) 30 ml INJECTION	Syringe Labels
2	1	1	1	1	10

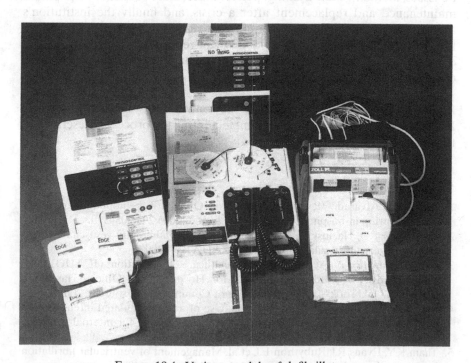

FIGURE 19.4. Various models of defibrillators.

defibrillator. In addition, the hands-free pads are safer to use for staff and patients, because there is less chance of electrical "arcing" or short circuit (particularly if the patient or the person delivering the shock is wet). The auto-analyze function tells the staff whether a shock is indicated; when a shock is recommended, the staff needs only to assess consciousness, and, if absent, defibrillate.

In high-traffic areas such as lobbies, corridors, and cafeterias, neither personnel nor equipment are readily available. We have placed emergency airway equipment (like a bag-mask device) and automatic external defibrillators to promote early intervention. Automatic external defibrillators are easy to use by lay personnel as visitors in an institution or the site, and who may possibly find themselves to be the first responder in a crisis.

Summary

To mount an effective emergency response, medication and equipment resources must be available, reliable, and organized in a way to make them easily usable. Staff must be trained adequately so that they know what their resources are and how to manage them. Standardizing the equipment and medications contributes to a safe system by improving a number of logistic issues, including staff training, performance, error reduction, equipment maintenance and replacement after a crisis, and finally the institution's ability to revise medication and equipment resources for crises. We believe that improving efficiency and reliability can reduce delays and errors, and contribute to the primary goal of improving patient outcomes following a crisis event.

Acknowledgments. We acknowledge the contributions of Jan Phillipps and Richard Snyder in developing and implementing the processes described in this chapter.

References

1. Abella BS, Alvarado JP, Myklebust H, et al. Quality of cardiopulmonary resuscitation during in-hospital cardiac arrest. *JAMA*. 2005;293:305–310.
2. Cummings RO, Hazinski, F. Guidelines for cardiopulmonary resuscitation and emergency cardiovascular care. *Currents.* AHA, Fall 2000.
3. Joint Commission on Accreditation of Healthcare Organizations (JCAHO). 2005 Comprehensive Accreditation Manual for Hospitals: The Official Handbook (CAMH). Oakbrook Terrace, Illinois: Joint Commission Resources; 2005.
4. Lighthall GK, Barr J, Howard SK, et al. Use of a fully simulated intensive care unit environment for critical event management training for internal medicine residents. *Crit Care Med*. 2003;31:2437–2443.
5. Tham KY, Evans RJ, Rubython EJ, et al. Management of ventricular fibrillation by doctors in cardiac arrest teams. *BMJ*. 1994;309:1408–1409.

20
Resident Training and the Medical Emergency Team

Geoffrey K. Lighthall

Introduction

Periodic re-examination of health care delivery systems have led to reforms aimed at improving the welfare and safety of patients. Medical Emergency Teams (METs) have emerged at the same time as resident work-hour restrictions have come into effect, public awareness of medical error has increased, and new models of residency program accreditation have been proposed (1,2). While well intentioned, the noted reforms and improvements in health care have not emerged as a coherent and user-friendly package. Concerns over medication error, for example, have led to directives for computer entry of drug orders, but this is not always compatible with a desire to maximize time at the bedside in the face of work-hour limitations. Likewise, the implementation of protocols and pathways that have provided higher quality of care may pose a threat to the concept of applying and individualizing basic and clinical science at the bedside. And while resident work-hour restrictions have been promulgated as a measure to improve patient safety, compliance with these new rules means even greater reliance on shift care or cross-coverage schemes, where there is greater likelihood that physicians will be responsible for patients with whom they have little familiarity. While numerous challenges abound in resident education, the question here is whether the implementation of a Medical Emergency Team (MET)—a classically patient-centered intervention—interferes with medical education, or whether there are ways in which medical education can be enhanced through the existence and operation of a MET.

Origins of the MET: A Solution to a Real Problem

The impetus to create Medical Emergency Teams comes from studies examining the quality of care and clinical decision making in patients who experienced cardiopulmonary arrest, or who had unplanned admission to an

217

intensive care unit (ICU). The studies were notable for demonstrating great variations in quality of care, and in particular, the widespread finding of care that was inadequate.

Studies evaluating patterns of ward care prior to ICU admission show a general lack of time urgency in evaluating and treating patients with abnormal vital signs and other forms of deterioration (3–5). Patients initially admitted to hospital wards (as opposed to ICU) had up to a 4-fold increase risk of mortality, suggesting that the nature of the care was a more significant determinant of the ultimate clinical trajectory than the admitting diagnosis (4). Both deterioration in the admitting condition and the development of new problems were key risks for a worse outcome.

In a study done by McQuillan et al., patients considered to have "suboptimal" care had twice the ICU mortality rate of the other groups (6). Areas considered problematic were: timing of admission (late), and management of oxygen therapy, airway, breathing, circulation, and monitoring. Reasons underlying the suboptimal care were "failure of organization, lack of knowledge, failure to appreciate clinical urgency, lack of experience, lack of supervision, and failure to seek advice." Our own experience in examining the dynamic decision making of house staff in a fully simulated ICU revealed similar deficiencies, including non-adherence to established protocols (7).

Two different studies of antecedents to cardiac arrest demonstrated that 75% to 85% of the affected patients had some form of deterioration in the hours prior to the cardiac arrest (3,8). Nearly one-third of such abnormalities persisted for greater than 24 hours prior to cardiac arrest, with a population mean of 6.5 hours (3). In one series, the majority (76%) of the disease processes eventually progressing to cardiac arrest were not considered intrinsically, rapidly fatal (8). In another series, over half of the cardiac arrests presented ample warning of decompensation: the majority of patients had uncorrected hypotension, and half of these had systolic blood pressures less than 80 mmHg for more than 24 hours (9). Other patients in this series had severe but correctable abnormalities such as hypokalemia, hypoglycemia, and hypoxemia. This collective experience suggests that quality of care, more so than the disease, may be responsible for the poor immediate survival of these patients. Inattention to or unawareness of a developing serious condition causes the additional problem of hasty decision making at the time of cardiac arrest. Once a cardiac arrest has occurred, the clinician's hand is forced, and ICU admission becomes mandatory for surviving patients in the absence of a do-not-resuscitate order.

Problems with establishing proper care were found to exist at multiple levels: nurses were not calling physicians for patients with abnormal vital signs or changes in sensorium; physicians did not fully evaluate these abnormalities when they were contacted; ICU consultants were not called in routinely, and senior level or consulting ICU caregivers did not obtain routine studies, such as blood gasses, hematocrit and electrolyte studies, that would have defined the patient's problem. In cases when laboratory studies were done, they were not always interpreted correctly, and when they were, therapy was not always initiated (5). All of the aforementioned studies were conducted in academic centers where junior team members are traditionally called to evaluate a patient and there is a varying degree of engagement by more senior staff members. Loss of valuable time in patient evaluation and stabilization may have been further compounded by attending staff that lack knowledge of seriously ill patients and their problems, and who lacked the skills to direct an appropriate resuscitation (6,10). Further, teaching hospitals have also increased their reliance on cross-coverage schemes, which also have been associated with a higher incidence of potentially preventable adverse events (11).

General Overview of a Medical Emergency Team

The MET's composition and scope will vary according to specific institutional needs and staffing patterns. Some have designed METs around the existing "code teams," while others use various combinations of critical care nurses and physicians. Ideally, the MET works best with some constancy in leadership and team membership. Having a team that draws on a smaller core of individuals over a wide range of times and schedules is a test of individual and institutional commitment, and poses a set of challenges that will not be dealt with here. Instead, the question of how to incorporate trainees into the team's operation will be considered. To provide one example, we are currently proposing a team with the following composition:

- Intensive care attending or senior critical care fellow as a leader
- Crisis nurse
- Anesthesiology resident or attending
- Internal medicine or surgery resident

The overall goals are: (1) perform a quick analysis of vital signs, ventilatory, and oxygen delivery status to assess the severity of acute and chronic conditions, (2) make timely decisions about triage, goals of care, or need for the involvement of other services (surgery, cardiac catheterization laboratories, etc.), and (3) rapidly stabilize respiratory and cardiovascular status prior to ICU transfer if needed. Moreover, the approach needs to be predictable and systematic.

This design reflects a desire to use the minimum number of people to accomplish all tasks related to the team goals: patient examination and historical investigation, invasive procedures including mechanical ventilation, analysis of laboratory values and clinical course, communication with consultants, and ongoing monitoring of patient and care plans until transfer to another setting. Additionally, the presence of an ICU attending physician assures proper supervision and backup for invasive procedures and airway management. Pharmacists, respiratory therapists, and electrocardiogram technicians can be summoned as needed without being part of every MET call. The primary caregiver or team would also be summoned to participate in evaluation and decision-making.

Concerns Over Implementing a Medical Emergency Team

While barriers to MET implementation are discussed in detail in Chapter 9, a brief discussion is needed here to understand the complexity of the barriers to implementing a teaching program that includes METs.

Acceptance and sustained success of METs has historically involved the cooperation and support of all major departments and services that interface with the team or its patients (12). In approaching department heads about instituting a MET, concerns that one should anticipate are: (1) whether the MET will move decision making authority away from the physician or the service with primary responsibility for a patient, and (2) whether the team's activity will deprive trainees of valuable patient care experience. We will examine how these concerns may have originated and critique the current state of affairs, and see that, at its core, the MET is more about restructuring resource delivery than about radical change.

One can understand, if not sympathize with, departments that are reluctant to accept an extra- or multi-departmental group caring for patients in their service. Yet interdepartmental cooperation frequently occurs at bedside, where the caregiving team is happy to relinquish significant portions of a patient's care management to a cardiologist, nephrologist, surgeon, or oncologist. Indeed, the latter specialties possess certain types of technology, protocols, and detailed knowledge of pathophysiology that can be key to the optimal care management and survival of a patient. In the context of specific organ-based derangements, it is rational to seek this type of support—so why not for critical illness as well? Intensive care may be poorly understood by other physicians, and mainly in narrow, stereotypic roles such as the use of mechanical ventilation, invasive monitoring, and hemodynamic support. In addition, the appearances of illnesses that permeate multiple systems do not present clear triggers for consultation with critical care specialists. To some extent, this is a fault of critical care specialists, who have not done the best job informing colleagues to the nature and spectrum of critical care (13). Likewise, criteria defining "critical illness" have been lacking. Unlike the patients with either myocardial infarction or anuria, it is difficult for physicians to identify when a constellation of nonspecific findings becomes a critical illness. Finally, without good feedback to ward medical teams as to the type of patients that end up in the ICU—and especially the ones that do poorly—intensive care has failed at creating demand for its services outside of the ICU.

Concern over lack of resident experience gained in caring for unstable ward patients probably comes from a fixation on the concept of the MET as an extension of ICU personnel to other patient care domains. However, most METs have some role for resident participation and the overall model is not rigid (12,14–17). Some teams have had the ICU resident participate, and others have used a senior ward resident on a rotating basis. In any case, the common denominator of nearly all MET systems is a concurrent summons of the primary ward team (18). Involvement of the primary team is beneficial to patients not only because it builds upon an existing relationship, but also because it creates a bridge of continuity where vital information can be passed on in the proper context. From a training perspective, having the primary ward team work with the MET not only maintains their exposure to interesting cases and proper care management, but also demands some agreement of care goals, and when there is no consensus, begs for an evidence-based settlement. Additionally, as MET team members, medical residents achieve cross-discipline training by caring for surgical patients, and surgery residents can gain valuable experience caring for medical patients. Since most METs have been developed outside the United States, the uninitiated can be confused by the description of some teams; teams are mostly composed of senior ICU nurses in the United Kingdom, senior residents and clinical fellows in Australia, and ICU nurses and physicians in the United States (19). Table 20.1 describes current resident involvement in different teams and the rough equivalent to postgraduate trainees in the United States (20).

Will a MET interfere with resident training, or more specifically, deprive the junior-level trainee of practical, problem-solving experience? Different types of arguments have been unconsciously incorporated into the culture of medical training: that it is the mission of residency training programs to provide experience and training to residents through the care of patients, and cognitive challenges and decision making are the payoffs for the investment of time, emotion, and hours of dull, unsatisfying work. Unfortunately, we are now learning that the current system has been hazardous to unstable patients, and the MET owes its genesis to the poor outcome of this population (3,8). Residents have other responsibilities and activities besides ward patient care (such as the operating room or clinic) and are not always available for evaluation of patient vital sign abnormalities. Instead, temporizing measures are instituted over the phone, and data and impressions gained from a bedside examination are frequently lacking. Valuable time is wasted as evaluations and decision-making proceeds slowly up a traditional hierarchy (3). Further, many resident teams feel that the care of

TABLE 20.1. Composition of different Medical Emergency Teams

Trainee Description (UK and Australia)	US equivalent	Bristow (15)	Bellomo (18)	Lee (17)	DeVita (19)	Goldhill (20)	Buist (14)
				Study author			
Intern	Subintern/intern						
Resident	Intern, early resident				2	X	
SRMO/registrar	Junior resident			MD use unclear			MD use unclear
Senior registrar	Senior resident/fellow	2	X				
Fellow/deputy consultant	Junior attending		X				
ICU faculty/consultant	Attending		as needed	X	leader	X	
ICU/CCU nurse		X	X		2	X	X
Specific mention of including primary team if available		X	X			X	X
Other personnel (resp. therapy, pharmacy, etc.)						X	

Key and abbreviations:

X = presence of house officer or staff member on team

2 = 2 members at the same training level (in 2 studies, a description of physicians on the team was not made)

SRMO = Senior resident medical officer

unstable patients is a test of their mettle, and that to solicit outside help is a sign of weakness. In many instances, the team's attending physician is never called to help with evaluation. Even when an one is summoned, they may not have the best understanding of how to prioritize diagnostic and stabilization efforts and organize and lead a multidisciplinary team, or possess the technical skills and knowledge required by the situation.

Medical training is structured around the concept of gradually increasing responsibility and decreasing supervision, and a belief in learning from mistakes. Given this, it is reasonable to consider whether a team-oriented approach to unstable patients undermines medical education by depriving residents of the ability to make and learn from their medical decisions. An argument could be made that there is little to be gained from allowing mistakes to occur (21). Observational studies in the intensive care unit as well as in a simulated environment have demonstrated that physicians make errors without even realizing that they occur (7,22); in the case of real patients, it is difficult to imagine how any educational benefit could result from such mistakes if the physician is unaware of them. When errors are detected, there is great variability among individuals, departments, and specialties in acknowledging errors and their sources. In one study on self-reported errors—despite 90% being associated with serious outcomes—only 54% of the house officers discussed their mistakes with an attending physician (23). In a more recent study of morbidity and mortality conferences in internal medical departments, cases containing errors were presented in less than half of the conferences, and were addressed as errors in only one-half of the applicable instances (24). By the authors' estimation, a substantive discussion of error would occur in the studied department's morbidity and mortality conferences only 7 times a year.

If one of the prime modalities of resident training is learning from mistakes, additional thought should be directed toward maximizing the yield of this process. Simulation training may be a superior alternative to practicing on patients—especially for development of crisis management skills (25–28). Simulation training for individuals and teams provides greater exposure to situations that generate errors, and allows residents to acknowledge errors immediately after they occur and to discuss them with peers and senior staff in a constructive, non-punitive environment (7,29). The use of simulation training as part of MET development will be discussed in greater detail below. To summarize here, the MET is not likely to interfere with the assimilation of knowledge and experience in residency training. There is good evidence that allowing too much independence in critical situations may create errors and hazards that are not known, caught, or discussed in a manner that maximizes the educational yield of each mistake. Resident participation in a MET rearranges resident responsibilities in a way that maximizes patient safety and survival, and may in part replace the ethically untenable system of "learning from mistakes" with one that does things the right way.

Procedures

Depending on design, a MET may differ from the current mode of ward care by having attending physicians or fellows involved early on in an evaluation and resuscitation. At first glance, this "top-heavy" approach may seem to deprive residents of valuable experience in performing procedures and evaluating bedside and laboratory data. Personal experience as a triage attending suggests that the opposite is true: when working with medical or surgical house staff to evaluate and stabilize patients in their care, the primary teams are typically pushed toward doing more—whether it is obtaining arterial blood gas studies, placing arterial or central venous catheters, or making changes in ventilatory or fluid therapy. Residents are actually encouraged to look deeper into the patient's problems and to understand more.

Not all critical care attending physicians are likely to participate in a MET; rather there is likely to be a self-selection bias toward those with a more hands-on approach to patient care. Having the MET led by a critical care-based faculty member or fellow is likely to bring to the bedside someone who is comfortable supervising and performing procedures, and who has the skills to back up the care by the primary team. To give a concrete example, our proposal for a MET includes a technology bundle that features a portable blood gas/chemistry analyzer, a portable monitor that can display invasive pressures and exhaled CO_2, and a portable ultrasound machine for analysis of cardiac structure and function. Thus, while the overall mode of care may be different for a ward emergency, the MET brings with it new and perhaps more advanced opportunities for patient evaluation and skill development.

Another example is central lines. Many of our residents on the ICU rotation complain that they get little experience placing central lines because the majority of patients have them placed in the operating room. However, these residents, hungry for experience, rarely place central lines on patients in the emergency room or in the intermediate care unit—even when indicated for safety reasons (for example, vasopressor administration) or by clinical evidence (for example, as a guide for fluid therapy in early sepsis) (30). With the loosening of critical care boundaries that would be seen with a MET, residents will learn more about different invasive procedures, their indication, and the interpretation of their data. Although unproven, we feel that based on this understanding, residents will actually perform more procedures than at present.

A Win-Win Situation

Many of the changes in health care delivery associated with METs are likely to facilitate the development and assessment of competencies now required by the Accreditation Council for Graduate Medical Education (ACGME) and the American Board of Medical Specialties. As part of the Outcomes Project, ACGME residency review committees have required accredited programs to develop competencies in 6 key areas: (2)

- Patient care
- Medical knowledge
- Practice-based learning and improvement
- Interpersonal and communication skills
- Professionalism
- System-based practice

Accordingly, residencies must define specific skills or knowledge for each competency and provide training to attain those objectives. Viewed as a whole, governing bodies not only expect trainees to assimilate medical knowledge in specific areas (as is still required to pass board examinations, qualify for fellowships, etc.) but also develop a more dynamic style of practice. For application of medical knowledge, this means the resident in training must be able to understand the natural history of a certain disease or finding, seek recent information that applies to the patient's case, critically evaluate the differences between the contexts of a given study and the clinical context of the current patient, and from this, synthesize a treatment plan. At the same time, a premium is attached to understanding patient needs and to develop models for shared decision-making. Finally, the resident is also required to attain some understanding of health care systems in general, and how their economics and structure impact the delivery of patient care.

Reading this description conjures up the image of an outpatient physician managing chronic illness with the struggles of balancing efficacy, cost, and complexity of treatment. However, ward emergency care also provides the opportunity to understand the interaction between individual needs and disease processes, care delivery systems, concepts of resource utilization and the culture of academic medicine. In fact, resident involvement in a MET will quite likely provide a reliable structure in which some of the competencies may be mastered, particularly those aspects of "patient care" that arise as urgent, life-threatening situations. The latter is an area of medicine where the stakes are very high and typically not accompanied by an equally high degree of faculty expertise, supervision, and mentorship. Creating a system—albeit a "top heavy" one—where patient care is enhanced by early expert intervention should be regarded as a win-win situation, even in the context of medical education.

How a Medical Emergency Team Can Teach Residents about Patient Safety

Emergency ward care also provides a microcosm of health care in which other competencies can be mastered. Practice-based learning requires not only evaluation of medical evidence in literature, but improvement in care based on the analysis of experience using a systematic methodology. As part of systems-based practice, residents are required to "effectively call on system resources to provide care that is of optimal value" (2). The existence of a MET reflects an institution's commitment to self-examination and its willingness to rearrange resources and disciplinary lines to create more efficient care and better outcomes for patients—but what is really learned from this? Some direct learning objectives can and should be built into MET operation, but a trainee will also benefit from the collective unconscious of an institution that encourages:

- Doing things the right way—placing a premium on patient safety over training
- Understanding the connection between events and errors, how sources of errors are analyzed, and how change results from this
- Understanding how safety underlies patient-system, doctor-patient, and doctor-system relationships and how institutional, cultural, and individual change has come from this focus
- Appreciating multidisciplinary teams and teamwork

While the MET aims to provide immediate service to patients in need, an educational component can be designed into its operation in a number of ways. First, the MET should engage in research that monitors patient outcomes and ensures that its calling criteria are properly aligned to the target patient population. Data from cardiac arrests, ICU admissions, quality assurance projects, and disease-specific treatments can be analyzed to understand patient care characteristics, and any gaps that need to be filled. Second, the MET should have routine debriefings (immediately after the event is best) with an emphasis on self-critique, team dynamics, and error analysis. Competency assessments can be designed into debriefings, and enhanced by the use of audio- or videotape analysis. Error analysis can provide important insight into whether improvements need to be made in technical training, teamwork, or organizational structure (31,32). The overall handling and discussion of errors and "near misses" is likely to increase the extent of error reporting if done in a proper manner. A system that that rewards admission of mistakes creates a healthy climate where there is a greater likelihood of identifying and correcting "latent" sources of future errors (29). Residents exposed to such a culture of safety may let this philosophy shape behavior and improve patient care in other settings.

In brief, the role of the resident is likely to change with the inception of a Medical Emergency Team. Despite what some may perceive as a loss of autonomy or independence with the change, a more favorable structure for patient care could be the product. Table 20.2 summarizes some differences one would likely see.

TABLE 20.2. Effect on Residents of a MET

Training Objective	Current Status	With MET
Patient evaluation and therapy	Relatively independent, gain sense of responsibility Bad habits may be reinforced No clear feedback on what was done correctly or not Heterogeneity in methods Process based on individual action	Get to see a refined operation Learn proven methods of evaluation Consistent method of analysis applied Can develop models for individual actions within framework of a team Latest evidence and methods likely applied Process based on multidisciplinary teamwork
Resident education and medical knowledge that address	Learn through experience Time-critical mistakes can be made while "learning by doing" Culture of "see one, do one"	See evidence-based methods applied strengths, weakness Debriefings allow appraisal of Would see development of curricula that address acute resuscitation Would receive some training on teamwork concepts
Patient safety	Occasional discussions roundson patient safety during rounds Different institutions are studying threats, or "near misses" Morbidity and mortality, QA conferences Culture of "see one, do one"	High-reliability organization concepts Provides a model for a "culture of safety" Allows design of a process that includes debriefings and open analysis of actions Potential for videotape review of real events Recognizes need for simulation and practice
Invasive procedures	Senior resident supervises (might not be that skilled) May be avoided due to lack of comfort or lack of expertise Other party performs the procedure Patient comfort and safety variable Unclear use of data from invasive lines	Expert may perform procedure if time is critical (resident gets to see procedure done right) Expert supervises resident during later procedures, (mistakes and technique lapses are corrected) Emphasis on comfort, speed, and safety Structured and systematic use of data, Patient benefits from procedure with potentially less risk

TABLE 20.2. *Continued*

Criteria for calling medical emergency team:
Airway Respiratory distress Threatened airway
Breathing Respiratory rate >30 breaths/min Respiratory rate <6 breaths/min Oxygen saturation <90% Difficulty speaking
Circulation Systolic blood pressure <90 mm Hg despite treatment Pulse rate >130 bpm
Neuroligic Unexplained decline in mental function Agitation or delirium Repeated or prolonged seizure
Other Concern about patient Uncontrolled pain Failure to respond to treatment Unable to obtain prompt assistance

Promoting Performance Standards: A Role for Human Patient Simulation

As opposed to a cardiac arrest team, the MET is charged with managing a wide array of conditions with greater diagnostic and therapeutic uncertainty. Therefore, the goals of the MET are best achieved by programs committed to additional training and continued re-examination of performance. From the outset, training activities should be geared toward managing critical conditions that commonly recur in the pre-arrest stage. Experience with antecedents to cardiac arrest and ICU admission has led to the development of a list of calling criteria that are designed to identify patients at risk (12,14,33). One such list, published by Buist et al. is reproduced below (14).

These different types of emergencies require different tasks and priorities, and the role of personnel will vary according to the situation. Non-technical aspects of patient care, such as teamwork, leadership, and task distribution, are probably best applied to real emergencies if they have been practiced at an earlier time. Medical simulation has been used to teach crisis management skills in a number of acute care professions, including critical care, and is a natural fit for MET training (7,30,34). As a training modality, human patient simulation guarantees the resident exposure to the desired case mix, and at no risk to the patient. Ideally, the MET will have periodic practice sessions to maintain competency, refine methods, and to incorporate new members. Scoring systems that rate individual performances in the management of specific patient emergencies have been developed and used in simulated patient scenarios, and may be applicable to the training and evaluation of MET teams as a whole (34,35).

As an operating principle, the MET should practice evidence-based medicine. Simulation training provides an opportunity for team members to discuss new diagnostic modalities and therapies and to rapidly incorporate them into team operations. There is certainly a basis for resident attendance and involvement in such activities, and this alone can provide some direct training experience in crisis management as well as engender some consistency in the evaluation of patients in uncontrolled settings.

The use of vasoactive and analgesic medicines in medical emergencies is vastly different from that in other settings, including advanced cardiac life support emergencies; our own work in ICU crisis simulation suggests that this remains an esoteric body of knowledge and a frequent source of error (7). A simulated environment is especially valuable in learning the use and pitfalls of these medicines for different types of patients and in dynamic situations. Most residencies lack direct skill development in crisis management, so, insofar as a MET can increase exposure to and assimilation of such skills, it should be regarded as another plus for the training of medical residents.

Summary

The need to train and develop house staff for independent practice may conflict with the needs of patients who require rapid stabilization. Finding a healthy balance between the 2, where the patient receives the best care possible, is a challenge to those in academic medicine. Increasingly, data suggests that the traditional models of resident training have in part failed to place the patient first. The contributors to this text believe that the implementation of Medical Emergency Teams will offset some of these shortcomings in care and improve the public accountability of medical education. The MET can also offer opportunities for the development of competencies in patient care for both trainees and established physicians. Likewise, the MET can provide an educational structure from which house staff can learn a great deal more about interdisciplinary teamwork, patient safety, and the responsiveness of health care to patient needs.

References

1. Kohn LT, Corrigan JM, Donaldson MS, eds. To Err Is Human: Building a Safer Health System. Washington, DC: National Academies Press; 2000.
2. Accreditation Council for Graduate Medical Education. Outcome project. Available at: http://www.acgme.org/outcome/. Accessed September 29, 2004.
3. Buist MD, Jarmolowski E, Burton PR, Bernard SA, Waxman BP, Anderson J. Recognising clinical instability in hospital patients before cardiac arrest or unplanned admission to intensive care. A pilot study in a tertiary-care hospital. *Med J Aust.* 1999;171:22–25.
4. Sax FL, Charlson ME. Medical patients at high risk for catastrophic deterioration. *Crit Care Med.* 1987;15:510–515.
5. Franklin C, Mathew J. Developing strategies to prevent in-hospital cardiac arrest: analyzing responses of physicians and nurses in the hours before the event. *Crit Care Med.* 1994;22(2):244–247.
6. McQuillan P, Pilkington S, Allan A, et al. Confidential inquiry into quality of care before admission to intensive care. *BMJ.* 1998;316(7148):1853–1858.
7. Lighthall GK, Barr J, Howard SK, et al. Use of a fully simulated intensive care unit environment for critical event management training for internal medicine residents. *Crit Care Med.* 2003;31:2437–2443.
8. Schein RM, Hazday N, Pena M, Ruben BH, Sprung CL. Clinical antecedents to in-hospital cardiopulmonary arrest. *Chest.* 1990;98:1388–1392.
9. McGloin H, Adam SK, Singer M. Unexpected deaths and referrals to intensive care of patients on general wards. Are some cases potentially avoidable? *J R Coll Physicians Lond.* 1999;33:255–259.
10. Hillman KM, Bristow PJ, Chey T, et al. Duration of life-threatening antecedents prior to intensive care admission. *Intensive Care Med.* 2002;28:1629–1634.
11. Petersen LA, Brennan TA, O'Neil AC, Cook EF, Lee TH. Does house staff discontinuity of care increase the risk for preventable adverse events? *Ann Intern Med.* 1994;121(11):866–872.
12. Bellomo R, Goldsmith D, Uchino S, et al. Prospective controlled trial of effect of medical emergency team on postoperative morbidity and mortality rates. *Crit Care Med.* 2004;32(4):916–921.
13. Franklin CM. Deconstructing the black box known as the intensive care unit. *Crit Care Med.* 1998;26:1300–1301.
14. Buist MD, Moore GE, Bernard SA, Waxman BP, Anderson JN, Nguyen TV. Effects of a medical emergency team on reduction of incidence of and mortality from unexpected cardiac arrests in hospital: preliminary study. *BMJ.* 2002;324:387–390.
15. Bristow PJ, Hillman KM, Chey T, et al. Rates of in-hospital arrests, deaths and intensive care admissions: the effect of a medical emergency team. *Med J Aust.* 2000;173:236–240.
16. Leary T, Ridley S. Impact of an outreach team on re-admissions to a critical care unit. *Anaesthesia.* 2003;58:328–332.
17. Lee A, Bishop G, Hillman KM, Daffurn K. The Medical Emergency Team. *Anaesth Intensive Care.* 1995;23(2):183–186.
18. Bellomo R, Goldsmith D, Uchino S, et al. A prospective before-and-after trial of a medical emergency team. *Med J Aust.* 2003;179:283–287.

19. DeVita MA, Braithwaite RS, Mahidhara R, Stuart S, Foraida M, Simmons RL; Medical Emergency Response Improvement Team (MERIT). Use of medical emergency team responses to reduce hospital cardiopulmonary arrests. *Qual Saf Health Care.* 2004;13:251–254.

20. Goldhill DR, Worthington L, Mulcahy A, Tarling M, Sumner A. The patient-at-risk team: identifying and managing seriously ill ward patients. *Anaesthesia.* 1999;54:853–860.

21. Pronovost PJ, Wu AW, Sexton JB. Acute decompensation after removing a central line: practical approaches to increasing safety in the intensive care unit. *Ann Intern Med.* 2004;140:1025–1033.

22. Landrigan CP, Rothschild JM, Cronin JW, et al. Effect of reducing interns' work hours on serious medical errors in intensive care units. *N Engl J Med.* 2004;351: 1838–1848.

23. Wu AW, Folkman S, McPhee SJ, Lo B. How house officers cope with their mistakes. *West J Med.* 1993;159:565–569.

24. Pierluissi E, Fisher MA, Campbell AR, Landefeld CS. Discussion of medical errors in morbidity and mortality conferences. *JAMA.* 2003;290(21):2838–2842.

25. Howard SK, Gaba DM, Fish KJ, Yang G, Sarnquist FH. Anesthesia crisis resource management training: teaching anesthesiologists to handle critical incidents. *Aviat Space Environ Med.* 1992;63(9):763–770.

26. Halamek LP, Kaegi DM, Gaba DM, et al. Time for a new paradigm in pediatric medical education: teaching neonatal resuscitation in a simulated delivery room environment. *Pediatrics.* 2000;106:E45.

27. Gaba DM. The future vision of simulation in health care. *Qual Saf Health Care.* 2004;13(suppl 1):i2–i10.

28. Reznek M, Smith-Coggins R, Howard S, et al. Emergency Medicine Crisis Resource Management (EMCRM): Pilot study of a simulation-based crisis management course for emergency medicine. *Acad Emerg Med.* 2003;10:386–389.

29. Lighthall G. The IMPES Course: Toward better outcomes through simulator-based multidisciplinary team training. In Dunn WF, ed. *Simulators in Critical Care and Beyond.* Des Plaines, Ill: SCCM Press; 2004:54–60.

30. Rivers E, Nguyen B, Havstad S, et al. Early goal-directed therapy in the treatment of severe sepsis and septic shock. *N Engl J Med.* 2001;345(19):1368–1377.

31. Helmreich RL. On error management: lessons from aviation. *BMJ.* 2000; 320:781–785.

32. Braithwait RS, DeVita MA, Mahidhara R, et al. Use of medical emergency team (MET) responses to detect medical errors. *Qual Saf Health Care.* 2004;13: 255–259.

33. Grenvik A, Schaefer JJ, DeVita MA, Rogers P. New aspects on critical care medicine training. *Curr Opin Crit Care.* 2004;10(4):233–237.

34. Boulet JR, Murray D, Kras J, Woodhouse J, McAllister J, Ziv A. Reliability and validity of a simulation-based acute care skills assessment for medical students and residents. *Anesthesiology.* 2003;99(6):1270–1280.

35. Gaba DM, Howard SK, Flanagan B, Smith BE, Fish KJ, Botney R. Assessment of clinical performance during simulated crises using both technical and behavioral ratings. *Anesthesiology.* 1998;89:8–18.

21
Teaching Organized Crisis Team Functioning Using Human Simulators

MELINDA FIEDOR, ELIZABETH A. HUNT, and MICHAEL A. DEVITA

Introduction

A recent report by the National Registry of Cardiopulmonary Resuscitation (NRCPR) of 207 hospitals within the United States revealed that the majority (86%) has an organized team to respond to in-hospital cardiac arrests (1). Despite the existence of these teams, there is mounting evidence that errors in the management of care for patients with in-hospital cardiac arrests and other medical crises may contribute to poor outcomes (2–8). Currently, no standards exist in terms of how such "code teams" are dispatched, how many members are on the team, or the team's composition. There are even fewer reports regarding the make-up of Medical Emergency Teams (METs). Training to enhance the quality of care delivered by crisis teams in hospitals is essential. Although the composition of these 2 types of hospital teams varies from place to place, the principles of team training remain the same, and are reviewed in this chapter.

The word "team" typically refers to a group of people that work together on a regular basis, in a coordinated and coherent fashion. Professional athletic teams provide an example of how a classic team functions: team members all have a *common goal* of winning their athletic events; they *practice together* regularly; individuals typically have 1 *designated role* or position that they play, and in which they become a true expert; team members often develop some type of shorthand to aid in *communication*; and the team typically functions best with a good *team leader* or captain.

Unique Aspects of Hospital Crisis Teams

Hospital crisis teams serve a critical purpose: to prevent death in suddenly critically ill patients. To succeed, they must function effectively and efficiently. Delays in action, miscommunication, and errors can increase the likelihood of a fatal outcome for the patient. Such a critical function should be the target of frequent and effective training programs, but ironically, training crisis teams is particularly difficult because of the dynamic nature of the teams. In many ways, crisis teams represent the antithesis of the well-trained athletic team and must overcome major barriers to function effectively.

The Ad Hoc Nature of Crisis Teams

Code teams are ad hoc teams—they consist of people who are brought together in a crisis, although previously they may never have worked together. Once the crisis is over, they return to their other activities and may not work together again. It seems impossible to train all of the possible combinations of a code team. A study by Pittman et al. of a cardiac arrest team revealed that 67% of team leaders had had no communication with the team members prior to the cardiac arrest event (9); 33% had "informal" communication prior, and only 7% had a debriefing session after the cardiac arrest (9).

The ad hoc nature of crisis teams makes it difficult to practice communication, organization, group problem solving, and the integrated functioning skills necessary for teamwork. The difference between a team that practices until they function like a well-oiled machine and the team whose members have literally never met becomes obvious when video recordings of crisis events are reviewed. Crisis team training programs must directly address the fact that the team that assembles for a crisis may not have worked together previously.

Simulation of Crises as Diagnostic Tool

Sullivan and Guyatt published one of the first studies of the use of cardiac arrest simulations in the hospital setting to identify deficiencies in the crisis team response (4). They concluded: "Mock arrests are an extraordinarily powerful means of revealing suspected and unsuspected inadequacies in resuscitation procedure and equipment, and in motivating physicians and administrators to correct the deficiencies rapidly" (4). Subsequent work by other teams has similarly revealed that simulation can be a powerful diagnostic tool in revealing inadequacies in a hospital's crisis response (5–8).

The mock code work by Dongilli et al. provides an example of applying crisis team training principles successfully as a diagnostic tool (6). Mock codes were run over several months in an adult hospital that is part of a 22-hospital health institution (6). The aim was to evaluate the first responders and the elapsed time until appropriate resuscitation maneuvers. Measurements included elapsed time: time to call the operator about the crisis, time to send a voice page to the code team, time to code pagers tones, and time to first responder arrival (6). Analysis of the results revealed that it took up to 4 minutes for the first responder to arrive at the crisis (6). In reviewing the hospitals' operator notification procedure, it was discovered that the operators received the call, entered information into the paging system, triggered the belt paging system (which requires 3 minutes to deliver the page alert), and then paged the code team on the overhead speaker system (6). This process caused an unnecessary delay in the time to the first responder's arrival to the crisis. Procedure was changed, and the operators were instructed to voice page the code team immediately after receiving the call and to set off the pagers afterwards (6). After this protocol change, time to arrival of the first responder at the next mock code was improved to 1 minute and 46 seconds, and has reliably remained around 90 seconds since (6).

Hunt performed a series of 34 surprise, multidisciplinary mock codes over a 3-year period at 3 hospitals that care for children (8). The mock codes consisted of scenarios of pediatric respiratory distress, respiratory arrest, or cardiopulmonary arrest (8). Evaluation revealed delays to the assessment of airway, breathing, circulation, administration of oxygen, initiation of chest compressions, and decision to defibrillate, as well as errors in leadership and communication (8). Hunt concluded that the study identified "targets for educational interventions to improve pediatric cardiopulmonary resuscitation and, ideally, outcomes" (8).

Crisis team training should focus on organizational skills, not on medical and nursing assessment and treatment skills. Required elements in a crisis team training session include well-written, simulated resuscitation scenarios and skillful debriefing that focuses on organization. General principles to follow for crisis team training scenarios include using life-like situations, having a specific learning objective or objectives for each scenario (or more accurately, each debriefing), and incorporating team quality improvement goals. In addition, real-life errors can be replicated to train teams to avoid similar mistakes. Finally, scenarios should be focused: they can be as short as 1 minute if the learning objective is to see how long it takes a person to recognize a crisis, request a MET response, and have the first responder arrive. On the other hand, if the goal is to focus on diagnosis and triage to an appropriate ICU, the scenario may require as long as 20 minutes.

In any case, one should not expect to use a simulator and suddenly be able to train teams. Team training requires an organized curriculum and effective teaching directed at achieving specific behaviors. This chapter will address some key elements in developing a crisis team training curriculum.

What to Teach

The first step in developing a curriculum for crisis team training is to create clearly defined educational objectives for the session. Although these objectives will vary slightly at each institution, based on identified deficiencies, the training must openly acknowledge the unique nature of crisis teams and provide a road map to enable the ad-hoc group to function well together. The following principles will invariably need to be covered: the team's goals, designated role assignment, communication, and leadership.

Goals of Crisis Teams

For crisis teams to function in an organized manner, they must devote time and effort to organization at the beginning of a crisis response. In our opinion, the major reason that crisis team responses tend to be disorganized is because individual members jump into medical and nursing actions prior to organizing the team. Teams are more likely to function well if the individuals have common goals, and they coordinate their efforts. Once organization has occurred, then medical and nursing interventions will proceed more efficiently.

The first and most important goal of the team is to deliver effective and efficient basic life support throughout the entire episode. This includes assessment of airway, breathing, and circulation, and if necessary rapid initiation of bag-mask ventilation and chest compressions, rapid defibrillation, and frequent reassessment. If the patient is in a shockable rhythm, the specific goal should be for the first shock to be delivered within 3 minutes of patient collapse.

The second goal is the effective and efficient delivery of appropriate advanced life support, including diagnosis of the underlying problem and delivery of definitive care. Finally, appropriate triage must occur.

Merely making team members aware of their overall goals and of the time intervals by which a specific resuscitation maneuver should be performed likely will be associated with better performance (10). In addition to the team goals, each individual member should be aware of the goals for their specific role, as each specific job, if done appropriately, will help meet the overall goals.

Designated Roles: Assignment and Definition

When a crisis occurs in the hospital, the worst-case scenario is to have no plan for dealing with it. This is very unlikely in the 21st century. However, it is surprisingly common for a hospital to make a concerted effort to determine who will carry code beepers and how they will be activated, and yet neglect to plan who will perform which resuscitation job, or even what the jobs are. Unfortunately, this often results in important jobs or resuscitation tasks being left undone—for example, a delay to the performance of chest compressions or placement of intravenous access.

The key to designing a crisis team response is to determine the specific roles and corresponding responsibilities that are desired, and then designate them ahead of time, during training. There are 2 effective approaches to role assignment. The first is to have very clear roles that need to be assumed; often it does not matter who assumes which role, only that each role is filled. The second approach is teach each person who carries the code beeper what their expected specific role will be when they arrive, so they know what they should do. If that role is filled while another remains open, the responders must recognize that circumstance and fill the empty role. Failure to do this may result in failure to perform key tasks and lead to patient harm.

Each institution also must determine how its team will be structured—that is, who will participate in the response. Organizing the team and choosing roles go hand-in-hand. One must be familiar with available personnel for a crisis team response and choose roles accordingly. For example, one institution may only have 4 available crisis team responders, while another may have 10. The latter team will be able to expand the number of available roles, i.e. having 2 crash cart managers instead of 1. Once it is clear how many people (and from which disciplines) are available to the team, assignment of the responsibilities for each role is the next step. Explicitly designating roles and responsibilities will remove the ambiguity that contributes to the chaos often seen during a crisis situation.

At the University of Pittsburgh, we have chosen 8 roles for our crisis team response. We initially used 6 members, but found repeated specific errors during training. We adjusted the team composition and added members until the training teams reliably succeeded in meeting preset task completion goals. We also decided that it is important that all team members are trained to assume any 1 of several roles that they are capable of performing. This cross training improves the team's flexibility and the understanding of the roles that other team members play, and failure to cross-train leads to errors of omission. For example, if a team has no anesthesiologists or intensivists, it is common that no one manages the airway; instead they wait for the airway expert to arrive, even though team members often possess sufficient skills to manage the airway until an expert arrives.

All members of the Medical Emergency Team—including residents, fellows, attending physicians, critical care nurses, respiratory therapists, and pharmacists—take part in crisis team training sessions at the WISER Simulation Center. These full-scale, human simulation training sessions have allowed us to analyze team function and have been the impetus for changes in team structure.

At the beginning of the team training sessions, MET members who have usually never worked together during a medical crisis are required to complete an online didactic program. Upon arrival to the simulation center, the facilitator reviews key concepts of the didactic, and orients the group to the simulator. They then participate in a simulated crisis scenario. We currently have 8 scenarios (including a "null" scenario in which the simulated patient is not in a crisis). We have observed that the first attempt by the team is invariably chaotic, and many important resuscitation tasks are either delayed or will not be performed at all. For example, after training over 500 Advanced Cardiac Life-Support trained individuals, only 1 team (usually 16 to 20 people participate in a crisis team training course) has successfully defibrillated ventricular fibrillation in under 3 minutes in their first simulator session; by the end of the training program, virtually all teams are successful. See Figure 21.1 for crisis task performance and Figure 21.2 for simulated survival during the training sessions.

During the training session, crisis team members familiarize themselves with *all* goals and the roles that they are individually capable of performing; we ensure this by not allowing any person to play the same role twice during training. After debriefing in which participants determine whether they assumed all the roles of our response, and whether they completed all the tasks associated with each role, they then move on to more simulations. The team participates in 4 simulations, with debriefings to assess role assignment, task responsibility, and team interaction. Because participants take on different roles in each simulation, they develop an understanding of how the team begins to function more effectively and efficiently when each role is filled and the responsibilities clearly defined. This "roles and goals"

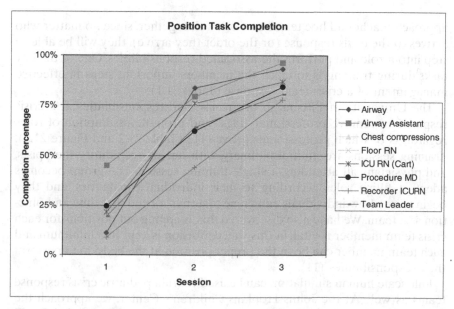

FIGURE 21.1. Performance improvement of role-related tasks from the first through the third sessions of a human-simulator crisis team-training program.

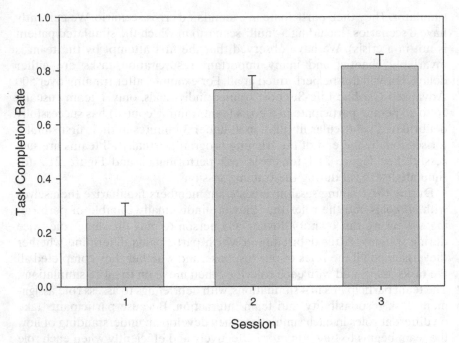

FIGURE 21.2. Overall team task completion rate during the first, second, and third scenario session of a 3-hour training program.

approach teaches ad hoc teams to work well together, since no matter who arrives to the crisis response (or the order they arrive), they will be able to step into a role and perform the associated responsibilities. One of the key tasks during training is to teach the members important steps in effective management of a crisis team response (Table 21.1).

The University of Pittsburgh has reclassified responsibilities at a crisis response to remove professional "tags" and promote assumption of roles regardless of which professionals arrive (11) (Table 21.2 and Figure 21.3). Training sessions are multidisciplinary, with nurses, respiratory therapists, and physicians all attending a single training session. The group becomes adept at filling roles according to their individual capabilities, and they begin to see how individuals can come together for the first time and function as a team. We have also discovered that mapping out positions for each crisis team member is vital; in this way, confusion is kept to a minimum and each team member can be in the proper position at the bedside to perform their responsibilities (11).

Full-scale human simulation can be used to train pediatric crisis response teams as well. At the Johns Hopkins Children's Center, we approach the team structure and function by training individuals on what their job will be upon arrival at every crisis they attend. We also avoid the term Pediatric

TABLE 21.1. Key lessons for crisis team training

Organize the team
Choose roles
Identify and complete responsibilities
Communicate data to relevant person
Analyze data
Diagnose patient
Treat patient

TABLE 21.2. Roles and goals of crisis team members

Roles	Goals
Airway manager (#1 in Fig. 22.3)	Manages ventilation and oxygenation, intubates if necessary
Airway assistant (#2)	Provides equipment to airway manager, assists with bag-maskventilation
Bedside assistant (#3)	Provides patient information including AMPLE*, medications delivery
Equipment manager (#4)	Draws up medications, supplies crash cart contents to appropriate team members
Data manager/recorder (#8)	Records vital signs, exam findings, test results, chart
Circulation (#6)	Evaluates pulses, performs chest compressions
Procedure MD (#7)	Performs procedures such as central lines, chest tubes, pulse check
Treatment leader (#5)	Analyzes data, diagnoses, and directs patient treatment

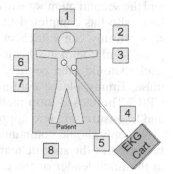

Team Roles and Goals

FIGURE 21.3. Graphic representation of team roles and goals. Numbers correspond to roles listed in Table 21.2.

Code Team, preferring instead Pediatric Rapid Response Team. The reason is that the team usually encounters a crisis, and not a cardiac arrest. The team has 10 members, in addition to the floor team, and each member has a specific role. The roles are defined in a hospital protocol, described to individuals during orientation and are practiced during various team-training sessions. For example, pediatric residents are trained to understand that during their internship year, any time they respond to a medical crisis their sole job will be to perform compressions if needed. The second-year pediatric residents are trained such that their job will be to defibrillate the patient if needed and otherwise assist with placement of vascular access.

In addition, there are monthly resuscitation training sessions for the residents rotating through the wards. They participate in a series of short mock codes and take turns practicing: 1) identifying themselves as a leader, 2) fulfilling the roles they will be expected to perform during actual events, 3) communicating during crises, and 4) performing important resuscitation tasks i.e. CPR, bag-mask ventilation, defibrillation, and placement of intraosseous needles.

Developing a method to ensure that every important resuscitation task will be completed at every crisis depends on creating: 1) clear role definitions, 2) a clear method for determining who will fill each role, and 3) training exercises to allow team members to practice filling the roles and completing the tasks as a cohesive unit.

Communication

Training to ensure effective communication is the next piece to organize. Closed-loop feedback communication is an important method: this term refers to the process whereby a team member will speak to another member and the second member will confirm hearing the message and confirm when he or she has completed the assigned task. For example, the team leader says, "Jimmy, can you check a pulse." Jimmy then states, "I will check the pulse" and completes his job by saying "I still do not have a pulse." The leader should then confirm receiving this information, "Okay there is no pulse, Jimmy please continue CPR." Jimmy confirms, "I am continuing CPR." The closed-loop method of communication serves to lessen chaos and to ensure safe and appropriate management of patient care.

Not only should communication occur in a closed-loop manner, it should be aimed at the specific team member who requires the information, such as the team leader or the crash cart manager; use of first names is important and effective. The team leader can then analyze data from the team members provided via closed-loop communication, assimilating the information and diagnosing the patient, and then again via closed-loop communication give instruction about appropriate patient treatment.

Simulation of cardiopulmonary arrests allows crisis team members to practice these communication skills. A particularly effective method is to allow code team members to visualize the effect of communication errors that occurred in the safe environment of the simulation center. For example, during a mock code of a patient in profound septic shock, a pediatric resident orders a 20 cc/kg bolus of normal saline, and when the blood pressure remains low, repeats the order 2 more times; at the end of the mock code, the resident believes the patient has received 60 cc/kg of normal saline. Upon discussion with the nurses, it becomes clear that they were almost done preparing the first bolus, but none of the fluid had actually been delivered. They had not even heard the second or third orders, and did not realize that the normal saline was a priority, believing that the antibiotics were more important.

Within a crisis team, there are "mini-teams" that have more specific functions, and communication channels must be developed within the group as well as among groups. The 3 mini-teams are the breathing team, the circulation and patient assessment team, and the diagnosis and treatment team. The breathing team consists of an airway manager and an assistant. They obviously must work closely together, and must have one-to-one communication independent of other communication. The circulation team is responsible for determining the presence and quality of circulation, and delivering both circulatory assistance and medications. They need to cross-check findings and coordinate tasks that might interfere with each other, like doing chest compressions, placing a central venous catheter, and placing defibrillator pads. Finally the diagnosis and treatment team must assemble all the data, make treatment decisions, and implement them. Recognition of the presence and role of these mini-teams can help improve communication. The goal of the emphasis on organization and communication is to foster a collective consciousness, in which team members coordinate to collect, transmit, and act on data as a group rather than as individuals. Such a goal has been described in the military for aircraft carrier flight crews, (12) but it is as yet not well described in the Medical Emergency Team literature.

Leadership

Multiple studies demonstrate that poor leadership during cardiopulmonary resuscitation efforts is associated with poor team function (3,13). Cooper and Wakelam observed actual cardiopulmonary arrests and used the Leadership Behavior Description Questionnaire (3). This study revealed that leaders who participated in tasks in a "hands-on" manner were "less likely to build a structured team, the teams were less dynamic, and the tasks of resuscitation were performed less effectively" (3). Marsch et al. studied simulated cardiopulmonary resuscitation efforts and observed that "absence of leadership behavior and absence of explicit task distribution were associated with poor team performance" (13).

While good leadership can help ensure good team functioning, a system must be in place to make sure that the team functions well even without an effective leader. For this reason team members should be taught to assume their roles without needing to be reminded to do it. However, simulation of cardiopulmonary arrests will allow the code team members to practice their leadership skills and actually see the effect of poor leadership. More importantly, training can allow leaders to practice until they can competently head a team.

At the University of Pittsburgh, we avoid using the "team leader" designation for several reasons. First, if there is a team leader, other participants hesitate to assume responsibilities until they are assigned, this in turn can lead to delays. Second, if the team leader is assigning roles and tasks, then the leader is not attending to the patient (he or she is caring for the team instead). Third, if the team leader responds late, key treatments may be delayed while people await the leader's arrival. Additionally, a hierarchical role structure assumed during codes may impede communication, especially when the team leader is perceived to be wrong. We choose a "flat" hierarchy: if everyone knows their roles and self-assigns, then the leader can attend to diagnostics and appropriate therapeutics. The terminology we prefer is "treatment leader" for the person who designates treatments, and "data manager" for the person who ensures all roles are assumed and obtains the data from each team member. The flat hierarchy aids communication and the crosschecking of data and treatment decisions. No study has yet been performed to determine what kind of team training results in best performance.

Debriefing

Debriefing is an essential component of crisis team training. Marteau et al. state there is a "well described tendency to invoke competence after success but not question it after failure." (14) Their data demonstrated that resuscitation experience without feedback increased confidence, but not competence (14).

The principles of debriefing include timeliness, objectivity, specificity, and balance. Timeliness means that debriefing is most effective for the learner if it occurs immediately after the scenario. This ensures that the experience is fresh in the minds of the trainees, allowing for the greatest learning from feedback and self-assessment.

Debriefing should be objective and specific. It should focus on particulars—not "you did a good job" but "you appropriately applied oxygen to the patient within 30 seconds." Debriefing can be made very specific using simulation and video recordings. Video review of team performance using an objective evaluation instrument allows exact and detailed debriefing.

Finally, debriefing should be balanced. Both successes and errors should be discussed. The key to successful debriefing is to be positive, even if an error is the learning point. The error should be noted, but the focus should be on correct actions. Prior to team training, it should be reinforced that errors will occur during the simulation scenarios just as they occur in the real world. Simulation, however, allows for errors to happen in a safe and educational environment. In the simulated setting, errors can be powerful instructional aids and provide motivation. At the University of Pittsburgh, we believe that it is difficult if not impossible to objectively debrief team members after a real crisis, especially if there is a bad outcome. First, they are not objective, balanced, and specific: there are no video and audio recordings upon which to base an objective assessment. Second, because a live person is involved, team members may have significant emotional or psychological responses to the event and the outcome that impair their ability to be objective or to learn.

What to Measure

Crisis team training is important for education, patient safety, and research. For each of these areas, training is most effective if its components can be measured. Measurement can identify deficiencies and demonstrate improvements, if they occur. The key is to measure the correct outcome.

If the aim of crisis team training is education, scenarios should be written with tasks centered on a specific educational goal, such as correct bag-mask ventilation. The measurement will ultimately be a dichotomous value, i.e. "yes" or "no," as to whether the skill was performed effectively. The results help to identify areas on which to focus during debriefing. Institutions may use this technique of successful skill completion to qualify individuals for privileges in a hospital. For example, anesthesiologists may have to successfully demonstrate difficult airway maneuvers in order to receive privileges in their institution.

If the goal of crisis team training is patient safety, measurement could be of patient outcome. However, since many of the outcomes we seek to avoid are rare, it may not be reasonable to look solely at changes in the rate of these outcomes. A second approach can be to observe adherence to desired procedures. For example, if simulation of airway management during a crisis increases the proportion of times that the team remembers to apply cricoid pressure during bag-mask ventilation, it is probable that aspiration events will be decreased.

Research using crisis team training can focus on combinations of the above. Measurement of successful tasks completed by a team member or the entire team can be compared before and after team training, as well as over time. Studies by Gaba et al. show that both technical and behavioral performance can be assessed via evaluation of videotapes of simulated crisis events (15). Their results show that cognition and crisis management behaviors vary considerably (15). This has been seen before and demonstrates the ability of simulation to be used as a "needs assessment tool."

Blum et al. describe the development of an anesthesia crisis resource management course (16). The course objectives were to understand and improve participant skills in crisis resource management and learn debriefing skills (16). Course usefulness, debriefing skills, and crisis resource management principles were highly rated by participants (16). It is interesting to note that course participants were eligible for malpractice premium reductions (16).

Conclusion

Data from both real and simulated events reveals that errors in the management of in-hospital cardiac arrests and other medical crises may contribute to poor patient outcomes (2–8). Successful crisis team training may improve the effectiveness and efficiency of crisis teams, and ultimately improve patient outcomes. Crisis team training should include: 1) clear delineation of the goals of the team, 2) designated role assignments of crisis team members, 3) communication training, and 4) leadership training. The training can be successfully achieved using simulation in combination with well-written scenarios, skillful debriefing, and specific measurements of deficiencies and achievements related to training.

References

1. Peberdy MA, Kaye W, Ornato JP, et al. Cardiopulmonary resuscitation of adults in the hospital: a report of 14 720 cardiac arrests from the National Registry of Cardiopulmonary Resuscitation. *Resuscitation.* 2003;58:297–308.
2. Abella BS, Alvarado JP, Myklebust H, et al. Quality of cardiopulmonary resuscitation during in-hospital cardiac arrest. *JAMA.* 2005;293:301–310.
3. Cooper S, Wakelam A. Leadership of resuscitation teams: 'Lighthouse Leadership'. *Resuscitation.* 1999;42:27–45.
4. Sullivan MJ, Guyatt GH. Simulated cardiac arrests for monitoring quality of in-hospital resuscitation. *Lancet.* 1986;2:618–620.
5. Palmisano JM, Akingbola OA, Moler FW, Custer JR. Simulated pediatric cardiopulmonary resuscitation: initial events and response times of a hospital arrest team. *Respiratory Care.* 1994;39:725–729.
6. Dongilli T, DeVita M, Schaefer J, Grbach W, Fiedor M. The use of simulation training in a large multihospital health system to increase patient safety. Presented at: International Meeting for Medical Simulation; January 2004; Albuquerque, NM.

7. Misko L, Molle E. Beyond the classroom—teaching staff to manage cardiac arrest situations. *J Nurses Staff Devt.* 2003;19:292–296.
8. Hunt EA. Simulation of pediatric cardiopulmonary arrests: a report of mock codes performed over a 40-month period focused on assessing delays in important resuscitation maneuvers and types of errors. Presented at International Meeting for Medical Simulation, 2004, Albuquerque, NM.
9. Pittman J, Turner B, Gabbott DA. Communication between members of the cardiac arrest team—a postal survey. *Resuscitation.* 2001;49:175–177.
10. Kinney KG, Boyd SY, Simpson DE. Guidelines for appropriate in-hospital emergency team time management: the Brooke Army Medical Center approach. *Resuscitation.* 2004;60:33–38.
11. Fiedor M, DeVita M. Human simulation and crisis team training. In: Dunn WF, ed. *Simulators in Critical Care and Beyond.* Des Plaines, Illinois: Society of Critical Care Medicine; 2004:91–95.
12. Weick KE, Roberts KH. Collective mind in organizations: heedful interrelating on flight decks. *Adm Sci Q.* 1993;38:357.
13. Marsch SCU, Muller C, Marquardt K, Conrad G, Tschan F, Hunziker PR. Human factors affect the quality of cardiopulmonary resuscitation in simulated cardiac arrests. *Resuscitation.* 2004;60:51–56.
14. Marteau TM, Wynne G, Kaye W, Evans TR. Resuscitation: experience without feedback increases confidence but not skill. *BMJ.* 1990;300:849–850.
15. Gaba DM, Howard SK, Flanagan B, Smith BE, Fish KJ, Botney R. Assessment of clinical performance during simulated crises using both technical and behavioral ratings. *Anesthesiology.* 1998;89:8–18.
16. Blum RH, Raemer DB, Carroll JS, Sunder N, Felstein DM, Cooper JB. Crisis resource management training for an anaesthesia faculty: a new approach to continuing education. *Med Educ.* 2004;38:45–55.

22
Information Systems Considerations: Integration of Medical Emergency Team Clinical Indicators

Lis Young, Jack Chen, and Kenneth Hillman

The Components to Implementing MET

There is increasing pressure within the health system to guarantee patient safety. This is not new. Serious adverse events have attracted widespread media attention lately and possibly reflect a growing international trend (1). Evidence of the magnitude of the problem began to emerge in the 1990s, signaled by the Harvard Medical Practict study (2,3). This seminal study found that 4% of patients suffer harm during their hospital stay: 70% of the adverse events resulted in short-lived disability, but 14% of the events led to death. When these figures were extrapolated across the United States, it was estimated that medical errors caused between 44000 and 98000 deaths annually.

The Quality in Australia Health Care Study (4) published in 1995, found a rate of adverse events of 16.6% among hospital patients, estimated to cause 10000 to 14000 potentially preventable deaths every year. Subsequent studies in New Zealand (5,6), the United Kingdom (7), Denmark (8), and Canada (9) have suggested adverse event rates of around 10%.

The reasons for such high rates of adverse events are many. Some are likely related to the increasing complexity of health care delivery, as well as patient vulnerability. Hospitals are increasingly caring for an aging population, in which co-morbidities and age-related frailty invariably increase the inherent dangers of complex operations, the side effects and interactions of polypharmacy, and the multiple therapeutic interventions to which these complex patients are likely to be subjected. The system's capacity to guarantee patient safety has not matched the increase in complex patient morbidity and high-risk therapeutic interventions.

Hospital infrastructure today is not very different from the one, which existed in the early part of the 19th century. Patients present with increasingly complex problems, yet they are admitted under the care of physicians who specialize in 1 organ disease. Coordination of care for patients with the complex medical problems of today, involving several specialist teams and expensive and sophisticated diagnostics, poses a mounting challenge to hospital administrators and clinical managers. The team responsible for the overall patient care tends to leave the day-to-day management to the less experienced doctors, who, on the other hand, are likely to be pursuing a specialty career path themselves. Thus, they tend to be less focused on acquiring and applying skills in the care of the critically ill patient with multiple organ problems. As a result, patients who may be deteriorating within hospital wards are managed by a staff that is relatively inexperienced and has inappropriate skills, and which is working within a system that does not have the capacity to respond rapidly and proactively to early warning signs (10,11). This situation is exacerbated by workforce issues related to an endemic shortage of nursing staff, which in the past would have had the time and the experience to remain vigilante while providing care for their patients.

The current system and staffing mix cannot meet the growing needs of a patient population with complex disease patterns and the associated high-risk, complex interventions. The adverse events that result from the gap between what patients require and what the hospital is able to provide are more likely related to deficiencies in system design and implementation and the relative scarcity of experienced staff, than to individual human errors or faulty products. For example, studies have attributed 15% of adverse drug events to system failures (12,13). The significance of system failure has been emphasized in the US Institute of Medicine's publication *To Err Is Human* (14). Using a system approach ensures that every component of patient safety is considered, rather than focusing on narrow and specific aspects of a problem.

The World Health Organization (WHO) states that patient safety includes 3 complementary actions: preventing adverse events, mitigating their effects when they occur, and making them visible.

The Medical Emergency Team (MET) system (15,16) provides a hospital-wide approach to patient safety consistent with the first two aims of WHO. The MET system offers intervention based on the principles of early identification and intervention for seriously ill hospital in-patients. The MET team is similar to the cardiac arrest team; the significant difference between them is the timing. The MET team intervenes before the patient suffers a cardio-respiratory arrest or serious complication (Figure 22.1).

Whatever the specific antecedents, associated events, or possible mistakes that lead to the deterioration of a patient's condition, the MET system ensures early identification of at-risk patients, and most importantly triggers a rapid response. The system has significant potential for mitigating complications of serious adverse events in patients who are critically ill. The MET system crosses the geographical and professional boundaries within the hospital and is patient-focused, thereby meeting the first two WHO objectives for patient safety: preventing and mitigating adverse events.

The third action recommended by WHO is visibility (17). Currently a widespread lack of awareness of the system issues associated with adverse

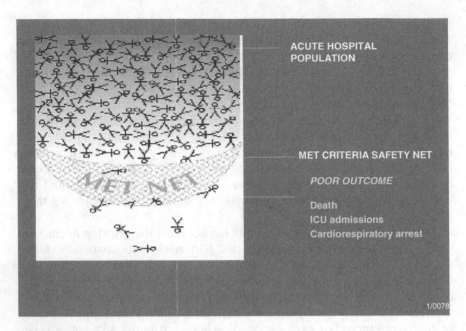

FIGURE 22.1.

events in hospitals prevails. Traditionally the emphasis has been on reporting events "upward," to committees and similar administrative and bureaucratic structures. This reporting is neither targeted nor specific, and significant potential for informing change and empowering staff at the clinical interphase is lost.

Current mandatory hospital reporting provides information on outcomes such as an unexpected return to the operating room, in-patient deaths, and patient complaints, as well as processes such as credentialing of medical staff and adherence to peer-review meetings.

The capacity for gathering data and turning it into information and targeted reporting has been hampered by several factors: a lack of robust, simple, and cost effective measures; reporting systems that are tailored to the audience; concerns relating to the possibility of breaching patient confidentiality; fear of professional liability; and a preoccupation with reporting "up" to those least able to adjust the system, rather than "down" to clinicians who—if empowered—can act on information about issues that lead to serious adverse events.

Merely collecting data is likely to simply result in a "data graveyard." The system must produce a visible and useful response for the users of the information. Within this context, the reporting system is as important as the response system. There has been an abundance of rhetoric about the serious nature of quality issues in hospitals (18,19), yet so far there is a paucity of validated, robust, and cost-effective indicators of the quality of the hospital itself (20).

System Integration of Clinical MET Indicators

The MET Indicators

When a systematic approach to improving patient safety is the aim, the key deliverable is the timely availability of the MET indicators at:

- The level of the patient
- The level of staff providing care for the patient
- The level of clinical and administrative managers

Both the collection and the reporting of the MET indicators must be adequately resourced. The criteria for adequate resource allocation is the demonstrated availability of reports to staff who provide care for the patient, and managers who are accountable for improving patient safety for critically ill patients. The MET indicators have been successfully integrated when MET outcomes are available as user-friendly reports across the hospital environment. Another way of ascertaining successful integration of clinical MET indicators is to demonstrate closure of the loop within the quality cycle that monitors the safety of critically ill patients. However, closure of the quality loop using timely, meaningful, and reliable information has remained elusive within clinical practice so far, in spite of a significant investment in quality assurance and the associated infrastructure in most hospitals.

The MET indicators are clinical indicators (Table 22.1) and reflect quality of care. They are universally distributed within the hospital environment: "Wherever there is a patient, there is a potential for a MET indicator." From a patient safety perspective, these indicators offer the opportunity of instituting universal monitoring of serious incidents across a hospital; timely feedback of clinical, quality indicators is the major draw of the MET system. Secondly, the MET provides high-quality, multipurpose data for monitoring trends in adverse events across the organization over time. When combined with other, existing clinical and administrative databases, a comprehensive picture of patient safety across hospitals can be made be available. The MET indicators (Table 22.1) embody the aims of the MET system: the prevention of potentially avoidable deaths and serious complications for the critically ill.

Implementing Clinical Indicators

Policy, hospital culture, and staff should all be part of the implementation plan for the clinical MET indicators (Table 22.2). The implementation should be aligned with the hospital's patient safety infrastructure, but the

TABLE 22.1. MET-related clinical indicators

Unexpected deaths	All deaths excluding those that have been categorized as "do not resuscitate"
Unexpected cardiac arrests	All cardiac arrests excluding those with explicit do-not-resuscitate orders
Unplanned admission to the Intensive Care Unit (ICU)	All admissions to ICU from the clinical areas where optimal monitoring is not part of patient care. For example, these would include general wards but not the emergency department, operating room, or the coronary care unit.

Although the criteria for an unplanned ICU admission aim to be generic, they may need modification and clarification within individual hospitals to allow for local variation in physical ward structures and their clinical functions.

preparedness of the hospital culture for systematic and standardized implementation of the MET performance indicators is equally important. A cultural assessment using off-the-shelf tools is the most cost-effective way to achieve this. A needs assessment of staff (medical and nursing) in regards to their awareness, knowledge, and skills in the collection of MET indicators is also essential (Table 22.2).

The MET Database

The MET indicators should be integrated into the information architecture supporting existing patient safety monitoring. At this stage the appropriate bio-statistical and epidemiological expertise should be available within the implementation team (Table 22.2). If such expertise is omitted from the setting-up phase, the organization might not reap the full benefit of the ongoing collection of MET indicators.

Data definitions and standards for the MET indicators should be aligned with local data standards. The data sources for extraneous data collection (data other than those data variables generated at the time of a MET call) need to be identified and appraised for completeness, accuracy, and ease of access. In instances of mixed data gathering (paper-based and electronic), a protocol for data extraction and data entry must be established. Accurate and reliable denominators for each key indicator are essential if an accurate and reliable monitoring system is to be established and maintained over time. Some relevant denominators at the hospital level include:

1. Total number of cardiac arrests (preferably updated monthly)
2. Total number of in-hospital deaths (preferably updated monthly)
3. Total number of do-not-resuscitate orders for all cardiac arrests and in-hospital deaths (should be captured over time within the hospital)

TABLE 22.2. Components of the MET system

MET clinical indicators	MET database	Clinician ownership	MET coordinator
Clinical MET indicators:			
1. Unexpected deaths—all deaths excluding those that have been categorized as "do not resuscitate"	Biostatistical, epidemiological, and health informatics expertise should be available within the implementation team during the setting-up phase.	Inform and consult widely across the hospital. Develop a plan to ensure that the staff has been systematically informed and consulted with.	Recruit MET coordinator(s) who has knowledge and skills in the care of the critically ill, as well as evaluation and research expertise.
2. Unexpected cardiac arrests—with all cardiac arrests excluding those explicit "do not resuscitate" orders	Develop data definitions and standards for the MET clinical indicators.	As part of the consultation process, identify the staff members who are opinion leaders, and those who are likely to take on the role of "change agents."	Provide training in MET data collection, reporting, and communication (MET results are sensitive-potential for "blame culture")
3. Unplanned admissions to the Intensive Care Unit (ICU)—all admissions to ICU from clinical areas where optimal monitoring is not part of patient care	Develop data definitions and standards for denominators, and other extraneous data variables relevant to MET reporting.	Based on the consultation process develop a change management plan including timeframes and a risk management strategy	Support and assist the MET coordinator(s) in engaging with the hospital culture across the entire environment.

TABLE 22.2. *Continued*

MET clinical indicators	MET database	Clinician ownership	MET coordinator
4. All MET calls ### Potentially preventable events are those with preceding MET criteria within 24 hours of the event, where no MET was called ###	Develop data dictionaries including standards for how data is collected: when, where, how, by whom. Select appropriate software that meets the local information technology department and liaise with its staff as well as other teams who are collecting patient safety data within the hospital.	Develop the user specifications for the MET reports, and liaise with the information technology staff to develop reporting formats that target specific audiences: e.g. daily or regular, frequent reports of identified information targeting clinicians at the point of patient care should be conveyed: "at a glance."	Support and assist the MET coordinator with developing and maintaining ownership of the MET clinical indicators and reports Integrate the MET coordinator into the existing quality assurance infrastructure, and patient safety infrastructure where one exists.
Some useful MET denominators: A. Total number of cardiac arrests. (preferably updated monthly) B. Total number of in-hospital deaths. (preferably updated monthly)	Agree on mode of data entry; develop processes for checking the validity, accuracy, and completeness of MET data over time.	Ensure that the appropriate level of expertise in epidemiology, statistics, and health informatics provide the algorithms that will deliver accurate and reliable trend reporting over time	Support and assist the MET coordinator(s) in closing the loop for the MET reporting: systematic capture of the issues and actions identified as a result of MET monitoring. A close alignment with hospital quality assurance staff may be a useful strategy that will ensure that MET reporting drive change within the hospital over time.
C. Total number of do not resuscitate "for all cardiac arrests and in"—hospital deaths should be captured over time. *(preferably updated monthly)*	Overall objective: develop and sustain a MET database to scientific standards as an integral part of clinical practice.		

Standardization of Data Collection

Current experience within the hospitals in the South Western Sydney Area Health Service, New South Wales, Australia (where the MET was conceived and developed) suggest that capturing a valid, accurate, and reliable denominator for do-not-resuscitate orders across the hospital environment is a critical success factor for MET. If the process of allocating a do-not-resuscitate status to individual patients is not clearly defined, agreed, and adhered to by all senior clinicians within the hospital, a standardized approach to the collection of do-not-resuscitate data may be particularly challenging. Furthermore documentation of do-not-resuscitate status for individual patients may not be systematically implemented across the hospital environment.

IT Requirements

The technical standards and the software used to create the MET database must be consistent with the local IT environment (Table 22.2). Particular attention should be given to user access (privileged). The level of technical security required to guard the confidentiality of this data must be negotiated and implemented with particular care.

System Integration in the Collection of MET Indicators

Embedding the data collection within the individual hospital environment represents a vital step for a robust and sustainable collection of MET indicators over time. The process should be based on well developed and easy-to-use data dictionaries and data collection methods. It is cost effective to train 2 or 3 clinical staff in data collection methods, standards, and reporting for a 600-bed acute hospital. The tools and manuals available to super trainers should be clear, exhaustive, and easy to apply within all hospital wards.

Reporting of Clinical MET Indicators

Timely, meaningful information is the hallmark of reporting aimed at driving change. In conjunction with the establishment of the database, the reporting needs for the MET indicators should be documented. An extensive consultation process that involves relevant staff across the hospital will procure the user specifications for regular, standardized MET reports (Table 22.2). Where hospitals are currently reporting on other clinical indicators (scorecards, control charts), MET reports should be integrated into them. A useful and effective process might be to identify and agree on: 1) which non-MET indicators are relevant for MET reporting, 2) how and when the indicators should be collected, and 3) who will assist with the integration of MET and other relevant patient safety indicators.

Clinical Ownership

The consultation with staff to identify reporting needs offers ample opportunity for engagement with key stakeholders and in the overall ward culture. An approach that balances the provision of information with staff consultation has the potential to nurture staff ownership of the clinical MET indicators across the hospital culture. The timetable for the MET indicator reports and the manner in which the reports are contextualized will vary with the objectives within the hospital. The message is best conveyed "at a glance"—this is pertinent for daily or regular, frequent reporting aimed at supporting clinicians in monitoring when, where, and why critical incidents occur. Clinicians include all health professionals who provide care for a patient who suffered a serious adverse event. The less frequent trend reporting (quarterly, biannually, and annually) provides more complex information based on the Liverpool experience; the more condensed information represented in trend reporting will benefit from the availability of an "interpreter," and an obvious candidate for this role is a MET coordinator. Staff working on related reporting within the hospital may also assist with "facilitated" dissemination of such information based on MET indicators.

The MET Coordinator

Establishing the database, developing the reports, and embedding the technical solution within the system of the local information technology environment require a multidisciplinary approach. As mentioned previously, knowledge and skills in data management, epidemiology, statistics, and health informatics are crucial in the setting-up phase. The integration of the knowledge generated through the collection, manipulation, and reporting of MET indicators is critical to successful incident monitoring. In Liverpool a MET coordinator performs this role. Dedicated staff resources that have experience in information management are the key. The MET coordinator must possess a mix of skills and competencies that include: experience in the care of the critically ill, data management and manipulation, and communication principles that enable a targeted approach to disseminating information about serious adverse events throughout the hospital.

Interpersonal skills and the ability to communicate information about serious adverse events while avoiding blame are important attributes of a MET coordinator. The coordinator is responsible for integrating the MET quality cycle into the overall hospital environment. The human resource requirements for a 600-bed, acute tertiary referral center are 2 full-time equivalent senior nursing staff (estimates based on the Liverpool MET system).

The 6 MET coordinators in South Western Sydney Area Health Service (6 hospitals) provide capacity for collecting and reporting the MET indicators daily throughout the year. Proof of universal monitoring of the hospital environment is critical to the successful implementation of MET at a system level. Over time, the key role of the MET coordinator is assisting hospital staff in identifying issues and the actions that will remedy factors that have contributed to serious adverse events reported via the MET system. Capturing the information in the form of timely feedback to the clinical environment poses the greatest challenge to a MET coordinator. Factors contributing to a serious adverse event may be at a system level, a staff level, or a patient level. MET indicators reflect the functioning—or nonfunctioning as it were—of a complex system providing care for critically ill patients in hospitals.

The range and the nature of the factors that contribute to an adverse event at these 3 levels of the system do not allow for standardization of data variables, such as would occur for quantitative MET reports. Rather, this data—capturing the issues and explaining the occurrence of serious adverse events—are of a qualitative nature. Collecting, reporting, and depicting trends of such qualitative information over time are evolving processes. Scoping of this task is best assessed on a regular basis to ensure that "a graveyard of comments and unstructured information" is not inadvertently created.

Providing synergy between the role of the MET coordinator and the hospital's overall quality assurance infrastructure may assist in a focused approach to the MET implementation. When addressing the task of managing a mixture of qualitative and quantitative information, one should be aware that the phase between quantitative and qualitative data still represents relatively uncharted territory within complex system monitoring. This area ought to be targeted as part of MET evaluation and research in the future.

Summary

Clinical MET indicators are simple, robust, and cost effective. First, they are the calling criteria for activating a MET response, and they constitute the outcomes for the MET intervention. Second, they are universally measured for all hospital patients, although the frequency of measurement depends on the ward. The last of the 4 MET calling criteria, "worry," encourages individual clinicians to apply and act on their professional experience and knowledge of the patients whom they care for. In the Liverpool experience (the cradle of MET) the "worry" criteria is a potent enabler for empowering staff to practice early identification of patients who are deteriorating within their ward.

Embedding the MET indicators within the local culture, communication flow, and information technology environment is best done as parallel but integrated tasks. This stage must be supported by a multidisciplinary implementation team that includes the relevant research expertise.

Sustainability can only be secured if senior and multi-skilled members of the staff are available in dedicated MET positions. Frequently, monitoring systems are conceived, developed, and ride on a wave of initial enthusiasm and individual leadership. The MET information coordinator guarantees the future of the MET system, ensuring that information is generated and knowledge about the incidence of serious adverse events among the critically ill is integrated into the organization at all levels.

Data collection, management, and reporting on both the processes and outcomes of the MET system are some of the duties and responsibilities of a MET coordinator. The coordinator should have expertise in caring for the critically ill patient, as well as knowledge and skills in data management and reporting. This is the lynch pin of the MET system, because the MET coordinator establishes and maintains clinician ownership of the MET indicators across the hospital environment.

References

1. Dyer C. Bristol doctors found guilty of serious professional misconduct. *BMJ.* 1998;316:1924.
2. Brennan TA, Leape LL, Laird NM, Hebert L, Localio AR, Lawthers AG. Incidence of adverse events and negligence in hospitalized patients: results of the Harvard Medical Practice Study I. *N Engl J Med.* 1991;324:370–376.
3. Leape LL, Brennan TA, Laird NM, et al. Nature of adverse events in hospitalized patients: results of the Harvard Medical Practice Study II. *N Engl J Med.* 1991;324:377–384.
4. Wilson RM, Runciman WB, Gibberd RW, Harrison BT, Newby L, Hamilton JD. The Quality in Australian Health Care study. *Med J Aust.* 1995;163:458–471.
5. David P, Lay-Yee R, Briant R, et al. Adverse events in New Zealand public hospitals I: occurrence and impact. *N Z Med J.* 2002;115:U271.
6. Davis P, Lay-Yee R, Briant R, et al. Adverse events in New Zealand public hospitals II: occurrence and impact. *N Z Med J.* 2003;116:U624.
7. Department of Health. An organization with a memory: report of an expert group on learning from adverse events in the NHS chaired by the Chief Medical Officer. Crownright. Department of Health, HMSO. 2000.
8. Schioler T, Lipezak H, Pedersen BL, et al. Danish adverse events study. Incidence of adverse events in hospitals. A retrospective study of medical records. *Ugeskr laeger.* 2001;163:5370–5878.
9. Baker GR, Norton PG, Flintolf V, et al. The Canadian adverse events study: the incidence of adverse events among hospital patients in Canada. *CMAJ.* 2004; 179:1678–1686.

10. McQuillan P, Pilkington S, Allan A, et al. Confidential inquiry into quality of care before admission to intensive care. *BMJ*. 1998;316:1853–1858.
11. Goldhill DR, White SA, Sumner A. Physiological values and procedures in the 24 hours before ICU admission from the ward. *Anaesthesia*. 1999;45:529–534.
12. Thomas EJ, Studdert DM, Runciman WB, et al. A comparison of iatrogenic injury studies in Australia and the United States I: context, method, casemix, population, patient and hospital characteristics. *Int J Q Health Care*. 2000; 12:371–378.
13. World Health Organization. Progress in essential drugs and medicine policy 1998–1999. WHO/EDM/2000.2: 2000.
14. Kohn LT, Corrigan JM, Donaldson MS, eds. *To Err Is Human: Building a Safer Health System*. Washington, DC: National Academies Press; 2000.
15. Lee A, Bishop G, Hillman K, Daffurn K. The Medical Emergency Team. *Anaesth Intensive Care*. 1995;23:183–186.
16. Hourihan F, Bishop G, Hillman KM, Daffurn K, Lee A. The medical emergency team: a new strategy to identify and intervene in high-risk patients. *Clin Intensive Care*. 1995;6:269–272.
17. World Health Organization. World Alliance for Patient Safety. Forward program 2005. France: WHO; 2005.
18. McGlynn E, Brook RH. Keeping quality on the policy agenda. *Health Aff*. 2001;20(3):82–90.
19. Becher EC, Chassin MR. Improving quality, minimizing error: making it happen. *Health Aff*. 2001;20:68–82.
20. Hillman K, Alexandrou E, Flabouris M, et al. Clinical outcome indicators in acute hospital medicine. *Clin Intensive Care*. 2000;11:89–94.

23
Evaluating Complex System Interventions in Patient Safety

JACK CHEN, LIS YOUNG, and KENNETH HILLMAN

Following the landmark reports from the Institute of Medicine (1) and other studies, numerous intervention programs have been introduced to improve hospital patients' safety (2–6). The evaluation of such a complex system of interventions continues to be a challenge—there is little robust evidence about the effectiveness of intervention programs aimed at system improvement (7). A rigorous evaluation of the systems for delivering health care presents a different challenge in evaluating single, simple interventions such as a new drug or a new piece of medical technology.

First, the paradigms must be decided on for the evaluation—whether quantitative or qualitative methods, or both. If the latter, what then is the sequence, what will the scope be, and how might the two methods be integrated? Secondly, the objectives of the evaluation must be clearly defined. Are we satisfied with knowing the final clinical outcomes of the intervention, or are we also interested in gaining new knowledge about the processes and their impact within complex systems? Health promotion experts have argued the importance of assessing all 3 aspects (8,9). The conceptual drawback of a singular focus on outcomes is the lack of knowledge about why the intervention did not produce the expected results.

In the case of the Medical Emergency Team (MET) intervention (10), the relevant clinical outcomes are assumed to be: unplanned admissions to the intensive care unit (ICU), unexpected deaths, and cardiac arrests. However, if the implementation of a MET system in a hospital does not produce these expected outcomes, how will we know whether the failure was due to specific factors—such as inadequate implementation, suboptimal calling criteria, a short study period, lack of skills on the part of the MET team, lateness of MET response—or if the whole concept just does not work? To understand the critical links is perhaps as important as assessing the clinical outcomes (Figure 23.1).

Other organizational characteristics, such as the value placed on patient safety, may also contribute to the effectiveness of the MET (11,12). The readiness of the hospital culture may be a very important dynamic, if the changes associated with the implementation of MET are to gain accep-

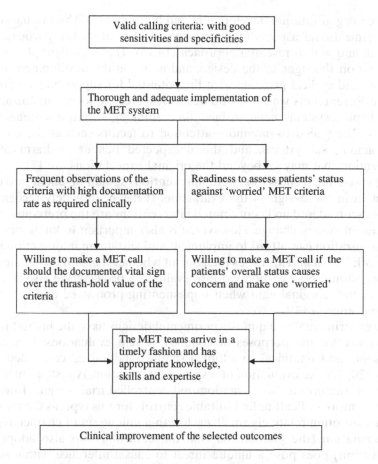

FIGURE 23.1. The critical links leading to successful MET outcomes.

tance: e.g. the need to modify the traditional balance of power between medical and nursing staff, a reconfiguration of interdisciplinary relationships, and the need to be proactive in accepting innovation within the local culture and context. All of these factors may impact upon both the processes and outcomes of a system intervention like MET, and so it is necessary to consider how they can be taken into account when evaluating the MET implementation.

An evidence-based approach to medicine tends to classify research evidence based on the design and the features of the evaluation. The single, large randomized controlled trial (preferably double-blind) is the ultimate gold standard. In randomized controlled trials, the emphasis is on the study's design and scale. This is very different from a research paradigm based on organizational development and learning (13). The evaluation of the organizational aspects of systems could also adopt the participatory research and action research approach (14,15). This paradigm places less emphasis on the rigor of the design, and more on the development of an iterative and cyclical program with the potential for supporting a learning culture. Researchers who lead and design research exploring organizations and complex systems need to base their thinking within a systems perspective. They need to pay more attention to factors such as the interactions among subsystems, and the unexpected benefit or harm of an intervention that may go beyond the original expectations (16,17).

The cost-effectiveness of system interventions should be taken into consideration in the design of the evaluation. It has been widely recognized that well-considered and coordinated interventions are the prerequisites to a successful system change. However, it is also important to know whether the organization can afford to implement and sustain an intervention such as the MET system. This raises the issue of whether a health economic perspective should be incorporated into evaluation projects. We also need to consider the marginal gain when implementing protracted and extensive system change (18,19).

The experimental and quasi-experimental designs have the highest internal validity for the purposes of complex system evaluations. It is often impossible and unethical to adopt a simple randomized controlled trial design (20) for the evaluation of a system intervention. A system intervention often requires a cluster randomized controlled trial design. However, it may be more difficult to find suitable controls for this type, as the number of units are often relatively small, each with a unique set of characteristics. Contamination (the phenomena that the control group also adopt the intervention) does pose a unique threat to causal inference within social intervention programs with a cluster randomized controlled trial or an experimental design. It is often very difficult, if not impossible, to prevent the control units from learning and mimicking the intervention applied to the experiment groups. This is especially true when the intervention has good face validity and is intuitively appealing. On the other hand, for a complex system intervention that targets structural, cultural, and behavioral change, not all the units within the experiment group will embrace the changes with the same willingness and commitment. Skepticism, ineptitude, and a dislike of the unknown may easily derail a great initiative. The very complexity of complex system interventions sends the researcher down a path fraught with challenges, relating to both the conceptualization and the implementation of a robust and useful evaluation. The third major hurdle is the large variation among hospitals in terms of their size and organizational characteristics. These attributes impact significantly on the cluster randomized controlled trials targeting hospitals. The greater the variation in these characteristics, the greater the number of hospitals required to achieve sufficient statistical power to test the primary and secondary outcomes (21). Due to the prohibitive costs incurred by this type of study, one frequently does not have reliable information on the variations or intraclass correlation coefficients (ICCs) (22) from previous research. Consequently researchers hesitate to embark on a study of this nature, for fear that there may be insufficient power to test the hypothesis. The power issue could become even more complicated, as there are often no reported crude ICCs (the ICCs calculated based on the whole sample or the control and the intervention group separately, without controlling for other covariates [23,24]). Moreover, the information for the conditional ICCs (after adjusting for key confounding factors such as hospital status—teaching, urban, or rural—in the multivariate analysis model) is even scarcer. If one mixes all of these hospitals, one may run the risk of comparing apples with oranges. A conditional model (conditional on the key confounding factors) could reduce this problem: a study that is underpowered based on the raw ICCs may have adequate power based on the conditional ICCs.

The fourth dilemma when evaluating a complex system intervention is the time dimension. Internalization of system change may often require a lengthy time frame to succeed, and this requirement translates into significant costs. For large-scale evaluation projects, such costs may become prohibitive, especially as they are already expensive and cumbersome compared with the conventional gold standard: a simple randomized controlled trial. This dilemma became very real for the researchers designing and implementing the Medical Early Response Intervention and Therapy (MERIT) study. The evaluation of the MERIT study involved a cluster randomized controlled trial, where 23 hospitals in Australia participated.

In studies such as the MERIT, there are many other associated challenges and difficulties: the plethora of databases, extracting and cleaning administrative data, the matching and linkage of administrative data with the study-specific data, and the multilevel nature of the data structure. Before embarking on such a large evaluation project, it was important to consider all of these conceptual and technical issues, and design a plan that was comprehensive yet achievable.

The MERIT Study: An Example of the Challenges in Conducting a Complex System Evaluation

The MERIT study's major aim was to evaluate the effectiveness of the MET system based on a cluster randomized controlled trial with 23 participating hospitals. The primary outcome was the aggregate of unplanned ICU admissions, potentially avoidable deaths, and cardiac arrests. Other sub-studies were incorporated into the design to systematically understand the processes and the impact of the intervention:

- A matched case-control study to explore the sensitivity and specificity of the MET calling criteria.
- A before-after repeat survey in MET hospitals to explore awareness of and attitudes toward the MET system; the willingness and the intent to call the MET team; the value the overall hospital culture assigned to patient safety; the readiness to change and possible resistance to innovations.
- The process and impact evaluation of components of the interventions (nurse education sessions and their participation rates).
- The systematic evaluation of the timing, assessment, and treatment provided by both cardiac arrest teams and METs within participating hospitals.
- Limiting discussions to design issues and the implications of the main MERIT project: the 23 hospitals, cluster randomized controlled trial.

The Design

Potential hospitals for recruitment into the study were identified using the Australian Hospital and Health Services Yearbook (25). Public hospitals with more than 20000 estimated annual admissions, that had an ICU and an emergency department as part of their service profile, and did not already have a MET system, were eligible. The director of the ICU or emergency department was contacted and invited to participate. Approval to participate was obtained from the human research ethics committee of each hospital.

Process and outcome measures were collected in all hospitals during a baseline period of 2 months. Midway through the baseline period, an independent statistician randomly assigned hospitals to either a standardized MET implementation or a control status. The randomization process was concealed from the panel of investigators and the participating hospitals. The randomization was stratified by teaching versus non-teaching status and blocked by number of hospital beds, using a group size of 4.

During the following 4-month period, an educational strategy was implemented to prepare hospitals for the introduction of the MET system (implementation period). Data collection continued during this period. At the end of the implementation period, the MET system was activated in the intervention hospitals only, where it was implemented and supported hospital-wide for the following 6 months (Figure 23.2). The control hospitals were unaware of what was happening in the intervention hospitals. The management and resuscitation committees in the control hospitals resolved that their cardiac arrest teams would continue to function as per normal for the duration of the study period—including the intervention phase. Process and outcome data were collected in all hospitals for the 6-month study period.

Prior to the start of the project, all the data collectors were trained by dedicated project staff based at the Simpson Center for Health Services

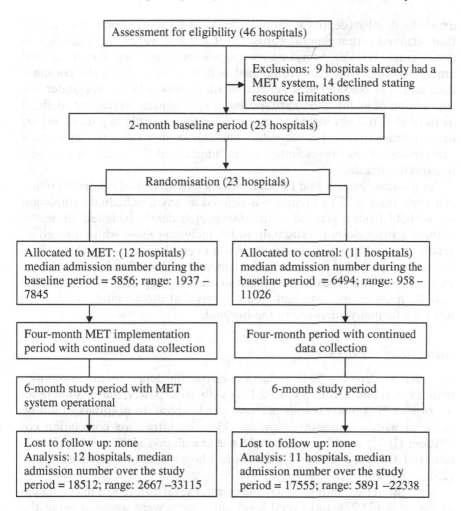

FIGURE 23.2. MERIT study flow diagram.

Research. The MERIT project was led from and coordinated by research staff at the center. A standardized data collection manual stipulated data standards, and scanable forms were used to capture primary data. Over the course of the study, 3 audits were carried out to ascertain data accuracy. The data audits targeted the accuracy of the project for specific data with reference to source documentation, accuracy of scanning techniques, and study outcomes.

The primary study outcome was the composite outcome of the incidence (captured events divided by the number of eligible patients admitted to the hospital during the study period) of cardiac arrests without a pre-existing do-not-resuscitate order, unplanned ICU admissions, and unexpected deaths (deaths without a pre-existing do-no-resuscitate order) that occurred within general wards. The ICUs, ICU-supervised high-dependency units (HDUs), operating rooms, post-operative recovery areas, and emergency departments were defined as non-general wards. The coronary care unit was considered a general ward, as was a HDU not under the supervision of an intensive care specialist. Thus general wards were defined as those that did not include monitoring of the critically ill patient as part of their duties of care. The secondary outcomes were cardiac arrests without pre-existing do-not-resuscitate orders, unplanned ICU admissions, and unexpected deaths.

A cardiac arrest was said to occur when a patient lacked a palpable pulse. An unplanned ICU admission was defined as any unscheduled admission to the ICU from a general ward. Unexpected deaths included all deaths without a prior do-not-resuscitate order, including those with a preceding cardiac arrest. If a patient had more than 1 event during a hospital stay, only 1 event was included in the composite measure. The following events were excluded from the study: events that had occurred in patients who were less than 14 years of age, who had died on arrival at the hospital, or who had not been formally admitted to the hospital.

Statistical Analysis

In order to detect a 30% reduction in the incidence of the composite primary outcome (from 3% to 2.1%) with 90% power, and assuming an average of 20000 admissions per year per hospital, 18 hospitals would be required with a 6-month follow-up (13). The intra-class correlation coefficient (ICC) used for the sample size calculation (ICC = 0.00127) was obtained from a previously published, 3-hospital non-randomized study (26).

A weighted t-test was used to assess cluster level differences in event incidence rates (21,27). Individual level differences were assessed using the Rao-Scott chi-square test in categorical variables, and the adjusted t-test for continuous variables (20).

Analytically weighted, multiple linear regression (weighted by the admission number of the study period) was used to adjust for stratification by teaching hospital status at randomization, and other differences in hospital (cluster) level characteristics (including baseline outcome variables) (6,28). A multi-level logistic regression model was used to adjust for the individual-level (gender, age) and cluster-level (bed number and teaching status) differences (29). A post-hoc exploratory analysis, using paired weighted t-tests, examined the difference in incidence rates between the study period and baseline.

The outcome-specific ICC and the design effect (22) were reported; these are measures used to adjust sample size in cluster randomized trials (24). The ICCs were derived from the null multi-level logistic regression model, with no independent variables. The design effects of the intervention effects (MET versus control) were calculated from the survey estimator logistic regression with the intervention effect only. The design effect in this context is the ratio of the standard error of the intervention effect from the model with adjustment for the cluster effect, to the standard error of the intervention effect from the model ignoring the cluster effect (30).

A p-value less than 0.05 was considered a statistical significance. All statistical analyses were conducted using Stata version 8.2 (30).

Discussion

So far, evaluations of the MET concept are limited. Three previous Australian studies suggest that the implementation of a MET system is associated with a reduction in the incidence of unplanned admissions to ICU, cardiac arrests, and deaths (26,31–33). Some important limitations in these studies include the use of historical controls and the lack of randomization.

The drawbacks to using historical controls are the difficulties in separating the efficacy (if any) from a secular trend or a regression to the mean. The seasonal effect, changes in case mix, potential investigator biases, and the Hawthorne effect could threaten the validity of the findings. These earlier studies were also conducted within relatively large hospitals (with over 300 hospital beds), and most of them were single-hospital based. Often these hospitals had an inspirational and charismatic clinical leader who championed the cause. Such factors limit the ability to generalize about the results, and given the small number of hospitals involved, it is not possible to gain any knowledge about the organizational characteristics and environmental factors that may have enabled or impeded the success of the system intervention. The information available on the implementation and the associated processes were insufficient to judge the weakest link of the implementation chain.

In comparing these earlier studies with the MERIT project, we should be aware that they used different outcomes. The calling criteria (upon which the MET was activated, see Table 23.1) applied within these studies also varied from the MERIT project. For example, Buist et al. (33) explored the incidence of cardiac arrests without a prior do-not-resuscitate order and the related deaths; their working definition of a cardiac arrest event was based on the cardiac arrest calls made via the switchboard. The primary endpoints of the Bristow et al. (26) study were all-cause mortality, cardiac arrests (including those with do-not-resuscitate), unplanned ICU/HDU admissions, as well as deaths without a prior do-not-resuscitate order; here, the definition of an unplanned ICU/HUD required that the patient was admitted to ICU/HDU for the same reason that he or she was admitted as an inpatient. The study by Bellomo et al. (31) explored the incidence of cardiac arrests and the related deaths, the number of post-cardiac-arrest bed days,

TABLE 23.1. The MET calling criteria

Airway	Threatened
Breathing	All respiratory arrests
	Respiratory rate <5
	Respiratory rate >36
	All cardiac arrests
Circulation	Pulse rate <40
	Pulse rate >140
	Systolic blood pressure <90
Neurology	Sudden fall in level of consciousness (Fall in general consciousness level of >2 points)
Other	Repeated or prolonged seizures
	Any patient you are seriously worried about that does not fit the above criteria

and the overall number of in-hospital deaths. It is worth noting that the study outcomes evaluated for MERIT are somewhat different from these definitions. For example, in the MERIT unplanned admissions to ICU are defined as those admitted to the ICU only, excluding those admitted to a HDU that was not supervised by an ICU specialist, as well as admissions to the ICU directly from an emergency department and operating room.

The decision whether or not to include do-not-resuscitate related patients as part of the outcome could influence the evaluation of the efficacy of the MET. If the investigators hope to demonstrate that the MET concept is effective as a pre-emptive effort to saving patients who exhibit signs of rapid deterioration, they may elect to include those patients without a prior do-not-resuscitate order in the primary outcome. Given that the evidence emerging from other studies suggest that an increasing number of do-not-resuscitate orders were issued at the time of a MET response to a medical emergency (34,35) there is good reason to advocate caution. Investigators were concerned that this practice could lead to the more severely ill being allocated a do-not-resuscitate "prematurely" to achieve an artificially improved outcome—e.g. the mortality rate for those without do-not-resuscitate. Thus in future studies, the rationale for including patients with a prior do-not-resuscitate should be scrutinized, and results of sensitivity analyses (with or without those with do-not-resuscitate) should inform the discussion wherever possible.

Another body of research, mainly from the United Kingdom, was triggered by the recommendations from the Audit Committee (36) and the Department of Health (37) based on the introduction of the outreach team concept there (34,38–42). The rationale for the outreach team service is similar to that of the MET, although the scope of the outreach service is much broader. There are 3 major aims:

1. Early identification of patients who are deteriorating, with the aim of either intervening to prevent an admission to ICU or securing a timely admission to ICU to achieve the best possible outcome for the patient.

2. Facilitated discharge, by supporting and assisting with the continued recovery of ICU patients discharged into the wards, as well as support for the patients and their family following hospital discharge.

3. Educate and support staff on the general wards and in the community in the application of critical care skills, as well as gather information about the process and outcomes of care for critically ill patients on the wards and in the community that will lead to improved critical care services for patients and their caregivers (37).

The broad scope of the outreach team concept poses even more challenges to evaluation and research efforts compared to the MET.

There are other important differences between the MET concept and the outreach team, such as the activation criteria for an intervention, which are structured very differently within the 2 systems. MET calling criteria were deliberately designed to be as simple and easy to implement as possible and include a subjective category, "worried". The intent behind the "worried" category is to empower individual staff to activate a MET call for patients who do not meet the simple, measurable MET criteria. In contrast, the criteria for activating the outreach team response are more structured and complex. The range of interventions that the outreach team can mount to address the needs of the deteriorating patient are also much broader than those provided by the MET (43). Again, the implications for any comprehensive evaluation efforts of this more complex intervention are substantial.

The results from UK-based literature are mixed. Pittard (41) found that the outreach team reduced the rates of emergency admissions to ICU, shortened the length of stay for patients admitted as an emergency to ICU, and produced a lower re-admission and mortality rates. Ball et al. (40) found that the implementation of an outreach team reduced readmissions to the critical care area and improved survival to discharge from hospital following discharge from critical care. However, these differences were not statistically different. Priestly et al. (39) found reduced in-hospital mortality following the implementation of an outreach team, but the results for length of stay in hospital were equivocal. Kenward et al. (34) did not demonstrate any significant improvement with respect to incidence rates of cardiac arrests, cardiac arrest excluding those with do-not-resuscitate and all-cause in-hospital mortality. The authors did find that about a quarter of the patients were designated a do-not-resuscitate status following a MET intervention (24-hour time window) compared with the 14% reported by Buist et al. (33). Each of the 4 studies involved 1 large hospital only. Three of them adopted a before-after design, while the fourth, Priestly used a well-crafted, ward-based, randomized, controlled trial design. The previously discussed limitations of the before-after design are pertinent to the 3 studies here. As for the fourth (Priestly), the possibility of contamination and investigator bias are relevant for the ward-based randomization, as are other technical issues such as the project design, and the complex statistical analyses.

Recent research in the United States has produced results from a study evaluating a hospital wide implementation of the MET concept. DeVita et al. showed a significant reduction in cardiac arrests (from 6.4 to 5.4 per 1000 admissions) following the implementation of a MET system. An overall increase in MET responses (from 13.7 to 25.8 per 1000 admissions) indicates how important time is, if the effectiveness of systems is to be measured. This study also found that the proportion of fatal cardiac arrests was similar before and after the increased use of the MET.

The above studies had a strong preference for a before-after design. They provide little, if any, evidence about the quality of the implementation. The process and impact evaluations were inadequate, and weaknesses in the design of the evaluation make causal inference relatively difficult within these studies. The studies also used different definitions and outcomes: some specifically excluded patients with a prior do-not-resuscitate, yet others used all the cases. There is also a lack of detail about how some of the data were defined and extracted. For example, it appears that all-cause deaths were extracted from the in-hospital, administrative databases, but the reliability and validity of the data were not described. Most of the studies were based within a single hospital, and hence it is hard to know how generalizable the results might be. Nor is it possible to link organizational characteristics to the outcome in a quantitative way.

The implementation of the MET system is complex. A hospital-wide system change is required, involving comprehensive re-education of clinical staff in resuscitation skills, as well as managerial support at all levels to achieve the relevant restructuring of operations and the associated cultural change. Most of the studies discussed here assessed the effect of a MET implementation conducted over a 1 to 2 year period. By comparison, the introduction of similar complex interventions such as a trauma systems have taken up to 10 years before any impact on mortality could be detected (47,48). Whether the MET system will produce similar improvements in the outcomes for critically ill patients over time remains a matter of conjecture.

Summary

The MERIT Study was designed to minimize the limitations of previous studies. However, many questions remain. We have completed the first round of our major analyses. We have assessed the process, the impact, and the outcomes of the study, paying special attention to possible contamination effects. We have explored the possible effects of hospital variation, and how these affected our sample size. We have addressed possible statistical artefacts by employing a comprehensive analysis strategy, and following an *a priori* designed, statistical plan as much as possible. We explored the possible relationships between organizational/contextual variables and the outcomes. We tried to understand not only whether on average the hospitals improved, but also why the results varied across hospitals. We also evaluated the unintended increase in do-not-resuscitate orders that resulted from the MET system intervention. The MERIT study can also provide some insight into process issues, based on the result of several sub-studies specifically designed to explore the processes and the impact of the MERIT project. Finally evaluating a complex system intervention such as MERIT requires careful planning and considerable commitment. It remains an enormous challenge and a daunting task.

References

1. Kohn LT, Corrigan JM, Donaldson MS, eds. *To Err Is Human: Building a Safer Health System.* Washington, DC: National Academies Press; 2000.
2. Institute of Medicine. Crossing the quality chasm: a new health system for the 21st century. Washington DC: National Academies Press; 2001.
3. Aspden P; Institute of Medicine (Committee on Data Standards for Patient Safety). Patient safety achieving a new standard for care. Washington, DC: National Academies Press; 2004.
4. Byers JF, White SV. *Patient Safety: Principles and Practice.* New York: Springer; 2004.
5. Child AP; Institute of Medicine (Committee on the Work Environment for Nurses and Patient Safety). Keeping patients safe transforming the work environment of nurses. Washington, DC: National Academies Press; 2004.
6. US Congress House Committee on Energy and Commerce. Patient Safety and Quality Improvement Act report (to accompany HR 663) (including cost estimate of the Congressional Budget Office). Washington, DC: US Government Printing Office; 2003.
7. Overit J. Safety deficiencies in healthcare—a review of research. Karolinska Institute Medical Management Center: 2004.
8. Green LW, Kreuter MW, Green LW. *Health Program Planning an Educational and Ecological Approach.* 4th ed. New York: McGraw-Hill; 2005.
9. Windsor RA. *Evaluation of Health Promotion, Health Education, and Disease Prevention Programs.* 3rd ed. Boston: McGraw-Hill; 2004.
10. Hillman K, Chen J, Brown D. A clinical model for Health Services Research—the Medical Emergency Team. *J Crit Care.* 2003;18:195–199.
11. Basanta WE. Changing the culture of patient safety and medical errors: a symposium introduction and overview. *J Leg Med.* 2003;24:1–6.
12. Cohen MM, Eustis MA, Gribbins RE. Changing the culture of patient safety: leadership's role in health care quality improvement. *Jt Comm J Qual Saf.* 2003;29:329–335.
13. Argyris C. *On Organizational Learning.* 2nd ed. Malden, Mass: Blackwell Business; 1999.

14. Howard JK, Eckhardt SA. *Action Research: a Guide for Library Media Specialists*. Worthington, OH: Linworth Pub; 2005.
15. Johnson AP. *A Short Guide to Action Research*. Boston: Pearson/Allyn and Bacon; 2005.
16. Jackson MC. Systems Thinking: Creative Holism for Managers. Chichester: Wiley; 2002.
17. Haslett T. Implications of systems thinking for research and practice in management. Caulfield East, Vic: Monash University, Faculty of Business and Economics; 1998.
18. Folland S, Stano M, Goodman AC. *The Economics of Health and Health Care*. 4th ed. Upper Saddle River, NJ: Pearson Prentice Hall; 2004.
19. Drummond MF, McGuire A. *Economic Evaluation in Health Care: Merging Theory With Practice*. Oxford: Oxford University Press; 2001.
20. Donner A, Klar N. *Design and Analysis of Cluster Randomization Trials in Health Research*. London: Arnold; 2000.
21. Kerry M, Bland JM. Statistical notes: sample size in cluster randomization. *BMJ*. 1998;316:549.
22. Kish L, Frankel M. Inference from complex samples. *J R Stat Soc*. 1974;36:1–37.
23. Simpson JM, Klar N, Donner A. Accounting for cluster randomization: a review of primary prevention trials, 1990 through 1993. *Am J Public Health*. 1995;85:1378–1383.
24. Campbell MK, Elbourne DR, Altman DG, group C. CONSORT statement: extension to cluster randomized trials. *BMJ*. 2004;328:702–708.
25. APN Business Information Group. Australian Hospital and Health Services Yearbook. 25th ed. Melbourne: APN Business Information Group; 2001.
26. Bristow PJ, Hillman KM, Chey T, et al. Rates of in-hospital arrests, deaths and intensive care admissions: the effect of a medical emergency team. *Med J Aust*. 2000;173:236–240.
27. Campbell MK, Mollison J, Steen N, Grimshaw JM, Eccles M. Analysis of cluster randomized trials in primary care: a practical approach. *Fam Pract*. 2000;17:192–196.
28. Johnston J, DiNardo J. *Econometric Methods*. 4th ed. New York: McGraw-Hill; 1997.
29. Hox J. *Multilevel Analysis: Techniques and Applications*. Lawrence Erlbaum Associates, Inc; 2002.
30. StataCorp. Stata statistical software: Release 8.2. College Station, Texas: Stata Corporation; 2003.
31. Bellomo R, Goldsmith D, Uchino S, et al. A prospective before-and-after trial of a medical emergency team. *Med J Aust*. 2003;179:283–287.
32. Bellomo R, Goldsmith D, Uchino S, et al. Prospective controlled trial of effect of medical emergency team on postoperative morbidity and mortality rates. *Crit Care Med*. 2004;32:916–921.
33. Buist MD, Moore GE, Bernard SA, Waxman BP, Anderson JN, Nguyen TV. Effects of a medical emergency team on reduction of incidence of and mortality from unexpected cardiac arrests in hospital: preliminary study. *BMJ*. 2002; 324:387–390.
34. Kenward G, Castle N, Hodgetts TJ, Shaikh L. Evaluation of a Medical Emergency Team 1 year after implementation. *Resuscitation*. 2004;61:257–263.

35. Parr MJ, Hadfield JH, Flabouris A, Bishop G, Hillman K. The Medical Emergency Team: 12-month analysis of reasons for activation, immediate outcome and not-for-resuscitation orders. *Resuscitation.* 2001;50:39–44.
36. Audit Commission. Critical to success: the place of efficient and effective critical care services within the acute hospitals. London: 1999.
37. Department of Health. Comprehensive critical care: a review of adult critical care services. London: Department of Health; 2000.
38. Hudson A. Prevention of in-hospital cardiac arrests—first steps in improving patient care. *Resuscitation.* 2004;60:113.
39. Priestley G, Watson W, Rashidian A, et al. Introducing critical care outreach: a ward-randomized trial of phased introduction in a general hospital. *Intensive Care Med.* 2004;30:1398–1404.
40. Ball C, Kirkby M, Williams S. Effect of the critical care outreach team on patient survival to discharge from hospital and readmission to critical care: non-randomized population based study. *BMJ.* 2003;327:1014.
41. Pittard AJ. Out of our reach? Assessing the impact of introducing a critical care outreach service. *Anaesthesia.* 2003;58:882–885.
42. Leary T, Ridley S. Impact of an outreach team on re-admissions to a critical care unit. *Anaesthesia.* 2003;58:328–332.
43. Ball C. Critical care outreach services—do they make a difference? *Intensive Crit Care Nurs.* 2002;18:257–260.
44. Braithwaite RS, DeVita MA, Mahidhara R, Simmons RL, Stuart S, Foraida M. Use of medical emergency team (MET) responses to detect medical errors. *Qual Saf Health Care.* 2004;13:255–259.
45. DeVita MA, Schaefer J, Lutz J, Dongilli T, Wang H. Improving medical crisis team performance. *Crit Care Med.* 2004;32(2 Suppl):S61–S65.
46. DeVita MA, Braithwaite RS, Mahidhara R, Stuart S, Foraida M, Simmons RL. Use of medical emergency team responses to reduce hospital cardiopulmonary arrests. *Qual Saf Health Care.* 2004;13:251–254.
47. Lecky F, Woodford M, Yates DW. Trends in trauma care in England and Wales 1989–97. *Lancet.* 2000;355:1771–1775.
48. Nathens AB, Jurkovich GJ, Cummings P, Rivara FP, Maier RV. The effect of organized systems of trauma care on motor vehicle crash mortality. *JAMA.* 2000;283:1990–1994.

24
Integrating MET into a Patient Safety Program

JOHN GOSBEE

Overview

Since at least the publication of the Institute of Medicine report *To Err Is Human* (1), most health care organizations have been struggling to find and eliminate hazards. Their struggle arises from the complex mixture of issues that plague any organization dealing with the seemingly easy problems to be solved by a new safety program. Many health care organizations soon realize they are dealing with organizational psychology issues that require tools from change management. Somewhat fewer facilities are aware of the problems ingrained in human factors engineering of systems, devices, and tools. We will define these terms and how they apply to Medical Emergency Teams (METs) throughout this chapter. A MET response is not just a wonderful tool to improve morbidity and mortality associated with hospital medical crises and cardiopulmonary resuscitation, it is also an indirect tool to address the struggles to improve quality and safety throughout a health care organization. Conceptually and empirically, most hospitals will likely need MET programs due to findings from human factors engineering and health care.

Creating and Sustaining Safety

The difficulty of creating and sustaining a patient safety program cannot be underestimated. Logistic and strategic questions quickly overwhelm the best and brightest: What are the most frequent or remediable adverse events that hurt and kill patients? Why did these adverse events occur? What can we do about the root causes of these events? What sources can provide effective remedies? Why are people so resistant to using safety remedies?

To answer these questions, hospitals have used safety methods required by regulatory organizations (e.g., Joint Commission on Accreditation of Healthcare Organizations (JCAHO)) or governments (e.g., state departments of health). These methods include root-cause analysis (RCA), failure mode and effect analysis (FMEA), and traditional quality improvement tools (2,3). These safety and quality approaches work best in organizations that are developing a so-called "high-reliability organization" (4). METs can complement RCA and FMEA activities that will be described more fully.

A MET can also provide the tangible proof that the organization is serious about the "safety culture" described for high-reliability organizations. Specifically, certain aspects of METs are especially suited to meet many of the criteria in a specific model of organizational change described by Rodgers (5), a model that has been accepted for many decades. This theory looks at factors such as perceived relative advantage, compatibility with existing values, and norms and trial-ability.

Definition and Relevance of Human Factors Engineering

The human factors engineering field is several decades old and has been applied in various organizations and domains when they face design, personnel, and policy issues such as those surrounding MET (6). Briefly, human factors engineering is the discipline that studies human capabilities and limitations and applies that information to safe, effective, and comfortable system design (7,8). It includes the design of tools, machines, and systems that take into account human capabilities, limitations, and characteristics. Ergonomics, usability engineering, and user-centered design are considered synonymous or closely related to human factors engineering, which is based on design-related aspects of several biomedical disciplines. From a systems perspective, a person is receiving input from a "clinical assessment machine," processing that input, and creating an output that goes to the "health care machine." Anthropometrics and biomechanics cover most of the physical aspects of input and output. The science of sensation and perception is related to input to the person. Cognitive psychology, which covers models and theories of human performance, memory, and attention, relates to the processing of the input and initiating the output.

Observations and studies regularly conclude that many design issues thwart even the best attempts at resuscitation and the application of critical care expertise (9). Some researchers have seen problems with using defibrillators—even those made for novices (10). Others have identified design problems with defibrillators, even when testing individuals like paramedics who use them often (11). The layout and human factors aspects of the medication drawers in many crash carts can add minutes of delay to well-intentioned and motivated clinicians and their ability to retrieve key medications (12). Lack of proper transitions of care and teamwork during and following resuscitation exists even in the best clinical care (13). The breakdowns and missed opportunities are accentuated by time pressure, design of devices, and even the layout and furnishings of the resuscitation area (14). All of this evidence points to the need to use METs to avoid or abort crises—even if the most highly skilled personnel and fully staffed settings are available.

MET as a Driving Force for a Patient Safety Program

For many reasons, METs can be a key driving force for a hospital safety and quality program. First, there are the difficulties and limitations of commonly used safety methods. Second, a MET is a broad-sweeping safety initiative that impacts and is visible to many sites in the health care organization, and to many types of professionals and personnel. Third, as a safety or quality activity, METs have the most successful change attributes that are cited in change management theory and practice.

Root Cause Analysis (RCA)

Most health care organizations perform many RCAs per year due to JCAHO requirements and the general standard of practice in the patient safety movement. The basics of the RCA include:

1. Deciding when to do an RCA
2. Figuring out what happened (e.g., people and devices involved, sequence of events)
3. Making decisions about root causes and contributing factors
4. Developing remedies or action plans, and approaches to measure effectiveness
5. Convincing and Selling to management and staff,, and then (hopefully) implementing the action plans

There may be more than 1 team or individual doing these general steps. Depending on the event to be studied, each general step might take hours or weeks to complete.

MET can aid all 5 general steps in the RCA process, but has the most effect on 2 troublesome steps: deciding when to do an RCA, and convincing, selling, and implementing action plans. When initiating an RCA on an adverse event, the hospital has to know several things besides just the severity of that specific event: what is the severity of events like the one in question, what is the frequency of this kind of adverse event, and how often is the event severe.

In a robust MET program, there are several adverse events that lead to the MET being called. Braithwaite et al. identified 31% of MET events that were associated with medical errors (adverse events and close calls) (15). In their hospital system experience, they found 18.4 events per 1000 hospital admissions. This is similar to the experience of Australian hospital systems (16), which reported 5 MET responses per 1000 admissions. Thus, most hospital systems could have a rather large body of knowledge about adverse events and close calls. This data would be several times larger than that obtained from auditing just cardiac arrest events, because crises seem to occur 5 to 10 times more frequently.

If the operators log all MET calls they make, the MET call itself provides 2 functions: it provides additional resources to prevent that patient from dying, and it enables creation of a database of crisis events to fuel patient safety reviews. Thus MET calls may help overcome perhaps the most difficult aspect of performing quality indicator activities: finding errors worth fixing. (People are notoriously poor at recognizing errors as they occur, or reporting them when they do recognize them.) As mentioned previously, the events detected by MET are quite diverse. This can aid in determining which of the many types of reported events upon which a hospital should do an RCA. Braithwaite et al. (15) identified 67.5% of the 114 adverse event–associated METs as diagnostic errors, such as incorrect or delayed diagnosis or delay or incorrect action following monitoring or test data. They also saw 59.6% related to treatment errors, including problems during or following surgery and medication administration. Finally, 26.3% of the MET events included problems arising from "prevention;" examples of prevention problems encompassed prophylactic treatment (e.g., anticoagulation for deep vein thrombosis) and telemetry monitoring issues for patients with hyperkalemia.

The richness and diversity of data from events or vulnerabilities that lead to MET can help the RCA team throughout their process. In short, people do poor root-cause analyses; some studies have demonstrated that developing accurate and specific root causes and contributing factors is problematic. Carroll et al. (17) looked at problem-investigation teams in nuclear power plants and chemical plants. In a quantitative analysis of 27 RCA teams at 3 different nuclear power plants, they found "a disappointing level of depth and completeness, insight, and clarity." The researchers were able to make some correlation between some attributes of the team members and the deeper and clearer RCAs. Their analysis found that "more training in teamwork" and "more varied plant experience" were the strongest positive predicting attributes. These attributes may be more widespread or likely to be increased in organizations that accept the central concepts behind MET processes, such as calling for help early (18).

Another troublesome step in RCA is the final one: convincing, selling, and implementing the action plans. Action plan implementation is the step where health care organizations and RCA teams discover how hard it is to change a system, and how resistant personnel can be if the organization has not embraced a culture of safety. It is difficult to convince managers and frontline personnel that 1 event or close call is serious enough for them to change. In essence, one must convince caregivers that their current work-flow is wrong and a new, untested work plan is better. With data from adverse events leading to the creation of a MET, and workflow changes directed at preventing repeats of actual near-death events, it is much more likely to change mindsets and practices.

For instance, an RCA about an empty oxygen cylinder almost being used during patient transport might result in an action to purchase cylinders with a more direct indication of contents (indicator valves). However the same problem that caused a near-death event from hypoxemia would more highly motivate not only the bedside caregivers, but also the administrators who oversee purchasing choices and materials management. Further-more, procurement committees will likely accept the additional cost if there was more than 1 event. Because METs tend to find similar types of errors, creating lists of similar events is not difficult. For example, if the orga-nization had 5 MET events that involved confusion over oxygen cylinder levels, the organization would be less likely to blame an individual and more likely to blame the system. Also, frontline respiratory therapists, pur-chasers, transport personnel, nursing staff, administrators, and physicians are more likely to become allies instead of naysayers if they know about all 5 events.

Failure Mode and Effect Analysis (FMEA)

Most health care organizations perform at least 1 FMEA per year due to JCAHO requirements and the general standard of practice in the patient safety movement. The general steps of a FMEA include (19):

1. Identifying and prioritizing a high-risk process
2. Flowcharting the process and subprocesses
3. For each subprocess, developing potential failure modes and prioritizing based on risk (risk priority is usually the product of severity, frequency, and detectability)
4. For each failure mode cause, identifying actions to remedy them
5. Convincing, selling, and then (hopefully) implementing the action plans

There may be more than 1 team or individual performing these general steps. Depending on the process to be studied, each general step might take hours or weeks to complete.

Much less has been written about the problems or shortcomings in apply-ing FMEA in health care (20). However, since FMEA shares many attrib-utes with RCA, many of the ideas and findings about the complementary role of the MET are likely true. In addition, some safety professionals think that there are many ways to inadvertently misuse FMEA as a safety tool (21). One could infer that data from the events preceding MET events and close calls seems invaluable for the FMEA team in all 5 general steps listed above.

For example the MET data can be used to develop realistic failure modes and failure mode causes. An FMEA team might only consider two failure modes in the monitoring and treatment of conscious cardiac care unit patients: 1) malfunction of physiologic monitors; and 2) the patient falling while getting out of bed. MET data would have provided them with a third failure mode such as that described by Braithwaite: bradycardia/asystole from delay in pacemaker placement. Or the team might not conceptualize the failure mode cause of "permanent pacemaker placement considered a low priority consult." Having a body of MET data associated adverse events and their causes will make the FMEA process more efficient.

The process of convincing and selling the action plan from FMEA is more difficult than RCA, since many health care personnel may not be motivated to change when no "real" event occurred. But just as the MET data helps sell and convince personnel to try and to accept action plans from RCAs (as described above), it will help promote FMEA action plans.

Safety Culture and High-Reliability Organizations

METs can also provide the tangible proof that the organization is serious about the safety culture described for high-reliability organizations. MET characteristics meet many of the criteria in 1 specific model of organizational change described by Rodgers (5). This model has been accepted and applied by many organizations for many years. The theory looks at 5 crucial factors for organizational change to occur:

1. Perceived relative advantage
2. Perceived as compatible with existing values and norms
3. Perceived low (or lack of) complexity
4. Trial-ability (ease of doing it on a trial basis)
5. Observe-ability (visibility of the change to non-experts)

As a contrast, one can see that the required safety method of RCA fares only average in each of the 5 organizational change factors. For those convinced that safety is an issue, they would positively perceive the relative advantage RCA (factor 1). However, many novices would see the several-hour process of RCA as burdensome when they believe the remedies, such as enforcing policies, are apparent in minutes of analysis. RCA is also perceived as somewhat compatible with existing values/norms (factor 2) and high complexity (factor 3). Since RCA team meetings often occur weekly and last 2 hours, busy clinicians would say that trialability is low (factor 4). Finally, as evidenced in Carroll's work (17), many RCAs result in training or policy changes that will not be viewed as really much of a change (factor 5).

MET comes out much better than RCA when judged against each of the 5 crucial factors for organizational change. The following analysis assumes that management of the organization is serious about rewarding, not punishing, providers for calling for help early. Providers see a large relative advantage to have an outside team deal with the clinical issues of their patient efficiently and effectively (factor 1). Certainly if an organization using MET has nearly the success with decreasing mortality and crisis code frequency as some US and Australian hospitals, the relative advantage will be clear to all stakeholders, from the boardroom to the classroom.

Calling for help early, accurate and reliable team communication, and teamwork are the hallmarks of high-reliability organizations as well as MET. Thus, Rodgers' second factor, compatibility of values and norms, will increase as the organization moves forward. In contrast, organizations that do not value teamwork and constructive critique will have dissonance with this crucial factor for change.

METs will have to be perceived as being of low complexity. This book contains many examples of the importance of making METs seamless with code teams, paging systems, and other hospital ward activities (see chapters 12, 17, and 18). Also, short lists of understandable, objective criteria for initiating METs increase organizational acceptance.

There are mixed aspects of METs when judging against the last 2 factors, trial-ability and observe-ability of success in organizational change (factors 4 and 5). Some providers are unaffected by changes in the organization due to MET implementation; for them, METs seem easy to try out. However, a MET trial may not seem so easy or non-threatening to personnel in critical care units, existing crisis code teams, and others who play a role in solving urgent or emergent problems. Fewer codes for acutely ill ward patients can be understood more easily by non-experts, if they are made aware of this. Changes in morbidity in critical care areas may not be as appreciated by some management. However, in many facilities quality and outcome measures of various types are now tracked by many non-direct care providers, so visibility of better outcomes would be higher and organizational change more likely in those settings of transparency.

Patient Safety Overall

General concepts discussed in patient safety communities include normalization of deviance and normalization of complexity—overly complex phrases that get at the observations in health care of something being out of place or hard to use. The general observations, if correct, also conspire to permit certain complication rates for procedures and patient interventions. Careful analysis of MET predecessors provides a stark set of data about how health care devices have grown overly complex, or standard policies needlessly convoluted. Once again, the attention of health care personnel is focused on these issues by the criticality of the event (respiratory or cardiovascular distress) and the fact that many of the events recur. Implementation of METs will tend to move the norm: instead of trying to prevent deaths, organizations have a tool to prevent crises, and to help prevent those crises that do occur from turning into a death. Calling for help early can be promoted to become the norm instead of the exception (22).

Conclusion

Using the prescribed patient safety tools of RCA or FMEA has only partially helped health care organizations with the struggle to find and eliminate system vulnerabilities. Organizations soon find that easy problems with easy answers are not common. Fortunately, METs provide a service that is complementary and supportive of other safety methods, since up to 30% of METs are associated with patient safety issues. METs are also needed since there are many ingrained problems with human factors engineering of systems, devices, and tools involved in resuscitation. That is, there are intransigent constraints to the maximum effectiveness in dealing with cardiopulmonary emergencies. Most important are the MET features that organizational theory and observation support as crucial success factors to turning an organization into a highly reliable one, with a solid safety culture.

References

1. Kohn LT, Corrigan JM, Donaldson MS, eds. *To Err Is Human: Building a Safer Health System*. Washington, DC: National Academies Press; 2000.
2. Bagian JP, Gosbee JW, Lee CZ, Williams L, McKnight SD, Mannos DM. VA's root cause analysis system in action. *Jt Comm J Qual Improv*. 2002;28:531–545.
3. Stalhandske E, DeRosier J, Patail B, Gosbee JW. How to make the most of failure mode and effect analysis. *Biomed Instrum Technol*. 2003;37: 96–102.
4. Weick KE, Sutcliffe KM. *Managing the Unexpected: Assuring High Performance in the Age of Complexity*. San Francisco: Jossey Bass; 2002.
5. Rodgers E. *Diffusions of Innovations*. 5th ed. New York: Free Press; 2003.
6. Sanders MS, McCormick EJ. *Human Factors in Engineering and Design*. 7th ed. New York: McGraw-Hill; 1993.
7. Gosbee JW, Lin L. The role of human factors engineering in medical device and medical system errors. In: Vincent C, ed. *Clinical Risk Management: Enhancing Patient Safety*. 2nd ed. London: BMJ Press; 2001.
8. Gosbee JW. Introduction to the human factors engineering series. *Jt Comm J Qual Saf*. 2004;30:215–219.
9. Donchin Y, Gopher D, Olin M, et al. A look into the nature and causes of human errors in the intensive care unit. *Crit Care Med*. 1995;23:294–300.
10. Mattei LC, McKay U, Lepper MW, Soar J. Do nurses and physiotherapists require training to use an automated external defibrillator? *Resuscitation*. 2002; 53:277–280.
11. Fairbanks RJ, Shah MN, Caplan S, Marks A, Bishop P. Defibrillator usability study among paramedics. In: *Proceedings of the Human Factors and Ergonomics*

Society 47th Annual Meeting. Santa Monica, CA: Human Factors and Ergonomics Society; 2004.

12. McLaughlin RC. Redesigning the crash cart: usability testing improves one facility's medication drawers. *Am J Nurs.* 2003;103:64A,64D,64G–64H.

13. Xiao Y, Hunter A, Mackenzie CF, Jeffries NJ, Horst R; The LOTAS Group. Task complexity in emergency medical care and its implications for team coordination. *Hum Factors.* 1996;38:636–645.

14. Xiao Y. Human and technology factors in coordination in emergencies. In: *Medicine, Technology and Human Factors in Trauma Care: A Civilian and Military Perspective.* Baltimore: National Study Center; 2001:16–21.

15. Braithwaite RS, DeVita MA, Mahidhara R, Simmons RL, Stuart S, Foraida M; Medical Emergency Response Improvement Team (MERIT). Use of medical emergency team (MET) responses to detect medical errors. *Qual Saf Health Care.* 2004;13:255–259.

16. Bellomo R, Goldsmith D, Uchino S, et al. A prospective before-and-after trial of a medical emergency team. *Med J Aust.* 2003;179:283–287.

17. Carroll JS, Rudolph JW, Hatakenaka S. Learning from high hazard organizations. In: Staw B, Kramer R, eds. *Research in Organizational Behavior.* Greenwich, CN: JAI Press; 2003.

18. Carroll JS, Rudolph JW, Hatakenaka S. Lessons learned from non-medical industries: root cause analysis as culture change at a chemical plant. *Qual Saf Health Care.* 2002;11:266–269.

19. ECRI. An introduction to FMEA. Using failure mode and effects analysis to meet JCAHO's proactive risk assessment requirement. Failure Modes and Effect Analysis. *Health Devices.* 2002;31:223–226.

20. DeRosier J, Stalhandske E, Bagian JP, Nudell T. Using health care failure mode and effect analysis: the VA National Center for Patient Safety's prospective risk analysis system. *Jt Comm J Qual Improv.* 2002;28:248–267.

21. Spath P. Worst practices used in conducting FMEA projects. *Hosp Peer Rev.* 2004;29:114–116.

22. Foraida M, DeVita MA, Braithwaite RS, Stuart SA, Brooks MM, Simmons RL. Improving the utilization of medical crisis teams (Condition C) at an urban tertiary care hospital. *J Crit Care.* 2003;18:87–94.

25
Are Medical Emergency Teams Worth the Cost?

DANIEL BROWN and RINALDO BELLOMO

Little information and evidence are available on the impact of change in hospital systems and their economic evaluation. The cost implications of system changes in resuscitation are not part of the previous literature or historical background of how hospitals provide emergency care to their in-hospital population. In an environment where return on investment and providing the best possible quality care at the lowest possible price is paramount, there is no answer to what that cost amount totals.

This chapter will attempt to provide some information on the cost implications of implementing a MET system using information obtained from 2 teaching hospitals and from the Medical Early Response, Intervention, and Therapy Study (MERIT). To understand costs, a quick explanation of the MET system and the background of its development are presented.

Adverse events occur in all hospitals, and the reasons for them may not always be evident (1). However, the cost to patients and the economy have been estimated in the millions of dollars, at a range of $95 to $4485 US per patient (2–5). These costs relate mainly to drug-related adverse events and errors. A study conducted in New Zealand found that the average cost for adverse events is $10264 NZ per patient; adverse events are estimated to cost the New Zealand health system $870 million NZ per year (6). In Australia, a study conducted in 1995 showed that between 10000 and 14000 Australians are likely to die of preventable deaths in acute care hospitals each year. The Quality in Australian Health Care Study found that adverse events would likely account for 3.3 million bed days and equate to $867 million AUS per year (7).

Issues of Financial Cost

If the MET system can identify these patients early and prevent them from having a cardiac arrest or being transferred to intensive care units (ICUs), what are the financial cost savings, and what are the monetary costs needed to ensure that its implementation is effective?

As already stated, the MET system needs to be implemented and adopted across the entire hospital system, and there are costs associated with its start up and maintenance. Ideally the MET system should have a coordinator, someone who sees that the system is implemented and monitored. In most large hospitals that have the MET system, this is usually a nurse who has critical care experience. It is the coordinator's responsibility to ensure that flyers, calling criteria wall charts, and identification badges are available, and that time is allotted in orientation programs to ensure that all new staff members are aware of the system and how to employ it. Using previous experiences, the cost of wall charts, flyers, identification badges, and other related items in a large hospital would equate to approx $7500. (Unless otherwise noted, costs are listed in Australian dollars, and the exchange rate at the time of writing is 1 AUD = 0.75 US$).

Depending on the hospital size, the coordinator position can be full- or part-time. A hospital with more than 400 beds would likely require full-time management. Hospitals larger than 800 beds may require more than 1 staff member to fill the role, and this may include another nurse or ICU fellow, or clerical support. The responsibilities include educating new staff, collecting data on MET calls, ensuring there is a roster of appropriately trained staff on duty 24/7, and organizing regular MET meetings. They may also need to review notes and disseminate the latest information on advanced resuscitation, and maintain the equipment used by the MET. The average cost of the coordinator position is around $47000 per year for a full time registered nurse at $24 per hour. It should be noted that the forecasting of costs for further staff has not been included and would certainly depend on the numbers of calls. A large hospital might need to employ a dedicated ICU fellow on the team (at least for a large part of the 24-hour cycle) to assist with research, while secretarial support to the MET coordinator may be required. A computer and printing costs for the year would add around $10000.

Most hospitals that use cardiac arrest teams have advanced resuscitation equipment available on every ward. This is not cost effective, as equipment maintenance is costly and checking the equipment is time consuming. It is also important to note that many hospitals use contracted external staff and so this equipment may go unchecked for some time (18). The MET takes its own equipment and relies on ward staff to provide basic life support until the team arrives with the necessary resuscitation equipment. It is important to note that all nursing and medical staffs in Australian hospitals are accredited each year on basic life support, so this system allows them to use the skills that they have already been taught. The MET system does not advocate the removal of advanced resuscitation equipment from critical care or high dependency areas of the hospital. The MET equipment comprises a trolley, bag and mask ventilation equipment, defibrillator, and a backpack containing circulation and respiratory packs, emergency drugs, and other consumables. Most large hospitals would require 2 of these setups in case there is more than 1 MET call at a time. The estimated cost of the MET equipment is approx $45000 with a further $8000 for consumables per year.

Allowing for part-time clerical support to assist the coordinator at a cost of approximately $23000 per year, the total start-up cost is around $133000 while the maintenance each year is approximately $83000.

Hospitals around the world spend millions of dollars to set up and maintain fire safety programs to provide patient safety. Yet the numbers of deaths from in-hospital fires is extremely low (19). Why not look at cheaper alternatives for fire safety and ensure that money is spent on an early warning system such as the MET? This is not to say that fire safety should not be ensured in hospitals, but simply that fire prevention is a patient safety issue that costs a lot and has very little measurable benefit.

The Data

In a 650-bed tertiary and referral hospital in South Western Sydney, Australia, an observational study was conducted over a 12-month period reviewing all the MET calls (for patients over 14 years of age) that had occurred to ascertain its economic impact. Although not published, the results show 855 MET calls on 625 patients; of these 625 patients, 477 remained on the ward, meaning that 148 patients were transferred to ICU. Of these ICU patients, 79 required ventilation. The study found that the ICU group stayed on average 5.9 days longer than those left on the ward. The average cost per day of an ICU bed in Sydney is just over $3122 (20), and if one multiplies that by the 6 days, the savings are $18737 per patient. Bristow et al. (15) has suggested that the MET may have the ability to prevent 60 patients per 10000 admissions from being transferred to ICU in a hospital with approximately 50000 separations (admissions) a year, as was the case in this study hospital. This would equate to 300 patients each year and a potential saving of $5.6 million a year. In a further recent study comparing the incidence of cardiac arrests in a large teaching hospital, the introduction of a MET system was associated with an 80% decrease in post-cardiac arrest ICU bed days and an 88% decrease in post-cardiac arrest hospital bed days (Figure 25.1 and 25.2) (17). This decrease represented a savings of approximately $3 million per year for cardiac arrest patients alone. In the same institution, the introduction of a MET system also reduced overall length of stay for patients having major surgery (Figure 25.3) (21). Given the yearly throughput of such patients in that teaching hospital, this would translate to savings of approximately $9 million annually. In the same study, unplanned ICU admissions in patients having major surgery were reduced by 44.4%, representing a further approximate saving

P<0.0001

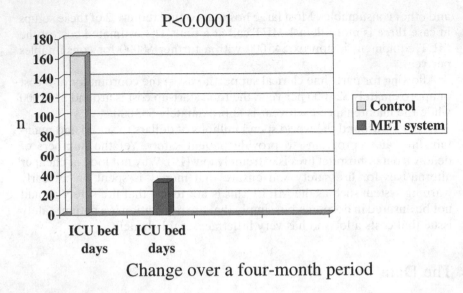

Change over a four-month period

FIGURE 25.1. Diagram illustrating the impact of the MET system on ICU bed days after cardiac arrest.

of $1 million. Given these observations, it is difficult to argue that the introduction of a MET system is too costly.

In addition, costs attributed directly to in-hospital cardiac arrest studied recently in the United Kingdom state that the average cost of resuscitation is just over £928. However, for the patients that survived more than 24 hours post-cardiac arrest the cost was £1589 (22). If these costs were similar in

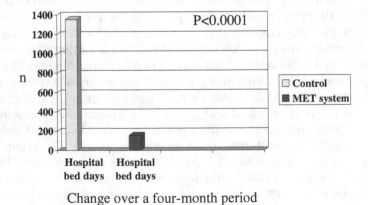

Change over a four-month period

FIGURE 25.2. Diagram illustrating the impact of the MET system on hospital bed days after cardiac arrest.

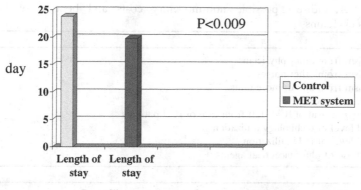

Change over a four-month period

FIGURE 25.3. Histogram illustrating the effect of the MET system on length of stay for patients having major surgery in a teaching hospital.

Australia, for the MET system to be cost effective in a large hospital it would need to prevent 55 cardiac arrests or 26 unplanned ICU admissions, or a combination of both. In the study quoted above (17) it prevented 133 cardiac arrests per year and also 133 unplanned ICU admissions per year.

There are non-monetary costs and non-monetary gains associated with METs as well. The non-monetary costs might relate to issues of hospital politics: for example, if the introduction of the MET does not occur along appropriate lines of broad consensus and information, some colleagues (medical or nursing) and/or specific units may become alienated and hostile. If execution is not inclusive, the same might happen. There might be a deskilling effect on junior staff. As argued elsewhere in this chapter and book, we believe this is not the case.

There are likely non-monetary savings associated with the MET, which are not easily assessed, and which go beyond improved patient outcomes. They include an effect on family complaints about the care received by their relative while in the hospital, an effect on medico-legal liability, and, in a competitive health care environment, an impact on the marketing of an institution to the community. The possible non-monetary costs and benefits are summarized in Table 25.1.

Does the MET System Have Flaws?

A common concern about the MET system is that it might "deskill" ward staff in relation to advanced resuscitation. But do ward staff have those skills in the first place, and if so how often do they ensure their skills are

TABLE 25.1. Indirect possible non-monetary costs and benefits of Medical Emergency Teams

Costs
Antagonism from other physicians
Antagonism from other nurses
Antagonism from one or more units
Deskilling of junior staff
Temporary removal of ICU staff from care of ICU patients
Increased level of technology utilization
Increased level of ICU utilization
Increased use of pharmaceutical agents

Benefits
Marketing advantage in a competitive health care environment
Decreased patient or family complaints
Greater medico-legal protection and decreased liability
Defense against litigation
Improvement in identification of patients requiring palliative care
Avoidance of unnecessary ICU admissions
Teaching of junior staff under safer circumstances
Decrease in job-related stress for ward nurses
Decrease in job-related stress for trainee doctors

maintained? We believe it would make more sense that ward staff should be trained to identify potentially critically ill patients through clinical observation, and then to alert appropriately trained members of staff who practice these skills on a daily basis.

Another concern is that the MET system may be turning many "unexpected deaths" into "expected deaths" simply by making more patients do-not-resuscitate status when the team arrives and evaluates the situation. This would decrease a hospital's unexpected death rate in an artificial way. On the other hand, if the MET system facilitates the making of appropriate, compassionate, dignified, and respectful end-of-life decisions, then we consider such changes desirable.

Conclusions

Available data suggests that the cost of implementing a MET system is relatively small, and that financial savings far exceed the costs. Other indirect non-monetary savings may also occur. More importantly, the data also suggests that METs save lives, prevent cardiac arrests, and decrease postoperative complications. We believe that the MET system is a cost-effective intervention for any modern hospital, provided it is implemented thoughtfully and according to the principles outlined in other chapters in this book. METs are clearly worth the cost and effort.

References

1. Kohn LT, Corrigan JM, Donaldson MS, eds. *To Err Is Human: Building a Safer Health System.* Washington, DC: National Academies Press; 2000.
2. Bates DW, Spell N, Cullen DJ, et al. The costs of adverse drug events in hospitalized patients. *JAMA.* 1997;277:307–311.
3. Classen DC, Pestotnik SL, Evans S, Lloyd JF, Buerke JP. Adverse drug events in hospitalized patients: excess length of stay, extra cost, and attributable mortality. *JAMA.* 1997;277:301–306.
4. Schneider PJ, Gift MG, Rothermich EA, Sill BE. Cost of medication-related problems at a university hospital. *Am J Health Syst Pharm.* 1995;52:2415–2418.
5. Senst BL, Achusim, LE, Genest RP, et al. Practical approach to determining costs and frequency of adverse drug events in a health care network. *Am J Health Syst Pharm.* 2001;58:1126–1132.
6. Brown P, McArthur C, Newby L, Lay-Yee R, Davis P, Briant R. Cost of medical injury in New Zealand: a retrospective cohort study. *J Health Serv Res Policy.* 2002;7:29–34.
7. Wilson RM, Runciman WB, Gibbert RW, Harrison BT, Newby L, Hamilton JD. The quality in Australian health care study. *Med J Aust.* 1995;163:458–471.
8. Daffurn K, Lee A, Hillman K, Bishop G, Bauman A. Do nurses know when to summon emergency assistance? Intensive Crit Care Nurs. 1994;10:115–120.
9. Hopkinson J. *Fire Safety Engineering in Hospitals.* Vision fm, Faber Maunsell, Issue 3;2004.
10. Bristow J, Hillman KM, Chey T, et al. Rates of in-hospital arrests, deaths and intensive care admissions: the effect of a medical emergency team. *Med J Aust.* 2000;173:236–240.
11. Bellomo R, Goldsmith D, Uchino S, et al. A prospective before-and-after trial of a medical emergency team. *Med J Aust.* 2003;179:283–287.
12. Bellomo R, Goldsmith D, Uchino S, et al. Prospective controlled trial of effect of medical emergency team on postoperative morbidity and mortaility rates. *Crit Care Med.* 2004;32:916–921.
13. Gage H, Kenward G, Hodgetts TJ, Castle N, Ineson N, Shaikh L. Health system costs of in-hospital cardiac arrest. *Resuscitation.* 2002;54:139–146.
14. Hillman K, Brown D, Daffurn K. *Implementing the Medical Emergency Team System into Your Hospital.* Liverpool: South Western Sydney Area Health Service Publication; 1999.

Index